Gamete Assessment, Selection and Micromanipulation in ART

Zsolt Peter Nagy • Alex C. Varghese
Ashok Agarwal
Editors

Gamete Assessment, Selection and Micromanipulation in ART

A Practical Guide

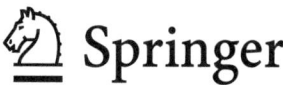

Editors
Zsolt Peter Nagy, MD, PhD,
 HCLD (ABB), EMB (ACE)
Scientific and Laboratory Director
Reproductive Biology Associates
Atlanta, GA, USA

Alex C. Varghese, PhD
Senior Embryologist
Montreal Reproductive Centre
Montreal, QC, Canada

Ashok Agarwal, PhD, HCLD (ABB),
 EMB (ACE)
Director, Center for Reproductive Medicine
Cleveland Clinic
Cleveland, OH, USA

ISBN 978-1-4614-8359-5   ISBN 978-1-4614-8360-1 (eBook)
DOI 10.1007/978-1-4614-8360-1
Springer New York Heidelberg Dordrecht London

Library of Congress Control Number: 2013946789

© Springer Science+Business Media New York 2013
This work is subject to copyright. All rights are reserved by the Publisher, whether the whole or part of the material is concerned, specifically the rights of translation, reprinting, reuse of illustrations, recitation, broadcasting, reproduction on microfilms or in any other physical way, and transmission or information storage and retrieval, electronic adaptation, computer software, or by similar or dissimilar methodology now known or hereafter developed. Exempted from this legal reservation are brief excerpts in connection with reviews or scholarly analysis or material supplied specifically for the purpose of being entered and executed on a computer system, for exclusive use by the purchaser of the work. Duplication of this publication or parts thereof is permitted only under the provisions of the Copyright Law of the Publisher's location, in its current version, and permission for use must always be obtained from Springer. Permissions for use may be obtained through RightsLink at the Copyright Clearance Center. Violations are liable to prosecution under the respective Copyright Law.
The use of general descriptive names, registered names, trademarks, service marks, etc. in this publication does not imply, even in the absence of a specific statement, that such names are exempt from the relevant protective laws and regulations and therefore free for general use.
While the advice and information in this book are believed to be true and accurate at the date of publication, neither the authors nor the editors nor the publisher can accept any legal responsibility for any errors or omissions that may be made. The publisher makes no warranty, express or implied, with respect to the material contained herein.

Printed on acid-free paper

Springer is part of Springer Science+Business Media (www.springer.com)

Preface

Appropriate assessment of oocytes and spermatozoa is a basic cornerstone of modern day IVF practice. It provides key information in selecting the treatment options for providing the best care for infertile patients to maximize the chance of successful outcomes. In addition to the well-established routine procedures, there are several recently developed evaluation methods which show great promise to advance accuracy of assessment and improve diagnostic value. Subsequently, choices and applications of micromanipulation techniques (including intracytoplasmic sperm injection or biopsy of polar body, cleavage or blastocyst stage embryo), using the most adequate instrumentations and procedures, are critical elements in the contemporary IVF laboratory. It requires not only abundant procedural experience but also a full and deep understanding of gamete and embryo physiology with adequate molecular insights.

Our textbook provides an excellent and detailed overview of well-recognized procedures of gamete assessment and micromanipulation, as well as a comprehensive presentation of novel techniques, approaches, and instrumentation. The textbook is unique in having a section dedicated to providing a comprehensive description of various micromanipulators available for the ICSI procedures. The unlimited theoretical and practical details provided by this book make it an indispensable resource to all professionals working in the field of assisted reproduction. The chapters are written by world-renowned experts on their field, with decades of practical experience and vast amounts of publication in the scientific literature.

We are thankful to Richard Lansing, executive editor, for his support and advice, and Kristopher Spring, Associate Editor and Margaret Burns, publishing manager, for their tireless efforts in reviewing and editing each of the manuscripts. Furthermore, we are grateful to all of the outstanding contributors for sharing their knowledge and submitting their manuscripts on time. Finally, we are indebted to our families for their love and support.

Atlanta, GA, USA	Zsolt Peter Nagy, MD, PhD
Montreal, QC, Canada	Alex C. Varghese, PhD
Cleveland, OH, USA	Ashok Agarwal, PhD

Contents

Part I Human Oocyte Evaluation in IVF

1. **Assessment of Oocyte Quality** 3
   Basak Balaban, Turgay Barut, and Bulent Urman

2. **Polarization Microscopy** 29
   Markus Montag, Maria Köster, and Hans van der Ven

3. **Cumulus Cell Gene Expression in Assessment of Oocyte Quality** 39
   Dagan Wells

Part II Sperm Evaluation and Selection

4. **Sperm Assessment: Traditional Approaches and Their Indicative Value** 49
   Margot Flint, Fanuel Lampiao, Ashok Agarwal, and Stefan S. du Plessis

5. **Sperm Assessment: Novel Approaches and Their Indicative Value** 63
   De Yi Liu, Harold Bourne, Claire Garrett, Gary N. Clarke, Shlomi Barak, and H.W. Gordon Baker

6. **Intracytoplasmic Morphologically Selected Sperm Injection** 73
   P. Vanderzwalmen, Magnus Bach, Batsuren Baramsai, A. Neyer, Delf Schwerda, Astrid Stecher, Barbara Wirleitner, Martin Zintz, Bernard Lejeune, S. Vanderzwalmen, Nino Guy Cassuto, Mathias Zech, and Nicolas H. Zech

7 **Sperm Testing and ICSI Selection by Hyaluronic Acid Binding: The Hyaluronic Acid-Coated Glass Slide and Petri Dish in the Andrology and IVF Laboratories** 93
Gabor Huszar

8 **Electrophoretic Sperm Separation** 121
Steven Fleming and John Aitken

9 **Magnetic-Activated Cell Sorting of Human Spermatozoa** 131
Enver Kerem Dirican

10 **Polscope-Based Sperm Selection** 145
Luca Gianaroli, Cristina Magli, Andor Crippa, Giorgio Cavallini, Eleonora Borghi, and Anna P. Ferraretti

Part III Micromanipulators and Micromanipulation

11 **Hydraulic Manipulators for ICSI** 157
Hubert Joris

12 **Research Instruments Micromanipulators** 167
Steven Fleming and Catherine Pretty

13 **Eppendorf Micromanipulator: Setup and Operation of Electronic Micromanipulators** 179
Ehab Abu-Marar and Safa Al-Hasani

14 **The Leica Microsystems' IMSI System** 187
Christiane Wittemer, Bruno Laborde, Frederic Ribay, and Stephane Viville

15 **Automated Robotic Intracytoplasmic Sperm Injection** 199
Zhe Lu, Xinyu Liu, Xuping Zhang, Clement Leung, Navid Esfandiari, Robert F. Casper, and Yu Sun

16 **Oocyte Treatment and Preparation for Microinjection** 209
Thomas Ebner

17 **Mechanism of Human Oocyte Activation During ICSI and Methodology for Overcoming Low or Failed Fertilization** 225
Dmitri Dozortsev and Mohammad Hossein Nasr-Esfahani

18 **Livestock Production via Micromanipulation** 237
Akira Onishi and Anthony C.F. Perry

19 **Assisted Hatching in IVF** 245
Itziar Belil and Anna Veiga

Part IV Biopsy Procedures on Oocytes and Embryos

20 Polar Body Biopsy 261
Markus Montag, Maria Köster, K. van der Ven,
and Hans van der Ven

21 Cleavage-Stage Embryo Biopsy 269
Alan R. Thornhill

22 Embryo Biopsy for PGD: Current Perspective 287
Steven J. McArthur, Don Leigh, Maria Traversa, James Marshall,
and Robert P.S. Jansen

**23 Microarrays and CGH for PGD of Chromosome Abnormalities
and Gene Defects** 303
Gary Harton and Santiago Munné

Part V Molecular Insights

**24 The Role of Mitochondria in the Establishment of Developmental
Competence in Early Human Development** 319
Jonathan Van Blerkom

**25 Nuclear and Cytoplasmic Transfer: Human Applications
and Concerns** 347
Josef Fulka Jr. and Helena Fulka

**26 Cytoskeletal Architecture of Human Oocytes with Focus
on Centrosomes and Their Significant Role in Fertilization** 359
Heide Schatten, Vanesa Y. Rawe, and Qing-Yuan Sun

**27 Molecular Mining of Follicular Fluid for Reliable Biomarkers
of Human Oocyte and Embryo Developmental Competence** 377
Jonathan Van Blerkom

Index 393

Contributors

Ehab Abu-Marar, MD IVF Unit, Department of Obstetrics and Gynecology, University of Schleswig-Holstein, Schleswig-Holstein, Lübeck, Germany

Ashok Agarwal, PhD, HCLD (ABB), EMB (ACE) Director, Center for Reproductive Medicine, Cleveland Clinic, Cleveland, OH, USA

John Aitken, PhD, ScD, FRSE ARC Centre of Excellence in Biotechnology and Development, University of Newcastle, Callaghan, NSW, Australia

Safa Al-Hasani, DVM, PhD IVF Unit, Frauenklinik, Lübeck, Schleswig-Holstein, Germany

Magnus Bach, Dip-Biol IVF Laboratory, IVF Centers Prof. H. Zech, Bregenz, Austria

H.W. Gordon Baker, MD, PhD, FRACP Melbourne IVF and Department of Obstetrics and Gynecology, Royal Women's Hospital, University of Melbourne, East Melbourne, VIC, Australia

Basak Balaban, BSc Assisted Reproduction Unit, American Hospital of Istanbul, Nisantasi, Istanbul, Turkey

Shlomi Barak, MD Melbourne IVF and Department of Obstetrics and Gynecology, Royal Women's Hospital, University of Melbourne, East Melbourne, VIC, Australia

Batsuren Baramsai, MD IVF Laboratory, IVF Centers Prof. H. Zech, Bregenz, Austria

Turgay Barut, MSc Assisted Reproduction Unit, American Hospital of Istanbul, Nisantasi, Istanbul, Turkey

Itziar Belil, BSc Department of Obstetrics, Gynecology, and Reproduction, Reproductive Medicine Service, Institut Universitari Dexeus, Barcelona, Spain

Eleonora Borghi, BSc Andrology Laboratory, SISMER, Bologna, Italy

Harold Bourne, M Rep Sci Reproductive Services/Melbourne IVF, The Royal Women's Hospital, East Melbourne, VIC, Australia

Robert F. Casper, MD Department of Obstetrics and Gynecology, University of Toronto, Toronto, ON, Canada

Nino Guy Cassuto, MD ART Unit, Drouot Laboratory, Paris, France

Giorgio Cavallini, MD Reproductive Medicine Unit, SISMER, Bologna, Italy

Gary N. Clarke, DSc Andrology Unit and Department of Obstetrics and Gynaecology, The Royal Women's Hospital, University of Melbourne, Carlton, VIC, Australia

Andor Crippa, PhD Andrology Laboratory and Genetics, SISMER, Bologna, Italy

Enver Kerem Dirican, PhD Department of Embryology, Memorial Hospital of Antalya, Antalya, Turkey

Dmitri Dozortsev, MD, PhD Reproductive Laboratories, Advanced Fertility Center of Texas, Houston, TX, USA

Stefan S. du Plessis, PhD Department of Medical Physiology, Stellenbosch University, Tygerberg, Western Cape, South Africa

Thomas Ebner, PhD IVF Unit, Landes Frauen and Kinderklinik Linz, Linz, Austria

Navid Esfandiari, DVM, PhD Andrology and Immunoassay Laboratories, Division of Reproductive Endocrinology and Infertility, Department of Obstetrics and Gynecology, University of Toronto, Toronto, ON, Canada

Anna P. Ferraretti, MD Reproductive Medicine Unit, SISMER, Bologna, Italy

Steven Fleming, BSc (Hons), MSc, PhD Assisted Conception Australia, Greenslopes Private Hospital, Brisbane, QLD, Australia

Margot Flint, MSc Department of Medical Physiology, Stellenbosch University, Tygerberg, Western Cape, South Africa

Helena Fulka, PhD Department of Biology of Reproduction, Institute of Animal Science, Prague, Czech Republic

Josef Fulka Jr., PhD Department of Biology of Reproduction, Institute of Animal Science, Prague, Czech Republic

Claire Garrett Melbourne IVF and Department of Obstetrics and Gynecology, Royal Women's Hospital, University of Melbourne, East Melbourne, VIC, Australia

Reproductive Services/Melbourne IVF, The Royal Women's Hospital, Melbourne, VIC, Australia

Luca Gianaroli, MD International Institutes of Advanced Reproduction and Genetics, SISMER, Bolgona, Italy

Gary Harton, BS, TS (ABB) Department of Molecular Genetics, Reprogenetics, LLC, Livingston, NJ, USA

Mohammad Hossein Nasr-Esfahani, PhD Royan Institute, Isfahan Fertility and Infertility Center, Isfahan, Iran

Gabor Huszar, MD Department of Obstetrics, Gynecology, and Reproductive Sciences, Male Fertility Program and Sperm Physiology Laboratory, Yale University School of Medicine, New Haven, CT, USA

Robert P.S. Jansen, MD CREI Sydney IVF, Sydney, Australia

Hubert Joris Vitrolife Sweden AB, Göteborg, Sweden

Maria Köster, DVSc Department of Gynecological Endocrinology and Reproductive Medicine, University of Bonn, Bonn, Germany

Bruno Laborde ART Centre, SIHCUS-CMCO, Schiltigheim, France

Fanuel Lampiao, PhD Department of Medical Physiology, Stellenbosch University, Tygerberg, Western Cape, South Africa

Don Leigh, PhD (UNSW) Sydney IVF, Sydney, Australia

Bernard Lejeune, MD, PhD IVF Laboratory, Centre Hospitalier Inter Régional Cavell (CHIREC), Bruxelles, Belgium

Clement Leung, BASc Department of Electrical and Computer Engineering, University of Toronto, Toronto, ON, Canada

De Yi Liu, PhD Melbourne IVF and Department of Obstetrics and Gynecology, Royal Women's Hospital, University of Melbourne, East Melbourne, VIC, Australia

Xinyu Liu, PhD Department of Mechanical Engineering, McGill University, Montreal, QC, Canada

Zhe Lu, PhD Department of Mechanical and Industrial Engineering, University of Toronto, Toronto, ON, Canada

Cristina Magli, MSc Research and Development, SISMER, Bologna, Italy

James Marshall, BAppSc (UTS) Sydney IVF, Sydney, Australia

Steven J. McArthur, BSc Sydney IVF, Sydney, Australia

Markus Montag, PhD Department of Gynecological Endocrinology and Fertility Disorders, University of Heidelberg, Voßstr. 9, Heidelberg, Germany

Santiago Munné, PhD Department of Molecular Genetics, Reprogenetics, LLC, Livingston, NJ, USA

A. Neyer, MSc IVF Laboratory, IVF Centers Prof. H. Zech, Bregenz, Austria

Akira Onishi, PhD Transgenic Pig Research Unit, National Institute of Agrobiological Sciences, Tsukuba, Japan

Anthony C.F. Perry, BSc, PhD Laboratory of Mammalian Molecular Embryology, Centre for Regenerative Medicine, University of Bath, Bath, UK

Department of Biology and Biochemistry, University of Bath, Bath, UK

Catherine Pretty, PhD Assisted Conception Services, Nuffield Health Woking Hospital, Woking, Surrey, UK

Vanesa Y. Rawe, MSc, PhD REPROTEC, Buenos Aires, Argentina

Frederic Ribay Leica Microsystems DSA/Clinical EU, Leica Microsystems SAS, Nanterre, France

Heide Schatten, PhD Department of Veterinary Pathobiology, University of Missouri-Columbia, Columbia, MO, USA

Delf Schwerda, MSc IVF Laboratory, IVF Centers Prof. H. Zech, Bregenz, Austria

Astrid Stecher, MSc IVF Laboratory, IVF Centers Prof. H. Zech, Bregenz, Austria

Qing-Yuan Sun, PhD State Key Laboratory of Reproductive Biology, Institute of Zoology, Chinese Academy of Sciences, Chaoyang, Beijing, China

Yu Sun, PhD Department of Mechanical and Industrial Engineering, University of Toronto, Toronto, ON, Canada

Alan R. Thornhill, PhD, HCLD The London Bridge Fertility, Gynecology and Genetics Centre, London, UK

Maria Traversa, BSc, MSc (Med) Sydney IVF, Sydney, Australia

Bulent Urman, MD Department of Obstetrics and Gynecology, American Hospital, Nisantasi, Istanbul, Turkey

Jonathan Van Blerkom, PhD Department of Molecular, Cellular and Developmental Biology, University of Colorado, Boulder, CO, USA

Hans van der Ven, MD Department of Gynecological Endocrinology and Reproductive Medicine, University of Bonn, Bonn, Germany

K. van der Ven Department of Gynecological Endocrinology and Reproductive Medicine, University of Bonn, Bonn, Germany

P. Vanderzwalmen, Bio-Eng. MSc IVF Laboratory, IVF Centers Prof. H. Zech, Bregenz, Austria

S. Vanderzwalmen, BSc IVF Laboratory, Centre Hospitalier Inter Régional Cavell (CHIREC), Bruxelles, Belgium

Anna Veiga, PhD Department of Obstetrics, Gynecology, and Reproduction, Reproductive Medicine Service, Institut Universitari Dexeus, Barcelona, Spain

Stephane Viville, Pharm D, PhD Department of Biology of Reproduction, Hospital of the University of Strasbourg, Schiltighein, France

Dagan Wells, PhD, FRCPath Nuffield Department of Obstetrics and Gynaecology, John Radcliffe Hospital, University of Oxford, Women's Centre, Oxford, UK

Barbara Wirleitner, PhD IVF Laboratory, IVF Centers Prof. H. Zech, Bregenz, Austria

Christiane Wittemer, PhD ART Centre, 8 rue des Recollets, 57000 Metz, France

Mathias Zech, MD IVF Laboratory, IVF Centers Prof. H. Zech, Bregenz, Austria

Nicolas H. Zech, MD, PhD IVF Laboratory, IVF Centers Prof. H. Zech, Bregenz, Austria

Xuping Zhang, PhD Department of Mechanical and Industrial Engineering, University of Toronto, Toronto, ON, Canada

Martin Zintz, PhD IVF Laboratory, IVF Centers Prof. H. Zech, Bregenz, Austria

Part I
Human Oocyte Evaluation in IVF

Chapter 1
Assessment of Oocyte Quality

Basak Balaban, Turgay Barut, and Bulent Urman

The identification of the viable human metaphase II oocyte is a controversial issue that has been subject to much debate in the last decade. The intricate and complex events during follicular maturation determine the capacity of the oocyte to undergo normal fertilization and subsequent embryonic development. Complete physiological maturation requires nuclear and cytoplasmic changes that need to be coordinately completed to ensure optimal cellular conditions. The asynchrony of nuclear and cytoplasmic maturation events may compromise oocyte quality, resulting in different oocyte dysmorphisms.

Starting from retrieval, cumulus–corona complex morphology and its relation with nuclear and cytoplasmic maturity of the oocyte have been studied over the years and correlated with different grading systems identified in the literature. With the application of intracytoplasmic sperm injection (ICSI) procedures that require mechanical and enzymatic elimination of the cumulus–corona cell layer, it became possible to identify and classify in detail the morphological deviations of the metaphase II oocyte. These deviations are either extracytoplasmic or cytoplasmic or a combination of both. Extracytoplasmic abnormalities include irregular-shaped oocytes, zona pellucida abnormalities, first polar body dysmorphisms and perivitelline space (PVS) deviations. Reported cytoplasmic abnormalities are cytoplasmic granularity and homogeneity, cytoplasmic viscosity and the presence of cytoplasmic inclusions (dark incorporations, spots, refractile bodies, vacuoles and smooth endoplasmic reticulum clusters [sERCs]).

While we are all eagerly awaiting for the most accurate and non-invasive way of assessing human oocyte viability, there is still no routinely applicable technique or

---

B. Balaban, BSc (✉) • T. Barut, MSc
Assisted Reproduction Unit, American Hospital of Istanbul, Guzelbahce St. No. 20, Nisantasi, Istanbul 34365, Turkey
e-mail: basakbalaban@superonline.com

B. Urman, MD
Department of Obstetrics and Gynecology, American Hospital, Nisantasi, Istanbul, Turkey

analytical device yet available to fulfil this goal. Hence, in vitro fertilization (IVF) clinics worldwide continue to select oocytes based on their light-microscopic morphology, thus making oocyte morphology evaluation schemes variable and highly subjective.

Morphological variations of the oocyte may result from intrinsic factors, such as age [1] and genetic defects, or extrinsic factors, such as medications used for controlled ovarian stimulation (COS) and the ovarian response to COS [2, 3].

This chapter aims to clarify the effect of different parameters on the morphological changes of the oocyte. These changes include; intrinsic factors (age [1], genetic defects) and extrinsic factors (COS protocols and ovarian reserve [2, 3]). There uses identifies morphological variations in oocyte evaluation schemes, as well as discuss morphological markers of oocyte quality/viability in relation to oocyte morphology. They are also used in attempting to determine whether morphological evaluation of the oocyte can be utilized for predicting the implantation potential of the derived embryo.

Effect of Ovarian Stimulation on Oocyte Quality and Morphological Appearance

Oocyte quality has been shown to be affected by ovarian stimulation regimens and hormonal environment changes which may result in the maturation of abnormal oocytes [4]. Majority (60–70%) of the oocytes retrieved from stimulated cycles exhibit one or more abnormal morphological characteristics [5].

There are very scarce data regarding the effect of different stimulation protocols, different gonadotropin preparations, the dosage and duration of medications employed for ovarian stimulation and oestradiol concentrations on the maturity and competence of oocytes. It has been recently shown that, no matter which stimulation protocol is used, pharmaceutical preparations of human gonadotropins used to induce the multiple follicular growth might influence the growing oocyte [6, 7]. Excessive ovarian stimulation and the resulting hyperestrogenic milieu may have detrimental effects on oocyte quality [8, 9]. This investigation suggests that amongst the cohort of recruited follicles, only the most sensitive to stimulation is likely to yield better quality embryos, whereas all the additional oocytes resulting from maximal stimulation might be of impaired quality. Alternatively, the reduction in pregnancy rate observed after maximal stimulation might be due to a direct effect of high serum oestradiol concentrations on the oocytes [10, 11] or on endometrial receptivity [11, 12]. Earlier studies suggested that high concentrations of LH during follicular phase of stimulation could have a negative impact on oocyte quality, pregnancy rate and the incidence of miscarriage [13–15]. Several studies examined the effect of polycystic ovarian syndrome on the maturation and quality of the oocyte, but the results were controversial [16]. Data from women with PCOS suggest that oocyte and embryo quality and implantation may be impaired in these patients treated with assisted reproduction [17]. This may be due to impaired gamete quality resulting from the high oestrogenic milieu or intrinsic problems. However, not all results are in agreement, and clinical outcome of PCOS patients appears to be equivalent to other infertility factors [5].

Most of the studies published so far examining the effect of clinical parameters on oocyte quality have been dependant upon oocyte maturity and quality rather than morphology [5]. Imthurn et al. [18] examined the effect of highly purified follicle stimulating hormone (HP-FSH) on nuclear maturity and morphological appearance of the oocyte in couples undergoing ICSI and compared the results with human menopausal gonadotropin (HMG) stimulation. Authors did not find any difference amongst the groups in relation to patient age, duration of stimulation, number of aspirated oocytes or maturity of the oocyte–cumulus complex. Rashidi et al. [2] also showed that nuclear maturity, oocytes with abnormal zona, polar body or cytoplasmic morphology were similar between the group of patients stimulated with either HMG or recombinant FSH.

Otsuki et al. [19] showed that the risk of producing oocytes with an aggregation of the sER is increased in patients with high levels of serum oestradiol on the day of human chorionic gonadotropin (HCG) administration. As the application of a short protocol seems to favour formation of sER clusters, this finding indicates that ovarian stimulation may directly influence oocyte appearance and quality, e.g. through recruitment of follicles that in vivo might have become atretic.

Similarly, PVS granularity, a dysmorphism that, not interacting with fertilization, cleavage behaviour and pregnancy outcome was increased in patients exposed to higher doses of gonadotropins [20].

Effect of Oocyte Morphology on Embryo Development and Implantation

Oocyte maturation consists of two separate processes: nuclear and cytoplasmic maturation, both of which should take place in a well-coordinated and synchronized manner in order to guarantee adequate oocyte quality [20]. In this context, nuclear maturity refers to the resumption of meiosis and the progression to metaphase II, the natural arresting point prior to ovulation [21]. Furthermore, full physiological maturation appears to require nuclear and cytoplasmic changes that need to be coordinately completed to ensure optimal cellular conditions [22]. The presence of a normal nuclear genetic material will not guarantee the potential of the oocyte to develop into a healthy embryo and foetus. While resumption of the first meiotic division takes place and the nucleus enters metaphase II stage, synchronously cytoplasmic maturation goes on achieving zonal ability to release calcium and cortical granules, mitochondrial changes, protein synthesis and cytoskeletal changes [23]. Absence of nuclear cytoplasmic coordination is seen in germinal vesicle (GV)-stage meiotically competent oocytes recovered from follicles at different stages of development, where the ability to support preimplantation development is achieved progressively during antrum formation [24]. The oocyte nuclear compartment is directly involved in the LH-mediated changes. These changes resume the meiotic process, which is undergoing germinal vesicle breakdown. When it reaches metaphase I and becomes characterized by the absence of the first polar body extrusion, some of the intermediate eggs may be fertilizable and arresting at the metaphase II (MII) stage. Disturbance or asynchrony of these two processes has been shown to result in different oocyte morphological abnormalities. A mature nucleus and cytoplasm are regarded as equally important for embryo development, and each is closely associated with oocyte morphology [25–27].

Correlation of Oocyte–Cumulus–Corona Complex Morphology with the Quality and the Maturity of the Oocyte

Apart from inducing the rupture of the follicle wall and triggering the conversion of the follicle into the corpus luteum, LH stimulation causes precise changes in the oocyte and the surrounding cumulus cells. Cumulus cells produce a viscoelastic extracellular matrix that accumulates in the intercellular spaces. This matrix, whose most characteristic component is hyaluronic acid, is organized into a mesh-like network that allows the preservation of a close contiguity between cumulus cells and the oocytes, despite the partial or total loss of intercellular coupling and contact between these cells [24].

Immature oocyte–cumulus–corona complex (OCCC) displays an unexpanded cumulus and a dense corona forming a compact layer of cells adhering to the zona pellucida of a prophase I (germinal vesicle-bearing) oocyte. The ooplasm cannot be seen through the cumulus mass associated with small parietal granulosa cells which appear in compact clumps [28]. In stimulated cycles, it is common to recover OCCC that display some degree of cumulus expansion but a compact corona layer or even an expanded cumulus–corona complex and nevertheless contain immature prophase I oocytes. If they are not recognized at harvest and are inseminated immediately, they will result in an absent or delayed fertilization. Under the stereomicroscope, a typical mature preovulatory OCCC displays an expanded radiating corona surrounded by the loose mass of cumulus cells, macroscopically visible [28] and mucified layer, due to the active secretion of hyaluronic acid in support of positive effects of cumulus–corona cells on oocyte development [29]. The sparse structure of these cells allows identification of the oocyte with a spherical, homogeneous ooplasm and sometimes the first polar body extruded in the PVS. Usually, however, cumulus and/or corona layers are dense in appearance and at times darkened, and the polar body cannot be observed [28].

Post-mature OCCC are believed to arise from cycles where there has been a premature attenuated LH surge or a delayed HCG administration. The cumulus displays clusters of darkened cells, while the corona is usually dark and tight. Degenerative or atretic OCCC, which form 3% at recovery, exhibit clear signs of

Table 1.1 Grading system for cumulus–oocyte complexes

Grade 1 (A)	Absent to sparse cumulus cells and 1–3 layers of corona cells
Grade 2 (B)	Dense cumulus cells and tightly packed corona cells
Grade 3 (C)	Expanded, fluffy cumulus cells and expanded corona cells
Grade 4 (D)	Expanded, scanty cumulus cells and expanded, often partially lost corona cells

Table 1.2 Grading system for oocyte maturity

Grade 1 (mature or preovulatory)	Expanded cumulus, very radiant corona, distinct zona pellucida, clear ooplasm, expanded well aggregated membrana granulosa cells
Grade 2 (approximately mature)	Expanded cumulus mass, slightly compact corona radiata, expanded well aggregated membrana granulosa cells
Grade 3 (immature)	Dense compact cumulus if present, very adherent compact layer of corona cells, ooplasm if visible with the presence of the germinal vesicle, compact and non-aggregated membrana granulosa cells
Grade 4 (post-mature)	Much expanded cumulus with clumps, radiant corona radiata yet often clumped, irregular or incomplete, very visible zona, slightly granular or dark ooplasm, small and relatively non-aggregated membrana granulosa cells
Grade 5 (atretic)	Rarely associated with cumulus mass, clumped and very irregular corona radiata if present, very visible zona, dark and frequently misshapen ooplasm, membrana granulosa cells with very small clumps of cells

abnormalities, e.g. oocytes with a dark and/or contracted irregular ooplasm, disrupted zona pellucida or empty zona surrounded by a retracted cumulus mass. It is recommended to discard these groups of OCCC and yielded oocytes from further culture and insemination [28].

There are very few studies in the literature that correlated OCCC morphology and oocyte quality since oocyte maturity at the time of retrieval is difficult to assess being obscured by a large cumulus mass infiltrated with abundant hyaluronic acid. Ng et al. [30], who used a modified grading system adapted by Wolf [31] (Table 1.1), showed that mature grade 3 cumulus–oocyte complexes (OCCC) were associated with higher fertilization rates. The pregnancy rate was higher in cycles when >50% of retrieved OCCC were grade 3 compared with cycles where ≤50% of OCCC were similarly graded [5].

A more recent study graded oocyte maturity on a scale from 1 to 5 based on the morphology of the ooplasm, cumulus mass, corona radiata and membrana granulosa cells [32] (Table 1.2). Grade 1 (mature) oocytes were included in the first group, whereas the second group consisted of oocytes graded from 2 to 5 (immature). This study showed that mature oocytes yielded higher fertilization rates. Although cleavage rates were similar in both groups, the percentage of poor morphology day 3 embryos from the immature group was significantly higher than from the mature group.

However, most of the studies published in the literature are based on the utilization of OCCC morphology for IVF cases where OCCC were not removed before fertilization check. The utilization of OCCC morphology for determination of good quality and mature oocytes is less likely to be applied nowadays as more and more IVF laboratories prefer microinjection as the method of fertilization, during which the maturity of the oocyte can more precisely be assessed following enzymatic and mechanical digestion of the OCCC.

A recent study by Engman et al. [33] similarly showed that for women undergoing ICSI, assessment of OCCC (oocytes–cumulus–corona complex) morphology is pointless; since there is no correlation between OCCC morphology, fertilization and cleavage rates. For conventional IVF, OCCC morphology may be useful for gamete selection if the couple wants to electively limit the number of oocytes to avoid creating surplus embryos for cryopreservation.

Morphological Dysmorphisms of the Metaphase II (MII) Oocytes and General View of Cytoplasmic and Extracytoplasmic Abnormalities

Removal of cumulus cells from oocytes of patients undergoing ICSI allows a more detailed observation of the 60–70% of all oocytes' morphological characteristics [24, 34]. Mature and good quality metaphase II oocyte is defined as: clear, moderately granular, homogenous and translucent cytoplasm without inclusions, small PVS, a clear to colourless and regular zona pellucida, perfectly spherical shape and an intact PBI [21, 24, 35–37]. However, the majority of the oocytes retrieved after ovarian hyperstimulation exhibit one or more variations of the described "ideal" morphological criteria [21, 35, 36, 38, 39]. Even in the very early years, it had been shown that 13% of unfertilized oocytes after IVF harboured morphological abnormalities [40].

Morphological deviations of metaphase II oocytes can be classified as intracytoplasmic and extracytoplasmic abnormalities. Most frequently observed cytoplasmically morphological variations are changes in colour, granularity of the cytoplasm presence of cytoplasmic inclusions such as vacuoles and sERCs and cytoplasmic incorporations. Extracytoplasmic variations are deviations from normal visualization of PVS, zona pellucida colour, first polar body morphology (fragmented or degenerated) [34, 41] and shape abnormalities [25, 35, 41, 42].

Cytoplasmic Abnormalities

Although the effect of cytoplasmic abnormalities on the clinical outcome had been controversial, evidence-based data on severe abnormalities agree on the point that embryos derived from oocytes with severe cytoplasmic abnormalities have reduced viability and implantation potential. One of the earliest studies by Xia et al. had shown that cytoplasmic abnormalities, such as dark cytoplasm, refractile bodies, dark incorporations, spots and single or multiple vacuolization and granulation in the cytoplasm, were correlated with fertilization and embryo quality [24, 35, 36]. The study by Serhal et al. also showed significantly lower fertilization rates, embryo cleavage rates and lower embryo quality in the group of oocytes with cytoplasmic inclusions [36, 43]. Therefore, it has been indicated even in the early years that cytoplasmic texture appears to be a very important characteristic for oocyte evaluation, and these cytoplasmic alterations may be a sign of oocyte immaturity [44].

Despite the presence of normal genetic material, ooplasmic factors play an important role in the fertilization process that could be compromised by cytoplasmic abnormalities [45]. Deficiency in cytoplasmic maturation could compromise all processes that prepare the oocyte for activation, adequate fertilization and embryo development. In addition, a disturbance or asynchrony of these two processes has been shown to compromise oocyte quality, resulting in different oocyte dysmorphisms [21, 44].

Given the data in the literature, it may be concluded that only severe cytoplasmic defects such as organelle clustering/centrally located granulation, appearance of sERCs and certain types of fluid-filled vacuoles should be considered as abnormalities, whereas slight deviations from the normal cytoplasmic structure should be accepted as normal oocytes with a phenotypically heterogeneous cytoplasm [46].

Cytoplasmic Granularity, Centrally Located Granulation and Cytoplasmic Viscosity

Cytoplasm changes, which accompany the oocyte growth, include mRNA transcription and protein synthesis [47, 48]. These processes are necessary for the meiotic maturation of oocyte, activation of the zygotic genome and blastocyst formation [49, 50]. Oocyte granularity is correlated with the localization of mitochondria and may represent domains of high ATP request that are necessary for the normal development of embryos [51, 52]. Slight or moderate granularity has been accepted as a normal feature of oocytes. It is conceivable that an increased viscosity of the cytoplasm may constrain cell organelles and/or pronuclei in their movement preventing the zygote from achieving alignment of both pronuclei or alignment of pronuclei with respect to the polar bodies, thereby severely impairing polarity and further preimplantation development [53, 54]. However, dense granularity focused in the centre of the oocyte is considered as a dysmorphism [5]. In correlation with these, Balaban et al. [42] showed similar fertilization rates and embryo quality in the group of embryos derived from oocytes with slight granular cytoplasmic appearance. Kahraman et al. [44] who studied condensed centrally located granulation in the oocyte cytoplasm also showed similar fertilization rates and embryo quality (4.2%) from embryos derived from such oocytes. However, the ongoing pregnancy rate was significantly decreased with higher abortion rates. It was also demonstrated in the same study that centrally located granulation is correlated with high chromosomal aneuploidy possibly being the reason for high abortion rates.

A more recent study by Rienzi et al. [55] showed that although fertilization rates of oocytes with cytoplasmic granularity or centrally located granular area are not affected, pronuclear morphology and embryo quality were affected by the presence of a centrally located granular area [55]. The authors suggested an MII oocyte morphological score (MOMS) including mainly cytoplasmic abnormalities and demonstrated that this grading system is predictive of the clinical outcome.

Cytoplasmic granulation and cytoplasmic viscosity appear to be in close correlation. It has been reported that granular areas are more viscous than the surrounding cytoplasm [56]. There is a lack of markers of increased cytoplasmic viscosity [57]. Ooplasm of higher viscosity is more likely to adhere to the spike of the injection pipette which could be seen in a limited number (~0.5 %) of injections after withdrawal of the glass tool. Persistence of the injection funnel after ICSI reflects a deficiency in cytoplasmic texture. Flux characteristics of cytoplasm are altered in the more viscous type which does not allow the oocyte to restore its original spherical shape as fast as seen in gametes with a more aqueous ooplasm. Since all oocytes involved show an injection funnel during ICSI, the observed difference in degeneration rate may be explained by a difference in cytoplasm fluidity. In other words, increased viscosity of the cytoplasm (persistent funnel) may keep it from leakage, whereas oocytes with more aqueous cytoplasm tend to leak more frequently after ICSI [56].

Another study by Loutradis et al. [58] showed that cytoplasmic viscosity impairs embryo quality, blastocyst formation rate, blastocyst quality, as well as the pregnancy and implantation rates [58].

Vacuolization

The presence of vacuoles or inclusions within the cytoplasm is considered to be a severe abnormality [19, 40, 59]. How cytoplasmic inclusions such as deficiency in cytoplasm fluidity and ooplasm vacuolization affects fertilization and further embryonic development processes remains unclear [60, 61]. This phenomenon could be related to cytoskeletal function and MII meiotic spindle structure [41, 60, 62]. Cytoplasmic defects lead to detrimental effects to pronuclear formation, as the cytoskeleton cannot function properly and the MII spindle can be displaced from its polar position [4].

Biological basis and possibly a genetic cause may result in either uncontrollable endocytosis or poor exocytosis and consequent vacuolar formation. Spindle visualization showed that macro vacuoles were not associated with spindle displacement. The presence of vacuoles and vesicles in the oocyte cytoplasm influenced the fertilization characteristics of oocytes negatively, even in the presence of top scores for other morphological characteristics [63]. De Sutter et al. [36] found a severely reduced fertilization rate in vacuolated oocytes (40%). Esfandiari et al. [46] also reported significantly lower fertilization rates for the group of oocytes with multiple vacuoles when compared with the oocytes with a single vacuole in the cytoplasm. Ebner et al. [64] recently analysed the actual influence of vacuolization (time of first appearance, number and size of vacuoles) on preimplantation embryo development up to the blastocyst stage. The authors [64] found that vacuoles in 3.9% of oocytes at collection, of which 66% had single, 21.3% had double and 12.7% had multiple vacuoles. Other studies [35, 37] suggest a slightly higher oocyte vacuolization rate (5, 7 and 12.4%, respectively).

Vacuoles arise either spontaneously [41] or by fusion of preexisting vesicles derived from SER and/or Golgi apparatus [65]. There was a significant relationship between the size of vacuoles (cut-off value 14 μm) and fertilization. The mean diameter of vacuoles in fertilized oocytes was 9.8 μm, compared with 17.6 μm for non-fertilized oocytes. The presence of membrane-bound vacuoles in the cytoplasm appears to be associated with a reduced fertilization rate [36, 60, 64].

It was demonstrated in the same study that vacuoles have a detrimental effect on embryo development as well, with significantly decreased rates of blastocyst formation from the group of embryos that were derived from oocytes with at least a single vacuole in the cytoplasm. In correlation with the previous findings, Rienzi et al. [55] also showed significantly lower fertilization rates in vacuoled oocytes. Besides lower fertilization rates, pronuclear morphology and embryo quality were reported to be similar between the group of fertilized oocytes with vacuolated cytoplasm or normal cytoplasmic texture. However, this study did not segregate the group of vacuolated oocytes according to their number or sizes.

It is very likely that a larger vacuole or multiple vacuoles will cause a much more detrimental effect to the oocyte than a small vacuole, since a larger portion of the cytoskeleton (e.g. microtubuli) cannot function as it is supposed to [21]. It has previously been demonstrated that extremely large cytosolic vacuoles physically displace the MII spindle from its usual polar position and thus might cause fertilization failure, as well as zygotic and embryonic arrest [41].

Macro vacuoles present within the ooplasm appear to have distorted oocyte cytoskeletal structure to such an extent that physiological processes involved in fertilization and embryogenesis were impaired, including sperm–oocyte signalling, sperm binding, meiotic resumption and embryonic cleavage [19, 41].

A novel solution to this problem could be to attempt the removal of the massive cytosolic vacuoles using modern micromanipulation techniques. However, vacuole drainage could result in a reduction in cytoplasmic volume, which in itself could be detrimental to embryonic development. Puncture and drainage of the vacuoles could also result in the leakage of intravacuolar fluid, which could contain toxic waste products that should have been exocytosed, into the surrounding ooplasm [66].

Appearance of Smooth Endoplasmic Reticulum Clusters

sERCs can also be defined as pronucleus sized slightly bulged/flat translucent vacuoles localized in the centre of the cytoplasm at the metaphase II stage and can be easily distinguished under inverted microscope from regular type of fluid-filled vacuoles (identical with perivitelline fluid [41]).

Intrinsic oocyte-specific defects of important molecular and cellular activities exist that are hardly detectable using conventional microscopic techniques. Electron microscopic studies stressed that cytoplasmic organization of normal-appearing oocytes is characterized by an apparently random distribution of cell organelles.

Oocytes showing deviations in fertilization or further development often display atypical distributions of cellular components [41]. A disk-like assemblage of the sER would represent such a cytoplasmic defect that could adversely influence competence [40]. It is presumed that these clusters arise by dilatation and fusion of sER saccules during maturational process of the gamete [41]. The relatively low frequency of this oocyte dysmorphism has kept several authors from analysing it separately [42, 43]. Others, however, scored between 1% and 3% of all analysed gametes to be sER cluster positive [37, 41, 60, 67].

These figures may be somewhat underestimated, since it became apparent from the findings of Otsuki et al. [19] that smaller clusters (e.g. 2–5 ptTi) cannot be detected without the help of an electron microscope. These smaller aggregations were exclusively found in presumed sER-negative oocytes (on the basis of light-microscopic analysis) of sER cluster-positive women [19], and thus, no bias was introduced into statistical analysis, as probably no sER-positive patients were missed. In addition, these smaller aggregations were exclusively situated in the cortical area of the ooplasm, and it is not clear whether they have the same detrimental effect as larger accumulations near the centre of the oocyte. It should be noted that the smallest aggregation detected in this prospective study was 5.1 µm in size and found in an egg with these clusters. Otsuki et al. [19] also showed that sER clusters are an exclusive anomaly of MII oocytes (not detected in prophase or metaphase I gametes) and tend to grow in diameter before disappearing approximately 16–20 h post-ICSI.

Otsuki et al. [19] studied the relationship between pregnancy outcome and sERCs in MII human oocytes. The presence of sERC in the cytoplasm significantly impaired embryo quality and was associated with a lower chance of conception even in sERC (oocyte-derived embryos from the same cohort that were transferred along with embryos derived from sERC (+) oocytes). Because Ca^{2+} release from sER plays a pivotal role in oocyte maturation, fertilization and early embryonic development [68] studies of Ca^{2+} signalling in sERC (+) oocytes may contribute to understanding of the cause and the effect of sERC [5]. In contrast, no relationship was found between the presence of sER in the oocyte cytoplasm and fertilization rate and pronuclear/embryo quality [55]. Besides these effects on embryo development and clinical outcome, they reported that one baby born in sERC-positive cycles was diagnosed with Beckwith–Wiedemann syndrome, a model imprinting disorder resulting from mutations or epigenetic events affecting the imprinted genes on chromosome 11p15.5. Questions arise as to whether inheritance of this disease is causally related to the use of assisted reproduction techniques [69, 70]. At present, there are no data concerning the relationship between sERC and the genomic imprinting defect. Currently, the correlation between sERC and imprinting disorders is not clearly known. It would be important to examine the unusual distribution pattern of the sERC formation that may be involved in the abnormal regulation of Ca^{2+} signalling.

Ebner et al. [71] recently showed that the appearance of sERC is significantly related to duration and dosage of the stimulation. Fertilization (58.9%) and blastulation rates (44.0%) were significantly lower in affected ova compared with unaffected counterparts (77.4 and 87.8%, respectively). Pregnancies in women with affected gametes were accompanied by a higher incidence of obstetric problems

($p < 0.01$) leading to a non-significant trend towards earlier delivery and significantly reduced birthweight ($p < 0.05$). This study recommended avoiding transfer of embryos/blastocysts derived from SER cluster-positive gametes and suggested to inform patients that even transfer of sibling oocytes without this anomaly involves a higher risk of detrimental outcome.

Meriano et al. [59] showed that the presence of sER in the oocytes significantly impairs clinical pregnancy and implantation rates despite similar fertilization and cleavage rates and embryo quality. Very importantly intracytoplasmic organelle clustering was the only significant repetitive abnormality in between other cytoplasmic and extracytoplasmic abnormalities that was found to be a negative predictor of pregnancy and implantation after ICSI.

It is clear that sERCs in human oocytes require future studies due to important functions of the sER in oocyte maturation and Ca^{2+} signalling for embryonic development. More research is needed to define the molecular and cellular mechanisms of organelle clustering [59].

Extracytoplasmic Abnormalities

The effect of extracytoplasmic abnormalities on clinical outcome is unclear. Although most of the published data in the literature did not show detrimental effects, there are still studies reporting controversial results. Extracytoplasmic abnormalities may be a physiological maturation-related phenomenon affected by hyperstimulation protocols and less stringent follicular selection [4]. One of the earlier studies had shown that extracytoplasmic abnormalities such as dark zona pellucida, zona pellucida thickness, large PVS or irregular shape of the oocyte are not related to fertilization rate and embryo quality after ICSI and commented that the oocytes showing such morphological deviations should be regarded as normal [35, 37, 72]. Results vary as to whether distinct oocyte dysmorphisms have any relation to fertilization and development rates, probably due to discordance in the scoring of these dysmorphisms [5]. Increased rate of degeneration after ICSI of oocytes with extracytoplasmic abnormalities is often noted [5, 35, 37, 73]. Although Ebner et al. [62] and Plachot et al. [74] have shown that extracytoplasmic abnormalities of the oocyte did not affect fertilization and embryo quality, both studies reported higher lysis rates after ICSI in the group of oocytes with outer layer abnormalities (fragile oolemma, dark zona pellucida, large PVS and shape irregularity). Outer layer abnormalities may be somehow related to sudden oolemma breakage pattern described by Palermo et al. [75].

Based on most of the published data, it is difficult to comment on only the effect of the extracytoplasmic abnormalities, since the grading systems used were mainly based on numerous factors including at least one additional cytoplasmic abnormality. Xia et al. [35] indicated that the main factor affecting fertilization and embryo quality was the characteristic of the cytoplasm which highly significantly decreased fertilization rates and embryo quality for the group of oocytes with cytoplasmic inclusions even without any extracytoplasmic abnormality. In contrast, there was a slight decrease in the fertilization rate and embryo quality in the group of oocytes without cytoplasmic inclusions but with extracytoplasmic abnormalities (fragmented first polar body, large PVS). Therefore, the main determinant for embryo developmental potential was found to be cytoplasmic properties rather than extracytoplasmic deviations. In line with these observations, Balaban et al. [42] showed that extracytoplasmic abnormalities of the oocyte such as dark zona pellucida, large PVS or shape abnormalities were not associated with a decreased fertilization rate or unfavourable embryo quality after ICSI [5]. It has been shown that the repetition of specific oocyte dysmorphisms from cycle to cycle is a negative predictor of pregnancy and implantation rates in ICSI [59]. However, none of the extracytoplasmic abnormalities such as large or granulated PVS or zonal abnormalities were found to be repetitive from one cycle to another [5].

Evaluation of First Polar Body Morphology

Recent studies investigated a possible correlation between PBI morphology and oocyte competence [76]. It has been claimed that PBI morphology assessment can be used to determine the post-ovulatory age of the oocyte [77]. The PBI morphology has also been suggested as a possible indicator of fertilization and embryo quality after ICSI [78, 79]. Ebner et al. [78] described five different morphological appearances of the first polar body. Grade 1 first polar bodies (round or ovoid and intact) differed from grade 2 first polar bodies (also round or ovoid and intact) in that the former has a smooth surface. Grade 3 (more than two fragments) and grade 4 (broken into two) first polar bodies were defined as fragmented, whereas grade 5 first polar bodies were characterized by their huge appearance being extruded to a similarly large PVS. ICSI to oocytes showing grade 1 and 2 first polar bodies resulted in higher fertilization rates and gave rise to higher quality embryos [39].

Embryo transfers selected on the basis of PBI morphology have been associated with increased implantation and pregnancy rates [78, 80]. Oocytes with an intact PBI of normal size undergo fertilization at a rate comparable to that of oocytes with a fragmented PBI (77.1 and 75.9%, respectively) but produce a significantly lower incidence of fragmentation in day 2 embryos (10.9 and 13.2%, respectively) and a higher blastocyst formation rate (54.9 and 42.2%, respectively) [81]. The presence of an abnormal PBI (degenerated or large) in the MII oocytes analysed was relatively rare (4.4%). However, this feature was associated with a significantly reduced fertilization rate. It has been suggested that a degenerated PBI may reflect an asynchrony between nuclear and cytoplasmic maturation [82]. Ebner et al. [81] showed that embryos with an intact first polar body group were associated with an increased rate of blastocyst formation when compared with the fragmented first polar body group [81].

In contrast to the studies indicated above, more recent studies came up to a conclusion that, as PBI formation is a dynamic procedure, fragmentation rates might differ within hours of culture, and therefore, the prognostic value of its evaluation can only be limited [79, 83, 84]. These studies were also able to demonstrate that there was no significant relation for fertilization rate, embryo quality or clinical outcome [79, 83, 84].

It has been reported in the same studies that PBI fragmentation is not related with the implantation potential of the resultant embryo [79, 83]. The PBI morphology, in particular degenerated and large (but not fragmented) polar bodies, may therefore be considered to be a marker of oocyte maturation disturbance [79, 85].

Verlinsky et al. [84] genetically analysed embryos derived from different polar body classes. No correlation was observed between polar body shape and genetic constitution; however, the only polar body group bearing a theoretical risk of chromosomal disorder considering the larger volume of ooplasm in huge polar bodies was not analysed [84]. The investigators also reported that the first polar body morphology was not associated with the chromosomally normality of the developing embryo. Verlinsky et al. [84] also detected first polar body morphology grading changes in terms of fragmentation in more than one-third of the oocytes studied. It appeared that morphology of the first polar body changes after a few hours of in vitro culture, and it can vary according to the time during which the observation is carried out. Therefore, the authors concluded that first polar body morphology assessment may not serve as a reliable marker of oocyte quality and competences.

Shape Abnormalities

Since most of the data in the literature examined extracytoplasmic abnormalities jointly, there is insufficient evidence-based analysis on the possible effect of shape abnormalities on embryo quality and viability, as well as the clinical outcome. Balaban et al. [42] reported that the incidence of irregular-shaped oocytes is around 3% within a whole cohort of oocytes retrieved. This study showed that out of 223 injected oocytes with shape abnormality, no significant difference was found in terms of fertilization and cleavage rates and embryo quality when compared with the group of oocytes with normal morphology. More recently, the study by Rienzi et al. [55] also demonstrated that the fertilization capacity of oocytes is not affected by the appearance of shape abnormalities.

Yakin et al. [86] demonstrated that similar fertilization, cleavage rates, cleavage stage embryo quality, blastocyst formation and quality could be obtained from the group of zygotes derived from oocytes with shape abnormalities when compared with group of zygotes derived from oocytes with normal morphology. More recently, Rienzi et al. [55] showed similar rates of fertilization, normal pronuclear morphology and cleavage stage embryo quality for the group of embryos obtained from oocytes with shape abnormalities.

Zona Pellucida Abnormalities

Abnormalities of zona pellucida can be described in different forms such as distorted, multi-layered, pigmented, hairy appearance, thinner or thicker than usual [28] or darker appearance. Zona abnormalities can appear in some oocytes as a "ghost" zona in which the top bilayer appears to detach or pull away from the bottom zonal bilayer [59].

The study by Balaban et al. [42] had shown similar fertilization, embryonic development, clinical pregnancy and implantation rates for the group of embryos derived from oocytes with dark zona appearance when compared with embryos obtained from oocytes with normal morphology [42]. More recently, the same group reported similar cryopreservation rates, and similar blastocyst formation, quality and hatching rates for the group of frozen–thawed embryos derived from oocytes with dark zona pellucida when compared with the frozen–thawed embryos derived from oocytes with normal morphology [87].

Palermo et al. [75] support the hypothesis that the hormonal environment during ovarian stimulation may affect the oocyte quality, e.g. oolemma behaviour as well as zona pellucida appearance. Any deviation from a presumed normal injection procedure (sudden and difficult breakage) could indicate a change in the three-dimensional structure of the outer shell, causing problems during the hatching process [88].

Low expression of the zona proteins by the growing human oocyte may indicate reduced developmental potential. In this respect, a German group [89] used polarization light microscopy to non-invasively analyse the texture and thickness of human zona pellucida by quantitatively measuring retardation magnitude and thickness of the three layers of the zona. In contrast to the middle and outer layer, the innermost one was significantly thicker and showed a nearly 30% higher light retardation in conception cycles as compared with cycles not resulting in pregnancy [21].

The same authors [89] observed that oocytes, with zona splitting, probably caused by mechanical stress during retrieval or denudation, were exclusively associated with non-conception cycles. An additional explanation would be that in these cases, the patterning of proteins may be temporarily interrupted during formation of the extracellular coat [21]. Though these types of ova usually show an ovoid shape, it has to be noted that the zona is responsible for the dysmorphism, and the oocyte, however, reveals a spherical shape. If both zona pellucida and oocyte are involved in distortion, corresponding embryos run the risk of developmental incompetence. If this shape dysmorphism runs throughout preimplantation development, theoretically, it will result in an atypical elongated embryo [21]. The thickness of the zona pellucida which influences sperm penetration varies from 10 to 31 µm and is not related to the cytoplasm diameter.

The oocytes are fertilized best in vitro when the thickness of the zona pellucida was less than 18.6 µm. The thick zona pellucida (22 µm and thicker) could be an indicator for the use of assisted hatching of embryos produced by ICSI from infertile patients [90]. The thickness of the zona pellucida had no influence on the embryo development after ICSI [91].

Cohen et al. [92] and Palmstierna et al. [93] suggested that patients transferred with embryos with thinner zona pellucida had a better chance of successful implantation and pregnancy compared with transferred with embryos with thicker zona pellucida [91]. Gabrielsen et al. [91] reported in their study that embryos with a minor variation in zona pellucida thickness had an implantation rate about 10%, which increased to 29% in embryos with higher zona pellucida variation. Palmstierna et al. [93] analysed that zona pellucida thickness variation exhibited high predictive values for pregnancy outcome and was thus considered an important indicator for good embryo quality [91].

Perivitelline Space Abnormalities: PVS Granularity and Large PVS

The PVS of human oocytes may vary in size (enlarged or not) and content (presence or absence of the grain) [35, 42]. It was estimated that oocytes with a large PVS developed worse after ICSI (37.5%) than those with a normal PVS (60.3%) [36].

The nature and origin of PVS granules still remains to be determined, but there is some evidence that this debris may derive either from coronal cell process remnants [94] or from an extracellular matrix [95]. Sathanathan [94] showed that oocytes with granularity in the PVS have an increased risk of developmental incompetence [94], and PVS granularity, considered to be an extracytoplasmic abnormality, may be a sign of gonadotropin overdose, since the percentage of oocytes with perivitelline granules was significantly higher in the high-dose (>45 ampoules) stimulated group compared with the low-dose (<30 ampules) stimulated group [20]. Earlier studies also indicated that in 15% of meiotically mature human oocytes, an incomplete and premature exocytosis of cortical granules can occur [41] and that PVS granularity may be a sign of gonadotropin overdose [20]. Other studies [95, 96] found that extracellular matrix compromising granules and filaments in the PVS are identical to the matrix observed between the cumulus and corona radiate cells. The study by Balaban and Urman [5] commented that PVS granularity may be a physiological maturation-related phenomenon that has no effect on fertilization and cleavage rates, embryo quality and the clinical outcome of assisted reproduction [5].

Early studies described that a large PVS could be related to oocyte over maturity [97]. The studies performed on the effect of large PVS appearance had been limited and controversial. Balaban et al. [42] showed that the appearance of large PVS has no detrimental effect on the fertilization rates, cleavage and embryo quality. In contrast, other studies demonstrated significantly decreased fertilization rates for injected oocytes with large PVS compared to oocytes with normal PVS. The study by Rienzi et al. [55] showed that the presence of large PVS is related to lower fertilization rate and higher incidence of abnormal pronuclear morphology. Besides these parameters, embryo quality was not affected by the appearance of large PVS.

Evaluation of Giant Oocytes

Giant oocytes can rarely be seen after hormonal stimulation for human assisted reproductive technologies. Although oocyte dysmorphism seems to have little effect on the rate of aneuploidy, giant oocytes which are usually diploid are more likely to cause triploidy after fertilization. Oocyte meiosis is very sensitive to endogenous and exogenous factors that may cause the production of oocytes with chromosomal abnormalities and, therefore, of abnormal zygotes. It is presumed that intra- and extrafollicular influences (perifollicular microvasculature, oxygenation, the presence of residues from cigarette smoke) may disturb maturation, leading to giant oocytes with an increased rate of aneuploidy [98].

Giant oocytes have been shown to be 30% larger in diameter than normal oocytes. The study by Balakier et al. [99] examined different morphological patterns amongst giant unfertilized and fertilized oocytes. All unfertilized oocytes appeared to be diploid and contained one or two metaphase plates (46 or 2×23 chromosomes) and one or two polar bodies. Fertilized giant oocytes exhibited either two or three pronuclei or two or four polar bodies. Both types of giant zygotes were reported to be capable of normal cleavage and development to blastocyst stage. However, chromosomal analysis of the embryos derived from these oocytes showed that they were all abnormal with numerical alterations indicative of ploidy change. Therefore, as these giant oocytes might be a possible source of human digynic triploidy, they should be excluded from transfer to avoid undesired miscarriages [99].

Recently, the study by Ebner et al. [29] also indicated that giant oocytes are produced either by lack of cytokinesis during mitotic division or by fusion of two oogonia and, consequently, are associated with a diploid set of genetic material. These mechanisms explain the binucleate state of immature giant eggs [100]. Since patients who developed giant gametes exhibited significantly higher levels of oestradiol and increased numbers of retrieved oocytes, this abnormality may be linked to ovarian stimulation [99]. The resulting zygotes from giant oocytes will have a triploid chromosomal set after DNA replication and be capable of normal cleavage and adequate blastocyst formation. Ebner et al. [29] also recommended excluding giant oocytes from transfer, even if they carry the regular number of two pronuclei. As a result of the evidence-based data, exclusion of giant oocytes from IVF trials is recommended. In case of fertilization, giant oocytes even with 2PN should be treated like multipronuclear zygotes.

Effect of Number of Morphological Abnormalities on Developmental Competence of the Oocyte

The effect of the number of morphological abnormalities of oocytes on the quality and the implantation potential of derived embryos has not been studied in detail. De Sutter et al. [36] showed that the fertilization rate and embryo quality of the oocytes with no abnormality, one or two or more abnormalities were similar. In a later study, Balaban et al. [42] demonstrated that the incidence of two abnormalities in a group of oocytes with morphological deviations was 26%, whereas this rate decreased to 6% for three abnormalities. Fertilization rate and embryo quality did not differ in the group of oocytes with no abnormality or one, two or three morphological abnormalities. In contrast, Loutradis et al. [58] showed a deleterious effect of the type and the number of only cytoplasmic abnormalities on the developmental potential of the oocyte and reported that the severity and the number of cytoplasmic defects have a deleterious effect on embryo quality. A more recent study on in vitro matured oocytes also showed that embryo quality was decreased in parallel to the number of the morphological abnormalities of the oocyte from which it was derived [97].

Yakin et al. [86] demonstrated that embryos derived from oocytes with multiple morphological abnormalities, especially when at least one single cytoplasmic dysmorphism is included, have a decreased blastocyst formation rate, and once the blastocyst is formed, the quality and hatching status is detrimentally affected. The same study also showed that aneuploidy rate of embryos derived from oocytes with multiple abnormalities including at least one cytoplasmic abnormality is significantly higher than the group of embryos derived from oocytes with single abnormality or normal morphological appearance.

Effect of Oocyte Morphological Abnormalities on the Cryopreservation Outcome

There are many published studies on the effect of abnormalities of oocyte morphology on embryo quality and viability. Whether morphological abnormalities of the oocyte influence cryosurvival and further development of derived embryos is not well known. The study by Balaban et al. [87] compared cryosurvival and progression to the blastocyst stage of 5,292 frozen–thawed embryos derived from normal and abnormal oocytes. The authors showed that the presence of a cytoplasmic abnormality of the oocyte significantly decreased cryosurvival. This detrimental effect was more pronounced in embryos derived from oocytes with vacuolar cytoplasm or with central granulation.

Furthermore, these embryos did not have the potential to develop into good quality blastocysts or reach the hatching stage. On the other hand, presence of a single extracytoplasmic abnormality of the oocyte did not affect cryosurvival and the potential to develop into good quality blastocysts. Grade 2 embryos derived from oocytes with irregular shape or a large PVS had decreased cryosurvival. However, when these embryos survived cryopreservation, their potential to develop into good quality blastocysts or to reach hatching stage was unaffected. Even if clinical outcome of frozen–thawed embryo transfer cycles in relation to oocyte morphology cannot be inferred from the results of this study as multiple embryo transfer was performed, it has been shown that the developmental behaviour of frozen–thawed embryos derived from multiple dysmorphic oocytes was similar when compared to results from the literature reported for fresh embryos [5, 21].

Different hypotheses might be introduced to explain the decreased cryosurvival and blastocyst development rates from morphologically good-looking embryos that are derived from oocytes with severe cytoplasmic defects. One of them is the increased rate of aneuploidy found in the embryos derived from such oocytes [40]. A more recent study by Yakin et al. [86] showed that cytoplasmic and multiple abnormalities where at least one cytoplasmic abnormality was included significantly impaired blastocyst development [86]. Although a 20% higher aneuploidy rate was found amongst embryos derived from these oocytes, the difference did not reach statistical significance.

An alternative hypothesis to explain reduced cryosurvival of embryos derived from oocytes with a non-homogenous cytoplasm may be prevention of dissemination of the cryoprotectant within the cell due to the presence of cytoplasmic vacuoles or centrally located granulation. Proper dissemination of the cryoprotectant within the cell is crucial for cryosurvival. It is important to note that, similar to the behaviour of fresh embryos derived from different types of morphological abnormalities, the presence of extracytoplasmic abnormalities alone does not affect blastocyst development despite decreasing cryosurvival. However, embryos derived from oocytes with vacuolar cytoplasm or central granulation do not seem to bear the potential to develop into good quality blastocysts or to reach the hatching stage after cryopreservation. These cytoplasmic abnormalities may be reflections of genetic, epigenetic or metabolic defects in the oocyte. Embryos with severe cytoplasmic abnormalities comprise around 5% of all embryos suitable for cryopreservation.

Women who have all of their excess embryos derived from oocytes bearing severe cytoplasmic abnormalities should be counselled about the reduced chance of these embryos developing into good quality blastocysts or reaching the hatching stage. It is difficult to assume that transfer of such an embryo will result in pregnancy. Cryopreservation and subsequent transfer of embryos derived from oocytes with severe cytoplasmic abnormalities should be avoided [87].

Genetic Constitution of Oocytes with Morphological Abnormalities

Based on the published data, it appears that the developmental potential of oocytes with severe cytoplasmic defects is significantly impaired. However, it is still not known for certain if these cytoplasmic dysmorphisms are a reflection of a developmental defect in the oocyte or if the dysmorphism itself is inhibitory to the eventual development of the oocyte and subsequent embryos. One of the possible reasons shown is the defective genetic constitution of these oocytes. Van Blerkom and Henry [41] showed that as many as half of the oocytes with dysmorphic phenotypes that arise early in meiotic maturation are aneuploid, with hypohaploidy being predominant. In contrast, cytoplasmic defects which occured at or after metaphase I are associated with a relatively low frequency (<15%) of aneuploidy which is comparable to that reported for oocytes with a normal cytoplasmic appearance [101]. Certain types of cytoplasmic abnormalities such as organelle clustering have also previously been shown to be associated with a high degree of aneuploidy and reduced oocyte and embryo metabolism [40].

Alikani et al. [37] analysed the relationship between variations found in oocyte morphology and aneuploidy as well as abnormal fertilization, embryo development and pregnancy and implantation rates. According to other authors [86], oocyte dysmorphism was not associated with a higher risk of aneuploidy in the developing embryo. Although statistically insignificant, oocytes with cytoplasmic dysmorphism and oocytes showing multiple morphological abnormalities were associated with lower fertilization and cleavage rates, as well as higher risk of aneuploidy in the derived embryos.

Kahraman et al. [44] showed that 53% of the embryos derived from the group of oocytes with centrally granulated cytoplasm were aneuploid. Although the genetic constitution of the oocytes displaying cytoplasmic abnormalities was studied, the fate of the oocytes with extracytoplasmic abnormality is not very clearly examined by earlier studies. A more recent study by Yakin et al. [86] demonstrated that although the aneuploidy rate of the group of embryos derived from oocytes with extracytoplasmic abnormalities (46.7%) was similar to the group of embryos derived from oocytes with normal morphology (41.8%), the aneuploidy rate for the group of embryos derived from oocytes with cytoplasmic abnormality was higher (60.0%) when compared with the group of embryos derived from oocytes with extracytoplasmic abnormality and the group of embryos derived from oocytes with normal morphology [86].

Yakin et al. [86] reported that embryos that developed from oocytes with normal morphology showed a lower (41.9%) aneuploidy rate when compared with embryos that have developed from oocytes with different types of morphological abnormalities in total (51.7%). However, this difference was not statistically different. When embryos were categorized according to the morphological abnormalities of the oocytes which they had been derived from, except the cytoplasmic abnormality group, all the other groups showed similar rates of aneuploidy. Embryos derived from oocytes with cytoplasmic and multiple abnormalities that contained at least one type of cytoplasmic abnormality showed the highest rate of aneuploidy (60.0 and 61.8%, respectively); however, the difference was still not statistically significant related to the low sample size in some study subgroups. As in this study no statistically significant differences for the chromosomal constitution of the normal group and morphological abnormality groups were found, the authors speculated that other defects like gene expression alterations may lead to failure in blastocyst formation. Wells et al. [102] demonstrated an association between certain forms of abnormal oocyte and zygote morphology and disturbances of gene activity.

Changes in oocyte mRNA associated with advancing maternal age have been reported, potentially linked to the well-documented age-related increase in oocyte aneuploidy. The application of the same technology has also revealed that morphologically abnormal preimplantation embryos frequently display atypical patterns of gene expression [103]. These findings suggest that the analysis of gene expression is a worthwhile approach for the identification of new viability markers [104].

It is well known that appropriate gene expression is vital for the regulation of metabolic pathways and key development events. The study by Wells et al. [102] examined the expression of nine genes in human preimplantation embryos and determined whether certain types of oocyte abnormalities such as granular cytoplasm, cytoplasm with condensed organelles or irregular shape are associated with altered gene activity. Altered BUB1 and BRCA1 gene expression was found in the condensed organelles group, whereas BUB1 alteration was observed for granular cytoplasm. No unusual expression of MAD2 was observed for the group of blastocysts derived from oocytes with irregular shape.

Fully validated microarray approaches involving the analysis of whole oocytes will be the near future applications for identifying oocytes destined to produce chromosomally normal, viable embryos with high likelihood for live birth [104].

Conclusions

After oocyte collection for assisted reproductive technologies, the oocytes display various aspects of maturation, integrity and viability. As there is still a lack of reliable and rapid biochemical, or molecular marker of their status, the best modality for evaluation of oocyte quality still remains to be direct microscopic observation of morphology [28].

Morphological assessment of human oocytes retrieved for ART remains to be a major tool in predicting IVF or ICSI outcome and should be further developed [28]. There are no clear and well-defined criteria for oocyte morphology evaluation as there are no widely accepted grading systems in effect. MOMS (metaphase II oocyte morphological scoring) should be introduced into human IVF laboratory practice, especially where oocyte selection before insemination is required. Moreover, universal MOMS could be used to unselect oocytes that have a lower chance to form a viable embryo for insemination (to reduce the creation of supernumerary embryos) as well as for cryopreservation [55].

Despite the fact that clear decisions for all types of morphological differences of human oocytes cannot be based upon data, some recommendations for specific abnormality types can be proposed.

Although results regarding the effect of only extracytoplasmic morphological deviations are still controversial, few studies were able to demonstrate their detrimental effect on the implantation potential of the embryo and further fate of the newborn. Therefore, in line with the published data, these types of oocyte dysmorphisms should perhaps not be considered as abnormalities but only a phenotypic deviation resulting from the heterogeneity of the oocytes retrieved.

In contrast to extracytoplasmic abnormalities, it is very clear that severe cytoplasmic deviations of the oocyte (organelle clustering also mentioned as sERCs, centrally severe granulation and excessive vacuolization) do impair the developmental and implantation potential of the embryo and may have important genetic consequences on the newborn [5, 19, 21, 105].

It can be concluded that morphological evaluation of the oocyte should be coupled with a detailed evaluation of the resulting embryo to reach a valuable conclusion regarding implantation and pregnancy. Certain morphological characteristics indicate a high likelihood of abnormality, and caution should be exercised when transferring embryos derived from such oocytes.

References

1. De Bruin JP, Dorland M, Spek ER, et al. Age-related changes in the ultrastructure of the resting follicle pool in human ovaries. Biol Reprod. 2004;70:419–24.
2. Rashidi BH, Sarvi F, Tehrani ES, et al. The effect of hMG and recombinant human FSH on oocyte quality: a randomized single-blind clinical trial. Eur J Obstet Gynecol Reprod Biol. 2005;120:190–4.
3. Ng EH, Lau EY, Yeung WS, et al. hMG is as good as recombinant human FSH in terms of oocyte and embryo quality: a prospective randomized trial. Hum Reprod. 2001;16:319–25.
4. De Cassia R, Figueira MS, Braga DPAF, et al. Metaphase II human oocyte morphology: contributing factors and effects on fertilization potential and embryo developmental ability in ICSI cycles. Fertil Steril. 2010;94(3):1115–7.
5. Balaban B, Urman B. Effect of oocyte morphology on embryo development and implantation. Reprod Biomed Online. 2006;12:608–15.
6. Recombinant Human FSH Study Group. Clinical assessment of recombinant human. Fertil Steril. 1995;63:77–86.
7. Huang FJ, Lan KC, Kung FT, et al. Human cumulus free oocyte maturational profile and in vitro development potential after stimulation with recombinant versus urinary FSH. Hum Reprod. 2004;19:306–15.
8. Pena JE, Chang PL, Chan LK, et al. Suprephysiological estradiol levels do not effect oocyte and embryo quality in oocyte donation cycles. Hum Reprod. 2002;17:83–7.
9. Baart EB, Martini E, Eijkemans MJ, et al. Milder ovarian stimulation for in vitro fertilization reduces aneuploidy in the human preimplantation embryo: a randomized controlled trial. Hum Reprod. 2007;22:980–8.
10. Hohmann FP, Macklon NS, Fauser BC. A randomized comparison of two ovarian gonadotropin-releasing hormone antagonist cotreatment for in vitro fertilization commencing recombinant follicle stimulating hormone on cycle day 2 or 5 with the standard long GnRH agonist protocol. J Clin Endocrinol Metab. 2003;88:166–73.
11. Fauser BC, Devroey P, Macklon NS. Multiple birth resulting from ovarian stimulation for subfertility treatment. Lancet. 2005;365:1807–16.
12. Macklon NS, Fauser BC. Impact of ovarian hyperstimulation on the luteal phase. J Reprod Fertil. 2000;55:101–8.
13. Howles CM, Macnamee MC, Edward RG, et al. Effect of high tonic levels of luteinising hormone on the outcome of in-vitro fertilization. Lancet. 1986;2(8505):521–2.
14. Homburg R, Armar NA, Eshel A, et al. Influence of serum luteinising hormone concentrations on ovulation, conception and early pregnancy loss in polycystic ovary syndrome. Br Med J. 1988;297:1024–6.
15. Regan L, Owen EJ, Jacobs HS. Hypersecretion of luteinizing hormone, infertility and miscarriage. Lancet. 1990;336:1141–4.
16. Franks S, Roberts R, Hardy K. Gonadotrophin regimens and oocyte quality in women with polycystic ovaries. Reprod Biomed Online. 2003;6:181–4.
17. Urman B, Tiras B, Yakin K. Assisted reproduction in the treatment of polycystic ovarian syndrome. Reprod Biomed Online. 2004;8:419–30.
18. Imthurn B, Macas E, Rosselli M, et al. Nuclear maturity and oocyte morphology after stimulation with highly compared to human menopausal gonadotrophin. Hum Reprod. 1996;11:2387–91.
19. Otsuki J, Okada A, Morimoto K, et al. The relationship between pregnancy outcome and smooth endoplasmic reticulum clusters in MII human oocytes. Hum Reprod. 2004;19:1591–7.
20. Hassan-Ali H, Hisham-Saleh A, El-Gezeiry D, et al. Perivitelline space granularity: a sign of human menopausal gonadotrophin overdose in intracytoplasmic sperm injection. Hum Reprod. 1998;13:3425–30.
21. Norbury C, Nurse P. Animal cell cycles and their control. Annu Rev Biochem. 1992;61:441–70.

22. Eppig JJ. Coordination of nuclear and cytoplasmic oocyte maturation in eutherian mammals. Reprod Fertil Dev. 1996;8:485–9.
23. Scott LA. Oocyte and embryo polarity. Semin Reprod Med. 2000;18:171–83.
24. Giovanni C, Elena S, Lucia S, et al. What criteria for the definition of oocyte quality? Ann N Y Acad Sci. 2004;1034:132–44.
25. Yang Y, Qingyun M, Xinjie C, et al. Assessment of the developmental competence of human somatic cell nuclear transfer embryos by oocyte morphology classification. Hum Reprod. 2009;24(3):649–57.
26. Hassan-Ali H, Hisham-Saleh A, El-Gezeiry D, et al. Perivitelline space granularity: a sign of human menopausal gonadotrophin overdose in intracytoplasmic sperm injection. Hum Reprod. 1998;13:3425–30.
27. Van Blerkom J. Occurrence and developmental consequences of aberrant cellular organization in meiotically mature human oocytes after exogenous ovarian hyperstimulation. J Electron Microsc Tech. 1990;16:324–46.
28. Mandelbaum J. Oocytes. Hum Reprod. 2000;15(4):11–8.
29. Ebner T, Moser M, Tews G. Is oocyte morphology prognostic of embryo developmental potential after ICSI? Reprod Biomed Online. 2006;12:507–12.
30. Ng Siu T, Chang T-H, Jackson TC. Prediction of the rates of fertilization, cleavage and pregnancy success by cumulus-coronal morphology in an in vitro fertilization program. Fertil Steril. 1999;72:412–7.
31. Wolf DP. Oocyte quality and fertilization. In: Wolf DP, editor. In vitro fertilization and embryo transfer. New York: Plenum Press; 1988. p. 129–38.
32. Lin Y-C, Chang S-Y, Lan K-C, et al. Human oocyte maturity in vivo determines the outcome of blastocyst development in vitro. J Assist Reprod Genet. 2003;20:506–11.
33. Engman L, Siano L, Schmidt D, et al. Outcome of in vitro fertilization in patients who electively inseminate a limited number of oocytes to avoid creating surplus embryos for cryopreservation. Fertil Steril. 2005;84:1406–10.
34. Veeck LL. Oocyte assessment and biological performance. Ann N Y Acad Sci. 1988;541:259–74.
35. Xia P. Intracytoplasmic sperm injection: correlation of oocyte grade based on polar body, perivitelline space and cytoplasmic inclusions with fertilization rate and embryo quality. Hum Reprod. 1997;12:1750–5.
36. De Sutter P, Dozortsev D, Qian C, et al. Oocyte morphology does not correlate with fertilization rate and embryo quality after intracytoplasmic sperm injection. Hum Reprod. 1996;11(3):595–7.
37. Alikani M, Palermo G, Adler A, et al. Intracytoplasmic sperm injection in dysmorphic human oocytes. Zygote. 1995;3:283–8.
38. Mikkelsen AL, Lindenberg S. Morphology of in-vitro matured oocytes: impact on fertility potential and embryo quality. Hum Reprod. 2001;16:1714–8.
39. Ebner T, Yaman C, Moser M, et al. Prognostic value of first polar body morphology on fertilization rate and embryo quality in intracytoplasmic sperm injection. Hum Reprod. 2000;15:427–30.
40. Van Blerkom J, Henry GH. Cytogenetic analysis of living human oocytes: cellular basis and developmental consequences of perturbations in chromosomal organization and complement. Hum Reprod. 1988;3:777–90.
41. Van Blerkom J, Henry GH. Oocyte dysmorphism and aneuploidy in meiotically mature human oocytes after ovarian stimulation. Hum Reprod. 1992;7:379–90.
42. Balaban B, Urman B, Sertac A, et al. Oocyte morphology does not affect fertilization rate, embryo quality and implantation rate after intracytoplasmic sperm injection. Hum Reprod. 1998;13:3431–3.
43. Serhal PF, Ranieri DM, Kinis A, et al. Oocyte morphology predicts outcome of intracytoplasmic sperm injection. Hum Reprod. 1997;12:1267–70.
44. Kahraman S, Yakin K, Donmez E, et al. Relationship between granular cytoplasm of oocytes and pregnancy outcome following intracytoplasmic sperm injection. Hum Reprod. 2000;15:2390–3.

45. Collas P, Poccia D. Remodeling the sperm nucleus into a male pronucleus at fertilization. Theriogenology. 1998;49:67–81.
46. Esfandiari N, Ryan EA, Gotlieb L, et al. Successful pregnancy following transfer of embryos from oocytes with abnormal zona pellucida and cytoplasm morphology. Reprod Biomed Online. 2005;11:620–3.
47. Sirard MA, Florman HM, Leibfried-Rutledge ML. Timing of nuclear progression and protein synthesis necessary for meiotic maturation of bovine oocytes. Biol Reprod. 1989;40:1257–63.
48. Kastrop PM, Bevers MM, Destree OH, et al. Protein synthesis and phosphorylation patterns of bovine oocytes maturing in vivo. Mol Reprod Dev. 1991;29:271–5.
49. Barnes FL, First NL. Embryonic transcription in in vitro cultured bovine embryos. Mol Reprod Dev. 1991;29:117–23.
50. De Sousa PA, Caveney A, Westhusin ME, et al. Temporal patterns of embryonic gene expression and their dependence on oogenetic factors. Theriogenology. 1998;49:115–28.
51. Blerkom J. Mitochondria in human oogenesis and preimplantation embryogenesis: engines of metabolism, ionic regulation and developmental competence. Reproduction. 2004;128:269–80.
52. Wilding M, Dale B, Marino M, et al. Mitochondrial aggregation patterns and activity in human oocytes and preimplantation embryos. Hum Reprod. 2001;16:909–17.
53. Edwards RG, Beard HK. Oocyte polarity and cell determination in early mammalian embryos. Mol Hum Reprod. 1997;3:863–905.
54. Garello C, Baker H, Rai J, et al. Pronuclear orientation, polar body placement, and embryo quality after intracytoplasmic sperm injection and in-vitro fertilization: further evidence for polarity in human oocytes. Hum Reprod. 1999;14:2588–95.
55. Rienzi L, Ubaldi FM, Lacobelli M, et al. Significance of metaphase II human oocyte morphology on ICSI outcome. Fertil Steril. 2008;90(5):1692–700.
56. Payne D, Flaherty SP, Barry MF, et al. Preliminary observations on polar body extrusion and pronuclear form score as a prognostic tool in IVF treatment. Hum Reprod. 1997;12:705–8.
57. Ebner T, Moser M, Sommergruber M, et al. Developmental competence of oocytes showing increased cytoplasmic viscosity. Hum Reprod. 2003;18(6):1294–8.
58. Loutradis D, Drakakis P, Kallianidis K, et al. Oocyte morphology correlates with embryo quality and pregnancy rate after intracytoplasmic sperm injection. Fertil Steril. 1999;72:240–4.
59. Meriano JS, Alexis J, Visram-Zaver S, et al. Tracking of oocyte dysmorphisms for ICSI patients may prove relevant to the outcome in subsequent patient cycles. Hum Reprod. 2001;16:2118–23.
60. Ebner T, Sommergruber M, Moser M, et al. Basal level of antimullerian hormone is associated with oocyte quality in stimulated cycles. Hum Reprod. 2006;21:2022–6.
61. Dozortsev D, Rybouchkin A, De Sutter P, et al. Human oocyte activation following intracytoplasmic injection: the role of the sperm cell. Hum Reprod. 1995;10:403–7.
62. Ebner T, Yaman C, Moser M, et al. A prospective study on oocyte survival rate after ICSI: influence of injection technique and morphological features. J Assist Reprod Genet. 2001;18:623–8.
63. Wilding M, Di Matteo L, D'Andretti S, et al. An oocyte score for use in assisted reproduction. J Assist Reprod Genet. 2007;24:350–8.
64. Ebner T, Moser M, Sommergruber M, et al. Occurrence and developmental consequences of vacuoles throughout preimplantation development. Fertil Steril. 2005;83(6):1635–40.
65. El Shafie M, Sousa M, Windt ML, et al. Ultrastructure of human oocytes: a transmission electron microscopy view. In: El Shafie M, Sousa M, Windt ML, Kruger TF, editors. An atlas of the ultrastructure of human oocyte. A guide for assisted reproduction. New York: Parthenon Publishing; 2000. p. 151–71.
66. Wallbutton S, Kasraie J. Vacuolated oocytes: fertilization and embryonic arrest following intra-cytoplasmic sperm injection in a patient exhibiting persistent oocyte macro vacuolization. Case report. J Assist Reprod Genet. 2010;27:183–8.
67. Corn CM, Hauser-Kronberger C, Moser M, et al. Predictive value of cumulus cell apoptosis with regard to blastocyst development of corresponding gametes. Fertil Steril. 2005;84:627–33.

68. Tesarik J. Use of immature germ cells for the treatment of male infertility. Hum Reprod Update. 1997;3:95–100.
69. Gosden R, Trasler J, Lucifero D, et al. Rare congenital disorders, imprinted genes, and assisted reproductive technology. Lancet. 2003;361:1975–7.
70. Maher E, Afran M, Barratt C. Epigenetic risks related to assisted reproductive technologies: epigenetics, imprinting, AR and icebergs? Hum Reprod. 2003;18:2508–11.
71. Ebner T, Moser M, Shebl O, et al. Gernot Tews prognosis of oocytes showing aggregation of smooth endoplasmic reticulum. Reprod Biomed Online. 2008;16(1):113–8.
72. Shen Y, Stalf T, Mehnert C, et al. Light retardance by human oocyte spindle is positively related to pronuclear score after ICSI. Reprod Biomed Online. 2006;12:737–51.
73. Hamamah S. Oocyte and embryo quality: is their morphology a good criterion? J Gynecol Obstet Biol Reprod. 2005;34:5S38–41.
74. Plachot M, Selva J, Wolf JP, et al. Consequences of oocyte dysmorphy on the fertilization rate and embryo development after intracytoplasmic sperm injection. A prospective multicenter study. Gynecol Obstet Fertil. 2002;30:772–9.
75. Palermo G, Alikani M, Bertoli M, et al. Oolemma characteristics in relation to survival and fertilization patterns of oocytes treated by intracytoplasmic sperm injection. Hum Reprod. 1996;11:172–6.
76. Choi T, Fukasawa K, Zhou R, et al. The Mos/mitogen-activated protein kinase (MAPK) pathway regulates the size and degradation of the first polar body in maturing mouse oocytes. Proc Natl Acad Sci U S A. 1996;93:7032–5.
77. Ritter-Eichenlaub U, Schmiady H, Kentenich H, et al. Recurrent failure in polar body formation and premature chromosome condensation in oocytes from a human patient: indicators of asynchrony in nuclear and cytoplasmic maturation. Hum Reprod. 1995;10:2343–9.
78. Ebner T, Moser M, Yaman C, et al. Elective transfer of embryos selected on the basis of first polar body morphology is associated with increased rates of implantation and pregnancy. Fertil Steril. 1999;72:599–603.
79. De Santis L, Cino I, Rabellotti E, et al. Polar body morphology and spindle imaging as predictors of oocyte quality. Reprod Biomed Online. 2005;11:36–42.
80. Balaban B, Urman B, Isiklar A, et al. The effect of polar body (PB) morphology on embryo quality, implantation and pregnancy rates. Fertil Steril. 2001;76:S11.
81. Ebner T, Moser M, Sommergruber M, et al. First polar body morphology and blastocyst formation rate in ICSI patients. Hum Reprod. 2002;17:2415–8.
82. Eichenlaub-Ritter U, Schmiady H, Kentenich H, et al. Recurrent failure in polar body formation and premature condensation in oocytes from a human patient: indicators of asynchrony in nuclear and cytoplasmic maturation. Hum Reprod. 1995;10:2343–9.
83. Ciotti PM, Notarangelo L, Morselli-Labate AM, et al. First polar body morphology before ICSI is not related to embryo quality or pregnancy rate. Hum Reprod. 2004;19:2334–9.
84. Verlinsky Y, Lerner S, Illkevitch N, et al. Is there any predictive value of first polar body morphology for embryo genotype or developmental potential? Reprod Biomed Online. 2003;7:336–41.
85. Verlhac MH, Lefebvre C, Guillaud P, et al. Asymmetric division in mouse oocytes: with or without MOS. Curr Biol. 2000;10:1303–6.
86. Yakin K, Balaban B, Isiklar A. Oocyte dysmorphism is not associated with aneuploidy in the developing embryo. Fertil Steril. 2007;88:811–6.
87. Balaban B, Ata B, Isiklar A, et al. Severe cytoplasmic abnormalities of the oocyte decrease cryosurvival and subsequent embryonic development of cryopreserved embryos. Hum Reprod. 2008;23(8):1778–85.
88. Ebner T, Moser M, Yaman C, et al. Prospective hatching of embryos developed from oocytes exhibiting difficult oolemma penetration during ICSI. Hum Reprod. 2002;17:1317–20.
89. Shen Y, Stalf T, Mehnert C, et al. High magnitude of light retardation by the zona pellucida is associated with conception cycles. Hum Reprod. 2005;20:1596–606.
90. Bertrand E, Van den Bergh M, Englert Y. Does zona pellucid thickness influence the fertilization rate? Hum Reprod. 1995;10(5):1189–93.

91. Gabrielsen A, Lindenberg S, Petersen K. The impact of the zona pellucida thickness variation of human embryos on pregnancy outcome in relation to suboptimal embryo development. A prospective randomized controlled study. Hum Reprod. 2001;16:2166–70.
92. Cohen J, Inge KL, Suzman K, et al. Videocinematography of fresh and cryopreserved embryos: a retrospective analysis of embryonic morphology and implantation. Fertil Steril. 1989;51:820–7.
93. Palmstierna M, Murkes D, Csemiczky G, et al. Zona pellucida thickness variation and occurrence of visible mononucleated blastomeres in preembryos are associated with a high pregnancy rate in IVF treatment. J Assist Reprod Genet. 1998;15:70–5.
94. Sathanathan H. Ultrastructure of the human egg. Hum Cell. 1997;10:21–38.
95. Dandekar P, Aggeler J, Talbot P. Structure distribution and composition of the extracellular matrix of human oocytes and cumulus masses. Hum Reprod. 1992;7:391–8.
96. Dandekar P, Talbot P. Perivitelline space of mammalian oocytes: extracellular matrix of unfertilized oocytes and formation of a cortical granule envelope following fertilization. Mol Reprod Dev. 1992;31:135–43.
97. Mikkelsen AL, Lindenberg S. Morphology of in vitro matured oocytes: impact on fertility potential and embryo quality. Hum Reprod. 2001;16:1714–8.
98. Plachot M. Genetic analysis of the oocyte—a review. Placenta. 2003;24:66–9.
99. Balakier H, Bouman D, Sojecki A, et al. Morphological and cytogenetic analysis of human giant oocytes and giant embryos. Hum Reprod. 2002;17:2394–401.
100. Rosenbusch B, Schneider M. Maturation of a binuclear oocyte from the germinal vesicle stage to metaphase II: formation of two polar bodies and two haploid chromosomal sets. Hum Reprod. 1998;13:1653–5.
101. Blerkom V, Henry G. Cytogenetic analysis of living human oocytes: cellular basis and developmental consequences of perturbations in chromosomal organization and complement. Hum Reprod. 1988;3:777–90.
102. Wells D, Bermudez M, Steuerwald N, et al. Association of abnormal morphology and altered gene expression in human preimplantation embryos. Fertil Steril. 2005;84:343–55.
103. Steuerwald N, Cohen J, Herrera RJ, et al. Association between spindle assembly checkpoint expression and maternal age in human oocytes. Mol Hum Reprod. 2001;7:49–55.
104. Patrizio P, Fragouli E, Bianchi V, et al. Molecular methods for selection of the ideal oocyte—review. Reprod Biomed Online. 2007;15:346–53.
105. Ebner T, Moser M, Shebl O, et al. Prognosis of oocytes showing aggregation of smooth endoplasmic reticulum. Reprod Biomed Online. 2008;16(1):113–8.

Chapter 2
Polarization Microscopy

Markus Montag, Maria Köster, and Hans van der Ven

The emerging field of cell biology in the nineteenth century was strongly influenced by advances in light microscopy. However, the use of polarized light at that time was rather low. In the first half of the twentieth century, Schmidt published a first systematic study of living animal cells and tissues and described the structure and development of skeletal and cellular components using polarization microscopy [1]. Later polarization microscopy was applied to study spindle dynamics in living cells [1–3]. Inoué and co-workers were the first to show the relationship between spindle retardance and microtubule density [4]. The introduction of video-enhanced microscopy greatly improved the sensitivity of polarized light microscopy [5].

Polarization Microscopy in Assisted Reproduction

The first investigation published on the application of polarized light in male gametes dates back to 1875, there Engelmann reported that the frog sperm tail shows birefringence, whereas the sperm head does not [6]. The very first photographic records of the spindle and astral birefringence in sea urchin zygotes were published in 1937 [7].

However, polarization microscopy only entered the field of reproduction in the late twentieth century, when advanced computer technology became available which allowed processing the huge amount of data generated in real-time imaging.

M. Montag, PhD (✉)
Department of Gynecological Endocrinology and Fertility Disorders,
University of Heidelberg, Voßstr. 9, 69115 Heidelberg, Germany
e-mail: markus.montag@med.uni-heidelberg.de

M. Köster, DVSc • H. van der Ven, MD
Department of Gynecological Endocrinology and Reproductive Medicine,
University of Bonn, Bonn, Germany

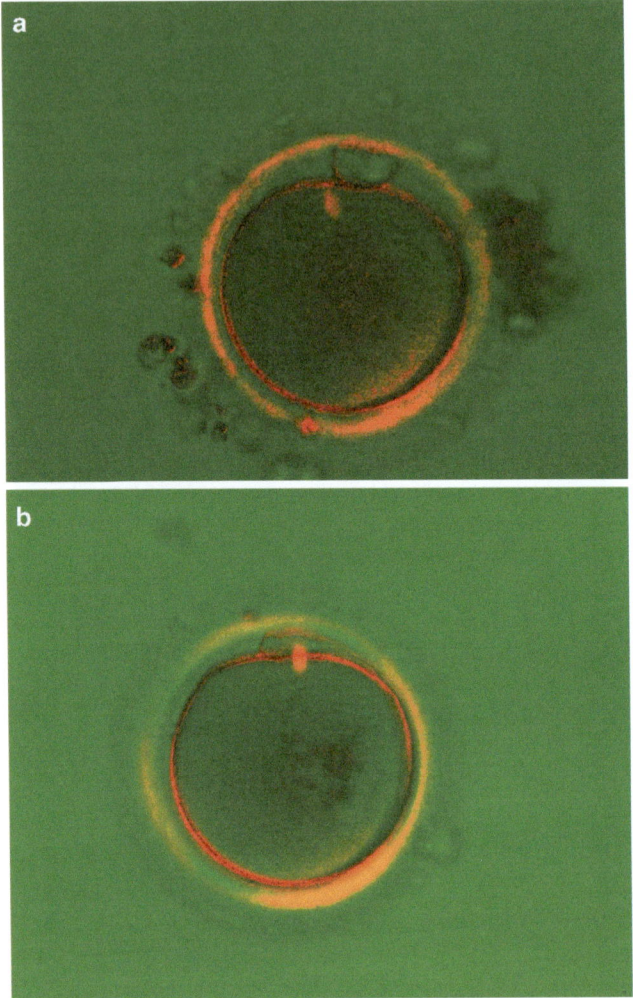

Fig. 2.1 Birefringence in human oocytes. The birefringence of the inner ring of the zona pellucida and the spindle underneath the polar body can be easily detected by polarization microscopy (**a**). In some oocytes, the spindle can be either absent or located at a different position. (**b**) An example of a spindle strand between the first polar body and the oocyte is shown

The new polarization microscope system used liquid crystals to modulate the polarization state and enabled real-time visualization of birefringent structures [8]. This type of instrument was the first with a proven applicability in assisted reproduction. The first publications on embryological specimens described the two elements within the mammalian oocyte which are birefringent: the zona pellucida [9] and the meiotic spindle [10] (Fig. 2.1a).

Spindle Imaging

Spindle Dynamics in the Meiotic Cell Cycle

The spindle is a highly dynamic structure, and especially during the progression of the meiotic cell cycle, the spindle disappears during the transition process in telophase I [11]. More detailed investigations on the course of the meiotic cell cycle were performed in human metaphase-I oocytes derived from stimulated cycles which were matured to metaphase-II in vitro [12]. This study showed that following the extrusion of the first polar body, the spindle formed a connective strand between the first polar body and the ooplasm prior to complete spindle disassembly (Fig. 2.1b). For a considerable time period, no spindle was detectable in the oocytes, followed by formation of the metaphase-II meiotic spindle which appeared underneath the first polar body approximately 115–150 min after extrusion of the first polar body from the oocyte. This study also showed that the presence of a first polar body by conventional light microscopy does not necessarily allow classifying an oocyte as metaphase-II.

Presence and Location of Spindles in Oocytes

As soon as spindle imaging was available in the IVF laboratory, the question arose whether it is relevant to locate the spindle during ICSI or not [10]. It became evident that the first polar body is not a reliable predictor of the location of the metaphase-II spindle. Rienzi et al. [13] reported that oocytes with a deviation of the spindle location from the position of the polar body of more than 90° showed lower fertilization rates, but that spindle position had no effect on embryo development, although another paper reported on the contrary [14]. Nowadays, it is believed that dislocation of the polar body from the spindle position may be a result of manipulation and stress caused during oocyte denudation [15], and therefore, the relevance of this point is unclear at the moment.

The relevance of the presence of the spindle for the outcome of ICSI was investigated in numerous publications with contradictory results in terms of fertilization rates, embryonic developmental competence on day 3, blastocyst formation rates, pregnancy and implantation rates (for references, see [16]).

A recent meta-analysis investigated the influence of the meiotic spindle visualization in human oocytes on the outcomes after ICSI [16]. The authors included ten published trials, although there was heterogeneity among some of the studies. The overall results showed for oocytes with a detectable spindle statistically higher fertilization rates, cleavage rates and embryo developmental rates up to the blastocyst stage. However, there was no benefit in terms of higher pregnancy or implantation rates.

Cryopreserved Oocytes

Polarized light microscopy was used to study the effect of cryopreservation on the spindle in metaphase-II oocytes. Using a conventional slow-freezing/rapid-thawing protocol, spindles reappear within 3 h after the thawing process in more than 50% of the oocytes [11, 17]. Using of a very efficient slow-freezing protocol with optimized sucrose concentrations, a reformation of the spindle was achieved in more than 80% of the frozen-thawed oocytes within 1 h after thawing [18].

Studies investigating the influence of oocyte vitrification on the spindle reported that spindles were found in 50% of the warmed oocytes, and in another 25%, the spindle appeared within the following 2 h [19]. Others reported that during the vitrification process, metaphase-II oocytes spindles remained present and did not disappear [20]. However, a temperature drop below 37 °C resulted in spindle depolymerization, whereas maintaining the temperature at a physiological point left the spindle intact and unaffected. These data show that the method of vitrification or slow freezing may have an influence on the spindle dynamics and may differ from lab to lab.

In Vitro Matured Oocytes

Spindle imaging is a good tool to follow the process of in vitro maturation and to decide on the optimal timing for ICSI in in vitro matured oocytes [21]. This is especially important if an in vitro maturation cycle is based on the presence of germinal vesicle (GV) stage oocytes, as oocytes matured from GV stage in vitro are not in synchrony during the following maturation process. Hence, timing of ICSI is of uttermost importance as in vitro matured oocytes do show a different time course compared to oocytes from stimulated cycles and develop faster [21].

Several publications have shown that the spindle of in vitro matured oocytes is very sensitive in regard to temperature [22]. Further, in vitro matured oocytes exhibit a high frequency of chromosome misalignments, probably due to spindle fragrance [23]. Like in oocytes from stimulated cycles, the location of the spindle is also positively correlated to the fertilization rates in in vitro matured oocytes [24].

Spindle Imaging and Laboratory Parameters

Spindle imaging is an ideal tool for quality assessment of certain laboratory parameters. Spindles are sensitive to pH and temperature, and it was shown that human spindles start to disintegrate at a temperature of 33 °C. Once disintegrated, spindle reassembly depends on how long it was exposed to the minimal temperature. Spindle reformation is very unlikely if the temperature dropped below 25 °C [25].

Exposure of oocytes in culture medium without stabilization of the pH in the medium also causes spindle disassembly within 8–10 min [26]. If spindle reformation after a pH shift is also dependent on a certain threshold is not known at present. Therefore, successful spindle imaging is a criterion that the settings for pH and temperature are correct and that manipulation of oocytes during the procedures preceding spindle imaging, like denudation and ICSI, did not lead to relevant changes.

Zona Imaging

Zona Birefringence and Zona Architecture

In conventional light microscopy, the zona pellucida of mammalian oocytes appears as a uniform layer surrounding the oocyte. However, polarization microscopy of hamster oocytes revealed a multi-layer architecture where three layers within the zona pellucida can be distinguished by their birefringent properties [9]. The inner zona layer exhibits the highest amount of birefringence, followed by a thin middle layer devoid of birefringence and an outer layer with a faint birefringence. The same characteristic pattern was also found in the zona pellucida of human oocytes [27]. How this relates to the known components of the zona pellucida, the zona proteins (ZP) and the embedded glycoproteins and polysaccharides is still unknown. It is commonly believed that the extent of birefringence of the inner zona layer is primarily an indication for the degree of order of the contributing structures within the zona during oocyte maturation.

Zona Imaging as a Prognostic Factor

Assessment of the zona pellucida by conventional microscopy and without the information of polarization microscopy cannot be used as a predictive factor for the success of ICSI [28]. However, Shen et al. found variations in the birefringence intensity of the inner layer of the zona pellucida among different oocytes by measuring zona thickness and intensity at three different positions of the entire zona. A further retrospective analysis showed that the mean zona birefringence intensity and thickness of the inner zona layer were higher among conception vs. non-conception cycles [29]. Using the same measuring approach like Shen et al., Rama Raju reported from retrospective data a correlation between zona birefringence and the potential of an embryo to develop to the blastocyst stage [30]. These studies stimulated further prospective investigations on the potential of zona birefringence imaging as a prognostic factor in ART.

Embryo Development and Pregnancy Outcome

One study investigated the intensity and uniformity of the zona inner layer's retardance in unfertilized metaphase-II oocytes by a non-invasive single observation prior to ICSI treatment [31]. Based on zona birefringence as the only selection criterion, two fertilized oocytes were selected for further culture and transfer. In this prospective study, implantation, pregnancy and live birth rates were significantly higher in cycles where the transferred embryos were derived from oocytes with high birefringence compared to those involving oocytes with low birefringence. Furthermore, embryo development on day 3 but not on day 2 was superior in embryos derived from high birefringent oocytes compared to embryos from low birefringent oocytes.

Meanwhile, two different approaches for automatic sampling of measurement values and automatic zona imaging have been presented [26, 32]. The first approach is based on the analysis of the radial orientation of glycoproteins in the inner zona layer [32]. The angular deviation of the radial orientated structures is greater if the inner zona layer is disrupted or less uniform and hence a characteristic for a presumably suboptimal oocyte. Data from a prospective clinical study supporting this theory are not yet available.

The second approach uses a software module which automatically detects the inner birefringent zona layer [26]. Following detection, a zona score is calculated in real-time based on the intensity and distribution of the birefringence at 180 measuring points. This enables an objective and user-independent score of the corresponding oocyte within a short observation time. It was shown that the results of automatic zona imaging were comparable to the data from the subjective study mentioned above [31].

In a prospective study, Ebner et al. used automatic zona imaging at the oocyte stage prior to ICSI and cultured embryos up to the blastocyst stage. When the automatic detection of the birefringence of the inner zona layer in the oocytes failed due to a heterogeneous intensity and thickness of the inner zona layer, the corresponding embryos showed significantly lower compaction rates and blastocyst formation rates. In addition, these embryos were significantly less involved in the initiation of a pregnancy. They concluded that the automatic zona score was a strong predictor of blastocyst formation rate [33]. In another prospective study, a positive correlation between zona pellucida birefringence score and implantation and pregnancy rates was reported [34–36]. This study showed for the first time that the miscarriage rate was higher in embryo transfer cycles where the transferred embryos were exclusively derived from oocytes with a low zona birefringence score.

Most of the studies conducted so far show that oocyte zona birefringence is a good predictive criterion for embryo implantation potential. Zona birefringence probably reflects the structural integrity of the zona pellucida. Oocytes with a high zona birefringence possess a very regular and optimal structured zona which is an indication for a good follicular development. Therefore, these oocytes may also have an optimal cytoplasmic potential which favors a good developmental competence for embryonic growth and implantation. Preliminary data indicate that different zona birefringent patterns (Fig. 2.2) correlate with different expression profiles of certain candidate genes in subpopulations of the cumulus-oophorus complex [35].

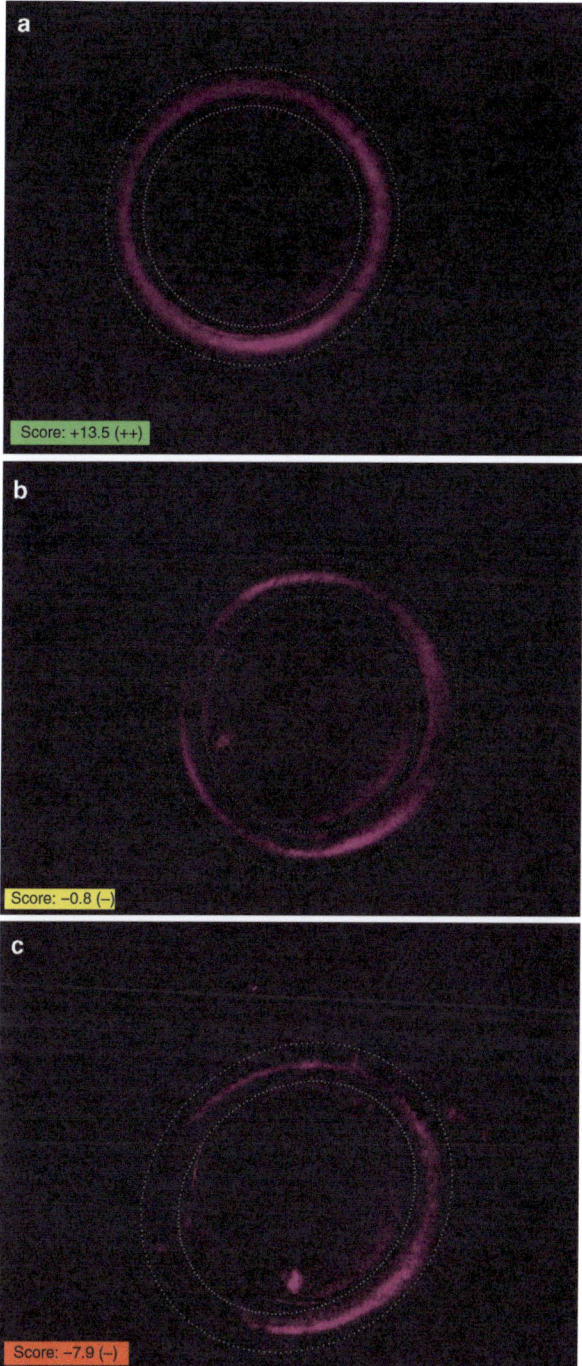

Fig. 2.2 Zona imaging by polarization microscopy. The different patterns of the birefringence of the inner zona layer can be automatically assessed and are characteristic for oocytes with a good (**a**), intermediate (**b**) or poor (**c**) embryo implantation potential

Summary

Polarization microscopy is on its way to become an important add-on in the laboratory for assessing the competence of gametes in assisted reproduction. The availability of polarization microscopes which can be used in the routine daily laboratory work is granted, and the use of this technique as a new tool in characterizing the developmental potential of oocytes could be proven by now in numerous studies. The applicability of polarization microscopy for classifying spermatozoa has been shown in some initial studies, too [36, 37], and this is an open field for further improvements. However, until to date most studies performed on the basis of polarization microscopy are more or less descriptive and/or comparative. What is really needed is the knowledge of the underlying physiological processes which result in the phenomenon which we describe. This may lead to improve laboratory practice as well as optimizing or individualizing stimulation protocols.

References

1. Schmidt WJ. Die Bausteine des Tierkörpers in polarisiertem Licht. Bonn: Cohen; 1924.
2. Inoué S. Polarization optical studies of the mitotic spindle. I. The demonstration of spindle fibers in living cells. Chromosoma. 1953;5:487–500.
3. Swann MM, Mitchison JM. Refinements in polarized light microscopy. J Exp Biol. 1950;27:226–37.
4. Sato H, Ellis GW, Inoué S. Microtubular origin of mitotic spindle form birefringence: demonstration of the applicability of Wiener's equation. J Cell Biol. 1975;67:501–17.
5. Inoué S. Video image processing greatly enhances contrast, quality and speed in polarization-based microscopy. J Cell Biol. 1981;89:346–56.
6. Engelmann TW. Contractilität und Dopperbrechung. Pflugers Arch. 1875;11:432–64.
7. Schmidt WJ. Die Doppelbrechung von Karyoplasma, Zytoplasma und Metaplasma. Berlin: Bornträger; 1937.
8. Oldenbourg R, Mei G. New polarized light microscope with precision universal compensator. J Microsc. 1995;180:140–7.
9. Keefe D, Tran P, Pellegrini C, Oldenbourg R. Polarized light microscopy and digital image processing identify a multilaminar structure of the hamster zona pellucida. Hum Reprod. 1997;12:1250–2.
10. Silva CS, Kapura K, Oldenbourg R, Keefe DL. The first polar body does not predict accurately the location of the metaphase II meiotic spindle in mammalian oocytes. Fertil Steril. 1999;71:719–21.
11. Rienzi L, Martinez F, Ubaldi F, et al. Polscope analysis of meiotic spindle changes in living metaphase II human oocytes during the freezing and thawing procedures. Hum Reprod. 2004;19:655–9.
12. Montag M, Schimming T, van der Ven H. Spindle imaging in human oocytes: the impact of the meiotic cell cycle. Reprod Biomed Online. 2006;12:442–6.
13. Rienzi L, Ubaldi F, Martinez F, et al. Relationship between meiotic spindle location with regard to polar body position and oocyte developmental potential after ICSI. Hum Reprod. 2003;18:1289–93.
14. Cooke S, Tyler JP, Driscoll GL. Meiotic spindle location and identification and its effect on embryonic cleavage plane and early development. Hum Reprod. 2003;18:2397–405.
15. Taylor TH, Chang CC, Elliott T, et al. Effect of denuding on polar body position in in-vitro matured oocytes. Reprod Biomed Online. 2008;17:515–9.

16. Petersen C, Oliveira JBA, Mauri AL, et al. Relationship between visualization of meiotic spindle in human oocytes and ICSI outcomes: a meta-analysis. Reprod Biomed Online. 2009; 18:235–43.
17. Bianchi V, Coticchio G, Fava L, et al. Meiotic spindle imaging in human oocytes frozen with a slow freezing procedure involving high sucrose concentration. Hum Reprod. 2005;20: 1078–83.
18. Sereni E, Sciajno R, Fava L, et al. A polscope evaluation of meiotic spindle dynamics in frozen-thawed oocytes. Reprod Biomed Online. 2009;19:191–7.
19. Chen CK, Wang CW, Tsai WJ, et al. Evaluation of meiotic spindles in thawed oocytes after vitrification using polarized light microscopy. Fertil Steril. 2004;82:666–72.
20. Larman MG, Minasi MG, Rienzi L, Gardner DK. Maintenance of the meiotic spindle during vitrification in human and mouse oocytes. Reprod Biomed Online. 2007;15:692–700.
21. Hyun CS, Cha JH, Son WY, et al. Optimal ICSI timing after the first polar body extrusion in in vitro matured human oocytes. Hum Reprod. 2007;22:1991–5.
22. Sun XF, Zhang WH, Chen XJ. Spindle dynamics in living mouse oocytes during meiotic maturation, aging, cooling and overheating: a study by polarized light microscopy. Zygote. 2004; 12:241–9.
23. Wang WH, Keefe DL. Prediction of chromosome misalignment among in vitro matured human oocytes by spindle imaging with the polscope. Fertil Steril. 2002;78:1077–81.
24. Fang C, Tang M, Li T, et al. Visualization of meiotic spindle and subsequent embryo development in in vitro and in vivo matured human oocytes. J Assist Reprod Genet. 2007;24:547–51.
25. Wang WH, Meng L, Hackett RJ, et al. Limited recovery of meiotic spindles in living human oocytes after cooling-rewarming observed using polarized light microscopy. Hum Reprod. 2001;16:2374–8.
26. Montag M, van der Ven H. Oocyte assessment and embryo viability prediction: birefringence imaging. Reprod Biomed Online. 2008;17:454–60.
27. Pelletier C, Keefe DL, Trimarchi JR. Noninvasive polarized light microscopy quantitatively distinguishes the multilaminar structure of the zona pellucida of living human eggs and embryos. Fertil Steril. 2004;81:850–6.
28. Ten J, Mendiola J, Vioque J, et al. Donor oocyte dysmorphisms and their influence on fertilization and embryo quality. Reprod Biomed Online. 2007;14:40–8.
29. Shen Y, Stalf T, Mehnert C, et al. High magnitude of light retardation by the zona pellucida is associated with conception cycles. Hum Reprod. 2005;20:1596–606.
30. Rama Raju GA, Prakash GJ, Krishna KM, Madan K. Meiotic spindle and zona pellucida characteristics as predictors of embryonic development: a preliminary study using polscope imaging. Reprod Biomed Online. 2007;14:166–74.
31. Montag M, Schimming T, Köster M, et al. Oocyte zona birefringence intensity is associated with embryonic implantation potential in ICSI cycles. Reprod Biomed Online. 2008;16:239–44.
32. Frattarelli JL, Miller KA, Fletcher-Holmes DW, et al. The use of quantitative birefringence imaging to assess oocyte competence. Hum Reprod. 2007;22 Suppl 1:i166.
33. Ebner T, Balaban B, Moser M, et al. Automatic user-independent zona pellucida imaging at the oocyte stage allows for the prediction of preimplantation development. Fertil Steril. 2010; 94(3):913–20.
34. Madaschi C, Aoki T, de Almeida Ferreira Braga DP, et al. Zona pellucida birefringence score and meiotic spindle visualization in relation to embryo development and ICSI outcomes. Reprod Biomed Online. 2009;18:681–6.
35. Van der Ven K, Montag M, Drengner C, et al. Differential gene expression profiles in cells of the corona radiata and outer cumulus oophorus in relation to oocyte competence. Hum Reprod. 2009;24 Suppl 1:i32.
36. Gianaroli L, Magli MC, Collodel G, et al. Sperm head's birefringence: a new criterion for selection? Fertil Steril. 2008;90:104–12.
37. Gianaroli L, Magli MC, Ferraretti A, et al. Birefringence characteristics in sperm heads allow for the selection of reacted spermatozoa for intracytoplasmic sperm injection. Fertil Steril. 2010;93(3):807–13.

Chapter 3
Cumulus Cell Gene Expression in Assessment of Oocyte Quality

Dagan Wells

Commentary

Cumulus Cell Biology and the Cumulus–Oocyte Relationship

The mature cumulus–oocyte complex (COC) is composed of the secondary oocyte, arrested at metaphase II following extrusion of the first polar body (PB), and surrounding cumulus cells (CCs). A unique characteristic of CCs is the presence of highly specialized cytoplasmic projections that pierce through the zona pellucida and form gap junctions at their tips with the oocyte [1]. This intimate association allows CCs to fulfill vital roles, supporting the maturation of the oocyte and relaying endocrine and other environmental signals.

Cumulus cells (CCs) originate from granulosa cells, the primary type of somatic cell in the follicle. Initiation of GC differentiation occurs upon follicular antrum formation, corresponding approximately to the end of the oocyte growth phase. In humans and other mammals, two anatomically and functionally distinct lineages are generated—mural GCs that line the wall of the follicle with primarily a steroidogenic role and the CCs, which encircle the oocyte [2, 3].

Cumulus cells undergo extensive proliferation prior to LH surge, and following the preovulatory LH surge, a cascade of events is initiated that leads to further proliferation and expansion [4, 5]. The competence to undergo expansion is a unique characteristic of CC differentiation [6], which has been shown to be critical for normal oocyte development, ovulation, and fertilization [7–9].

CCs are known to metabolize the bulk of glucose consumed by the COC, supplying metabolic intermediates like pyruvate, mainly via glycolysis, to the oocyte

---

D. Wells, PhD, FRCPath (✉)
Nuffield Department of Obstetrics and Gynaecology, John Radcliffe Hospital,
University of Oxford, Level 3, Women's Centre, Oxford OX3 9DU, UK
e-mail: Dagan.Wells@obs-gyn.ox.ac.uk

(for a detailed review on role of glucose metabolism in the oocyte, refer to Sutton-McDowall [10]). Other substrates of low molecular weight such as amino acids and nucleotides are passed to the growing oocyte for its own synthesis of macromolecules as well as ribosomal and messenger RNA from the GCs/CCs.

The nutritional support, trafficking of macromolecules, and dissemination of endocrine signals that this system allows may be particularly important for oocytes due to the avascular nature of the granulosa layer (reviewed by Johnson and Albertini [1, 11]). This communication is so crucial that genetic deletion of the oocyte specific gap junctional subunit, connexin-37, leads to female sterility in mice, resulting from a lack of mature follicles, failure to ovulate, and development of numerous inappropriate corpora lutea.

The role of CCs in supporting in vivo oocyte development as well as IVM [12, 13] has led increasing numbers of researchers to study these cells. Not only do investigations in this area promise to shed light on the biology of the follicle and the mechanisms promoting oocyte competence, but it is also possible that new biomarkers of oocyte potential may be identified.

One important component of the follicular environment, relevant to oocyte viability, is oxidative stress. Antioxidants produced by CCs, such as superoxide dismutases (SOD), are postulated to protect the oocyte from damage caused by reactive oxygen species. SOD levels in CCs have been noted to decrease with advancing female age, and higher SOD activities were associated with successful outcomes in assisted reproduction techniques [14]. Glutathione S transferases are another class of enzymes known to protect cells from reactive oxygen species. In a study by Ito et al. [15], GSTT1 (glutathione S transferase theta 1) was shown to be a good indicator of age-related infertility. Not only does this data emphasize the influence of oxidative stress on oocyte viability, it also suggests that SOD and GSTT1 might serve as potential biomarkers of prognostic significance.

Other studies have indicated that apoptosis rates are elevated for CCs associated with morphologically abnormal oocytes [16]. An increase in CC apoptosis has also been associated with immaturity of human oocytes, impaired fertilization [17], suboptimal blastocyst development [18], and poor IVF outcomes [19, 20]. It may be that abnormal/poor-quality oocytes induce apoptosis in the associated CCs. Alternatively, CCs with high levels of apoptosis, perhaps symptomatic of a suboptimal follicular environment, may lead to impaired oocyte development. Whatever the explanation, these observations highlight the interdependence of the oocyte and its CCs and suggest that certain elements of CC biology may serve as indicators of oocyte viability.

Gene Expression Studies of Human Cumulus Cells: Identifying New Biomarkers of Oocyte Quality

With appropriate methods, it may be possible to detect and decode molecular alterations in the CCs associated with differences in oocyte viability [21]. For example, patterns of gene expression reflect processes occurring within a cell at a given moment in time, including the cell's responses to environmental challenges. Thus, patterns of gene activity in CCs may reveal much concerning the conditions within the follicle during the final stages of oocyte maturation. Several groups have utilized emerging transcriptomic techniques to gain a better understanding of follicle biology and to try and identify novel biomarkers of oocyte competence [22–29] (see Glossary).

CCs are constantly responding to the intrafollicular environment to ensure optimal oocyte development, adjusting gene expression in order to maximize oocyte support and minimize damage caused by extrinsic factors (e.g., reactive oxygen species). An ongoing study of the CC transcriptome in our laboratory has indicated that the follicular microenvironment might even play a role in the origin of oocyte meiotic chromosome abnormality, one of the main causes of oocyte incompetence. The study revealed that cumulus cells associated with aneuploid oocytes have characteristic deviations in their gene expression profile [29] (Fragouli, Wells, and Patrizio, unpublished data). Abnormally expressed genes include several involved in pathways related to cellular stress (e.g., hypoxia, nutritional deprivation), suggesting an association between aneuploidy and suboptimal environment. Some genes involved in hormonal response also displayed abnormal expression, potentially providing a link between the increased frequency of aneuploidy and the altered hormone levels seen with advancing age. Furthermore, a number of genes with roles in apoptotic pathways showed distorted expression levels, in keeping with previous studies suggesting an association between CC proliferation and/or apoptosis and poor IVF outcomes [17–19, 30].

Gasca and colleagues [23] attempted to identify potential regulators and marker genes involved in oocyte maturation by screening human oocytes and CCs using microarrays [23]. Their study identified a number of potentially significant genes involved in processes such as cell cycle checkpoints and DNA repair, including *BARD1, RBL2, RBBP7, BUB3 and BUB1B*. Appropriate expression of these genes may have relevance to oocyte quality, although this remains to be conclusively proven.

Another microarray study, conducted by Assou et al. reported patterns of CC expression associated with embryo morphology and pregnancy outcome. These included upregulation of *BCL2L11* (involved in apoptosis) and *PCK1* (involved in gluconeogenesis) and downregulation of *NFIB* (a transcription factor). The researchers proposed that these three genes might be useful biomarkers for the prediction of pregnancy [28].

Feuerstein et al. [25] assessed the expression of six genes chosen because their expression is induced by the LH peak (*STAR, COX2* and *AREG*) or because of known roles in oocyte lipid metabolism (*SCD1* and *SCD5*) or in gap junctions (*Cx43*). With the exception of *Cx43*, all of the genes displayed increased expression in CCs after resumption of meiosis. Nuclear maturation of the oocyte was associated with increased expression of *STAR, COX2, AREG, SCD1* and *SCD5* in CCs. Interestingly, mRNA transcript levels of these genes were lower and distributed over a narrower range in CCs enclosing oocytes, achieving blastocyst development at day 5/6 than in CCs enclosing oocytes unable to develop beyond the embryo stage.

Further potential markers of oocyte competence identified by gene expression studies include *PTGS2* (prostaglandin-endoperoxide synthase; cyclooxygenase), *HAS2* (hyaluronic acid synthase 2), and *GREM1* (gremlin 1) [31]. CCs associated with oocytes that produced high-quality cleavage-stage embryos were found to have greater numbers of transcripts compared to CCs from oocytes that produced poor-quality embryos (expression of *PTGS2* and *HAS2* was sixfold higher; *GREM1* was 15-fold higher). Complementary results were obtained for *GREM1* and *HAS2* by Cillo and colleagues, suggesting that the measurement of transcripts from these genes in CCs might complement morphological evaluation and provide a useful tool for selecting oocytes with greater chances of fertilization and development in vitro [24].

Altered expression of several genes has been correlated with early cleavage post-fertilization, a feature generally considered to be a positive indicator of IVF outcome. The function of these genes suggest a role for hypoxic conditions (*CXCR4, GPX3, DVL3, HSPB1*) or delayed oocyte maturation (*CCND2, TRIM28, DHCR7, CTNND1*) in non-early cleavage embryos [26]. Not only do these results shed light on aspects of follicle biology that might predispose to late/early cleavage, but as with the studies discussed above, they also provide a set of markers that might assist oocyte selection.

A further set of markers of oocyte/follicle competence were reported by Hamel et al. [27] who performed experiments with the aim of identifying cumulus/granulosa cell genes specifically expressed in follicles that produced a pregnancy. They created a DNA microarray composed of cumulus/granulosa cell expressed sequence tags from subtracted libraries (cumulus/granulosa cells from women who became pregnant versus cells from those who did not). Altered expression of the *CDC42, 3bHSD, SERPINE2, FDX1* and *CYPA191* genes was significantly associated with competent follicles that resulted in pregnancies. These correlations were confirmed with quantitative PCR analyses [27].

Conclusion

The various studies seeking to characterize the CC transcriptome have yielded a wealth of novel data, including a detailed catalog of the genes expressed in CCs. Importantly, a number of genes displaying differential activity, apparently related to oocyte competence, have been identified. Quantification of the mRNA transcripts from such genes, or the proteins they produce, may provide new insights into oocyte (and embryo) competence, not possible using conventional techniques. Clinical trials aimed at assessing the potential of CC-based strategies of oocyte quality assessment are now underway. In the near future, diagnostic approaches based upon analyses of cumulus cells may revolutionize the way in which oocytes and embryos are selected for uterine transfer during IVF treatments, potentially leading to increases in fertilization, implantation, and clinical pregnancy rates. If markers of aneuploidy can also be identified, as initial data suggests, a reduction in the rates of miscarriage and aneuploid syndromes (e.g., Down syndrome) are also anticipated. A noninvasive preconception test for aneuploidy would overcome some of the most important technical and ethical difficulties facing preimplantation genetic screening [29].

Acknowledgment Dagan Wells is funded by NIHR Biomedical Research Centre Program.

Glossary

Downregulated/underexpressed Cases where fewer mRNA transcripts are found. Gene expression is reduced (i.e., the gene is less active).

Gene expression A complete set of all of the genes (i.e., the entire genome) is present in all cells. However, only a fraction of these genes are active in a cell at any given moment. Genes which are being actively transcribed, producing mRNA and ultimately proteins, are said to be "expressed."

Microarray A method for simultaneously quantifying the number of transcripts from large numbers of genes (typically thousands or tens of thousands of genes simultaneously assessed).

mRNA transcripts The molecules that serve as intermediates between genes (made of deoxyribonucleic acid, DNA) and the proteins they produce. The DNA sequence of a gene is transcribed into a messenger RNA (ribonucleic acid) copy, which is subsequently translated into a polypeptide.

Real-time PCR A method of quantifying the number of mRNA transcripts from individual genes. Real-time PCR is generally considered the most accurate method for quantifying gene expression but only allows analysis of small numbers of genes at a time.

Transcriptome The sum total of all mRNA transcripts found within an individual cell or tissue. The characterization of the transcriptome reveals all of the genes expressed (i.e., active).

Upregulated/overexpressed When two different samples are compared, some genes may be found to have differences in the number of mRNA transcripts. If a sample contains a greater number of mRNA transcripts than expected, the gene is said to be upregulated or overexpressed (i.e., it is more active).

References

1. Albertini DF, Combelles CM, Benecchi E, Carabatsos MJ. Cellular basis for paracrine regulation of ovarian follicle development. Reproduction. 2001;121:647–53.
2. Chian RC, Lim JH, Tan SL. State of the art in vitro oocyte maturation. Curr Opin Obstet Gynecol. 2004;16:211–9.
3. Gilchrist RB, Lane M, Thompson JG. Oocyte-secreted factors: regulators of cumulus cell function and oocyte quality. Hum Reprod Update. 2008;14:159–77.
4. Scherzer J, Ghuman SPS, Pope M, Routly JE, Walter I, Smith RF, Dobson H. Follicle and oocyte morphology in ewes after treatment with insulin in the late follicular phase. Theriogenology. 2009;71: 817–28.

5. Lin YH, Hwang JL, Seow KM, Huang LW, Chen HJ, Tzeng CR. Effects of growth factors and granulosa cell co-culture on in-vitro maturation of oocytes. Reprod Biomed Online. 2009; 19:165–70.
6. Diaz FJ, O'Brien MJ, Wigglesworth K, Eppig JJ. The pre-granulosa cell to cumulus cell transition in the mouse ovary: development of competence to undergo expansion. Dev Biol. 2006;299:91–104.
7. Elvin JA, Clark AT, Wang P, Wolfman NM, Matzuk MM. Paracrine actions of growth differentiation factor-9 in the mammalian ovary. Mol Endocrinol. 1999;13:1035–48.
8. Chang H, Brown CW, Matzuk MM. Genetic analyses of the mammalian transforming growth factor beta superfamily. Endocr Rev. 2002;23:787–823.
9. Vanderhyden BC, Macdonald EA, Nagyova E, Dhawan A. Evaluation of members of the TGFβ superfamily for the oocyte factors that control mouse cumulus expansion and steroidogenesis. Reprod Suppl. 2003;61:55–70.
10. Sutton-McDowall ML, Gilchrist RB, Thompson JG. The pivotal role of glucose metabolism in determining oocyte developmental competence. Reproduction. 2010;139(4):685–95.
11. Johnson MH. Ovarian function in the adult. In: Johnson MH, Everitt BJ, editors. Essential reproduction. 6th ed. Oxford: Blackwell; 2007. p. 82–91.
12. Vanderhyden BC, Armstrong DT. Role of cumulus cells and serum on the in vitro maturation, fertilisation and subsequent development of rat oocytes. Biol Reprod. 1989;40:720–8.
13. Ebner T, Moser M, Sommergruber M, Shebl O, Tews G. Incomplete denudation of oocytes prior to ICSI enhances embryo quality and blastocyst development. Hum Reprod. 2006;21:2972–7.
14. Matos L, Stevenson D, Gomes F, Silver-Carvalho JL, Almeida H. Superoxide dismutase expression in human cumulus oophorus cells. Mol Hum Reprod. 2009;15:411–9.
15. Ito M, Muraki M, Takahashi Y, Imai M, Tsukui T, Yamakawa N, Nakagawa K, Ohgi S, Horikawa T, Iwasaki W, et al. Glutathione S-transferase theta 1 expressed in granulosa cells as a biomarker for oocyte quality in age-related infertility. Fertil Steril. 2008;90:1026–35.
16. Yang YJ, Zhang YJ, Yuan L. Ultrastructure of human oocytes of different maturity stages and the alteration during in vitro maturation. Fertil Steril. 2009;92:396.e1–6.
17. Host E, Gabrielsen A, Lindenberg S, Smidt-Jensen S. Apoptosis in human cumulus cells in relation to zona pellucida thickness variation, maturation stage and cleavage of the corresponding oocyte after intracytoplasmic sperm injection. Fertil Steril. 2002;77:511–5.
18. Corn CM, Hauser-Kronberger C, Moser M, Tews G, Ebner T. Predictive value of cumulus cells apoptosis with regard to blastocyst development of corresponding gametes. Fertil Steril. 2005;84: 627–33.
19. Nakahara K, Saito H, Saito T, Ito M, Ohta N, Takahashi T, Hiroi M. The incidence of apoptotic bodies in membrana granulosa can predict prognosis of ova from patients participating in in-vitro fertilization programs. Fertil Steril. 1997;68:312–7.
20. Oosterhuis GJE, Michgelsen HW, Lambalk CB, Schoemaker J, Vermes I. Apoptotic cell death in human granulosa-lutein cells: a possible indicator of in vitro fertilization outcome. Fertil Steril. 1998;70:747–9.
21. Patrizio P, Fragouli E, Bianchi V, Borini A, Wells D. Molecular methods for selection of the ideal oocyte. Reprod Biomed Online. 2007;15:346–53.
22. Fragouli E, Bianchi V, Delhanty J, Patrizio P and Wells D (2007) Gene expression analysis of human oocytes: towards a non-invasive diagnosis of meiotic aneuploidy. Hum Reprod. 22(Suppl 1):i32, O-078.
23. Gasca S, Pellestor F, Assou S, Loup V, Anahory T, Dechaud H, De Vos J, Hamamah S. Identifying new human oocyte marker genes: a microarray approach. Reprod Biomed Online. 2007;14:175–83.
24. Cillo F, Brevini TAL, Antonini S, Paffoni S, Ragni G, Gandolfi F. Association between human oocyte developmental competence and expression levels of some cumulus genes. Reproduction. 2007;134:645–50.
25. Feuerstein P, Cadoret V, Dalbies-Tran R, Guerif F, Bidault R, Royere D. Gene expression in human cumulus cells: one approach to oocyte competence. Hum Reprod. 2007;22:3069–77.

26. Van Montfoort APA, Geraedts JPM, Dumoulin JCM, Stassen APM, Evers JLH, Ayoubi TAY. Differential gene expression in cumulus cells as a prognostic indicator of embryo viability: a microarray analysis. Mol Hum Reprod. 2008;14:157–68.
27. Hamel M, Dufort I, Robert C, Gravel C, Leveille MC, Leader A, Sirard MA. Identification of differentially expressed markers in human follicular cells associated with competent oocytes. Hum Reprod. 2008;23:1118–27.
28. Assou S, Haouzi D, Mahmoud K, Aouacheria A, Guillemin Y, Pantesco V, Rème T, Dechaud H, De Vos J, Hamamah S. A non-invasive test for assessing embryo potential by gene expression profiles of human cumulus cells: a proof of concept study. Mol Hum Reprod. 2008;14:711–9.
29. Wells D, Fragouli E, Bianchi V, Borini A, Patrizio P. Identification of novel non-invasive biomarkers of oocyte aneuploidy. Fertil Steril. 2008;90 Suppl 1:S35.
30. Gregory L. Ovarian markers of implantation potential in assisted reproduction. Hum Reprod. 1998;4:117–32.
31. McKenzie LJ, Pangas SA, Carson SA, Kovanci E, Cisneros P, Buster JE, Amato P, Matzuk MM. Human cumulus cells granulosa cell gene expression: a predictor of fertilisation and embryo selection in women undergoing IVF. Hum Reprod. 2004;19:2869–74.

Part II
Sperm Evaluation and Selection

Chapter 4
Sperm Assessment: Traditional Approaches and Their Indicative Value

Margot Flint, Fanuel Lampiao, Ashok Agarwal, and Stefan S. du Plessis

The basic semen analysis plays a pivotal role in the diagnosis of male infertility and makes a significant contribution to the diagnostic process in andrology, gynaecology and clinical urology [1]. In 1902, the man considered to be "the founding father of modern andrology", Edward Martin, proposed that an analysis of a semen sample should be incorporated into all infertility assessments [2, 3]. Following this suggestion, in 1956, the scientist John MacLeod advanced the basic semen analysis from beyond a mere observation and introduced the importance of certain sperm parameters such as morphology and motility [2, 3].

The present day examination includes the analysis of certain established semen parameters which can provide key information about the quality of a patient's semen and the functional competence of the spermatozoa [1]. A semen analysis including sperm assessment is a valuable diagnostic tool in assessing possible disorders of the male genital tract and the secretory pattern of the male accessory sex glands. This information can help to determine the reproductive capacity of the male and can be used in conjunction with the partner to indicate the impact of male genital pathophysiology in the assessment of a couple's prospect for fertility. The World Health Organization (WHO) has provided both reference values, based on the semen of fertile men, and a multi-step manual for a semen analysis. The traditional analysis is essentially performed in three functional steps: pre-analytic, analytic, and post-analytic phases [4, 5]. The WHO manual is generally accepted as the standard reference that establishes uniformity in laboratory procedures [6]. It is furthermore useful

---

M. Flint, MSc (✉) • F. Lampiao, PhD • S.S. du Plessis, PhD
Department of Medical Physiology, Stellenbosch University, Tygerberg 7505,
Western Cape, South Africa
e-mail: mf@sun.ac.za

A. Agarwal, PhD, HCLD (ABB), EMB (ACE)
Director, Center for Reproductive Medicine, Cleveland Clinic, Euclid Avenue 9500,
Cleveland, OH 44195, USA

Lerner College of Medicine of Case Western Reserve University, Cleveland, OH, USA

in providing essential ranges and lower limits of normality from which prognosis of fertility or diagnosis of infertility can be extrapolated by the clinician [7]. The parameters outlined by the WHO include the following: assessment of sperm characteristics and the physical and biochemical analysis of semen [1]. The reference values provided by the latest WHO manual are based on retrospective and prospective analysis of semen samples from hundreds of males from different countries whose partners had a time-to-pregnancy (TTP) of less than 12 months [8, 9]. Semen parameters can vary greatly among individuals; therefore, laboratories should interpret these result values together with clinical information of the patient. Interpretations of results are also challenging as different laboratories base their analysis on their own particular "reference values", and hence, lack of standardization is often a dilemma [7]. With regard to assisted reproductive technology (ART), semen parameters from analyses that fall into the 95% confidence interval (CI) are not necessarily guarantees of fertility [8]. A basic semen analysis can show diverse irregularities or deviations from the standard reference values. A follow-up investigation can then be carried out in order to assess specific sperm functions and prepare a diagnosis.

Despite the relevance of a semen analysis, it still has limitations in its diagnostic potential. It must be remembered that semen is naturally heterogeneous, and the composition is influenced by several variables, for example, infection, accessory sex gland functioning and the period of sexual abstinence [6]. All of these confounding elements can result in deviation from the standard reference values of the semen parameters and can subsequently alter their indicative value. The limitations of analyses have been described as the problem that it is "a visual observation of a continually variable biological product" [6]. It must be considered that there is no strict feedback system that controls the composition of semen. Consequently, variation may occur among individuals, countries and even between consecutive samples obtained from the same patient [6, 9]. Certain factors are also responsible for potentially altering the results of a semen analysis, such as the time period from collection to analysis [10]. The traditional semen analysis is an extremely valuable laboratory procedure. However, the crucial step is remembering that each variable alone is neither a powerful sole discriminator nor a predictor of fertility status and must therefore be considered in the context of other variables [11]. While measurements made on the whole population of ejaculated spermatozoa cannot define the fertilizing capacity of the few spermatozoa that reach the site of fertilization, the semen analysis nevertheless provides essential information on the clinical status of the individual [8].

It must also be noted that it is impossible to characterize a man's semen quality from evaluation of a single semen sample. It is therefore advisable to examine at least two or three samples before making any conclusions.

The Standard Semen Analysis

The traditional spermiogram is a test which can provide information on several levels. It can assess whether or not a patient is to be considered "normal" based on the quality of his semen and whether or not the degree of this impairment would

Table 4.1 The different macroscopic and microscopic evaluations performed during the traditional semen assessment/analysis

Macroscopic evaluations	Microscopic evaluations
Liquefaction	Motility
Appearance	Concentration
Viscosity	Morphology
Volume	Vitality
pH	Non-specific cellular elements

Table 4.2 The lower reference limits (fifth centile and their 95% confidence intervals) for semen parameters

Parameter	Lower reference limit
Semen volume (mL)	1.5 (1.4–1.7)
Total sperm number (10^6/ejaculate)	39 (33–46)
Sperm concentration (10^6/mL)	15 (12–16)
Total motility (PR + NP, %)	40 (38–42)
Progressive motility (PR, %)	32 (31–34)
Vitality (live spermatozoa, %)	58 (55–63)
Sperm morphology (normal forms, %)	4 (3.0–4.0)
pH	≥ 7.2
Peroxidase-positive leukocytes (10^6/mL)	<1.0

Data from WHO [8]; and Cooper et al [9].

compromise his fertility status [12]. Secondly, the test can pinpoint an abnormality such as teratozoospermia and can therefore offer a diagnosis [12]. Despite the option of computer-aided semen analysis (CASA), a semi-automated technique, the manual analysis of semen parameters is still an extremely effective indicator of the quality and composition of semen [11].

The methods described in this text (Table 4.1) are the ones most commonly used in the andrology setting and is only intended as guidelines. They should not necessarily be taken as obligatory, but it is however important to note that all aspects of semen collection and analysis must be done by properly standardized procedures if the results are to provide valid and useful information. The lower reference limits (fifth percentile and their 95% CI) for the semen parameters measured by these respective analyses are shown in Table 4.2.

Sample Collection

Correct sample collection is important as the results of laboratory measurements depend on it. It is well described that the collection method and the time since the last sexual activity can influence semen quality [13–16]. It is also known that during ejaculation, the first semen fractions voided are more sperm rich as opposed to the later fractions that predominantly consist of vesicular fluid [17].

For the collection of semen for diagnostic or research purposes, it is important to give the man clear instructions concerning the collection of the sample. It must be emphasized that the sample needs to be complete, and if loss of any fraction occurs, it must be reported. The sample should be collected after a minimum of 2 days and a maximum of 7 days of sexual abstinence by means of masturbation and ejaculated into a clean wide-mouth container. It is advisable that the sample is collected near the laboratory in order to limit temperature fluctuations and time between collection and analysis. The specimen container must be kept between 20 and 37°C prior to ejaculation and left at either ambient temperature or in an incubator at 37°C while the semen liquefies in order to avoid large changes in temperature that may affect the spermatozoa. It is furthermore important to label the sample thoroughly and record all applicable information in a report. This may include the patient's name, date, period of abstinence, time of collection, interval between collection and start of analysis and completeness of sample amongst others.

Macroscopic Evaluation

The variables that are traditionally assessed during the macroscopic evaluation of a semen sample include liquefaction and appearance, viscosity, volume and pH (Table 4.3) [11]. Inter-patient variability may result in deviations from the normal reference values with a macroscopic assessment. However, ductal obstruction and/or vas/epididymal defects are often the most common reasons for abnormalities of these parameters [11]. Macroscopic analysis should begin preferably at 30 min, but no longer than 60 min after ejaculation.

Liquefaction and Appearance

During sperm collection, the entire ejaculate is collected in one container, where spermatozoa are trapped in coagulation developed from proteins of seminal vesicle origin. This coagulation is subsequently liquefied by the actions of prostatic proteases [17, 18]. Semen naturally liquefies within 60 min if the sample is left at room temperature, and it is normal for semen to begin liquefying after 15 min. The process of liquefaction is significant as it allows for immobilized sperm to become motile [8]. Gelatinous masses may be present in the sample which does not liquefy in the expected period after ejaculation. This phenomenon appears to have no clinical significance [8]. However, it must be recorded in a routine analysis if certain semen samples are not able to liquefy within the required period. Action is then required in order to induce the process of liquefaction through enzymatic digestion or mechanical manipulation of the sample using repeated pipetting [8]. Incomplete liquefaction can be indicative of a disturbance of the accessory sex glands, in particular, the seminal vesicles and prostate. Fibrin, a protein which forms the meshwork of a clot, is responsible for the coagulation of semen directly after ejaculation. Fibrinolysin, a proteolytic enzyme produced by the prostate, acts to degrade the fibrin, which liquefies the congealed semen within 5–15 min. Therefore, if semen fails to liquefy, it can be indicative of a glandular dysfunction of the prostate [19].

Table 4.3 Summary of the clinical significance of various parameters performed during a routine semen analysis

Routine parameter	Abnormality	Clinical significance (indicative of)	References
Coagulation/liquefaction	Absence of coagulation	Agenesis of the vas deferens	[1, 11]
	No liquefaction	Dysfunctional prostate	
Colour/appearance	Yellow	Jaundice; drugs	[1, 2]
	Red-brown	Haemospermia	
Volume	High volume	Inflammation/dysfunction of accessory sex glands	[1, 2, 11]
		Prolonged abstinence period	
	Low volume	Partial retrograde ejaculation	
		Ejaculatory duct obstruction	
		Short abstinence period	
Viscosity	Hyperviscosity/hypoviscosity	Dysfunctional accessory sex glands	[1, 11]
pH	High pH (>7.8)	Dysfunctional prostate and seminal vesicles	[3, 8]
	Low pH (<7.2)		
Sperm concentration	Low concentration	Short abstinence period	[3, 4, 8, 9]
		Incomplete collection	
Morphology (normal forms)	Teratozoospermia	Abnormal spermatogenesis	[3, 5, 8, 41]
Vitality/viability (live)	Non-viable	Abnormal spermatogenesis	[3, 8]
		Dysfunctional prostate and seminal vesicles	
White blood cells	Leukocytospermia	Male genital tract infection	[1–3, 6, 8]

The typical appearance of a normal semen sample is a grey-opalescent colour [8]. If a patient has used certain drugs, consumed vitamin supplements or is suffering from jaundice, then the semen may present with a yellow colour [1]. Semen with a red-brown appearance, known as haemos-permia, is indicative of the presence of erythrocytes in the ejaculate [1, 8].

Viscosity

The viscosity of a semen sample is estimated by aspirating it into a plastic pipette (±1.5 mm diameter) and allowing the semen to drop by gravity and observing the length of any thread formed. A sample is considered normal if it leaves the pipette in small discrete drops. A sample with abnormal viscosity will have drops which form a thread of more than 2 cm long [8]. Viscosity can also be measured by dipping a glass rod into the sample and examining the length of the thread that forms upon removing the rod. If it exceeds 2 cm, it is yet again regarded as abnormal or hyperviscous. Hyperviscosity has been shown to be associated with a lower percentage of motile spermatozoa [20] and is indicative of a deficiency in the functional activity of the accessory sex glands. Changes in the viscosity of semen suggest impairment in both the seminal vesicles and the prostate [1, 21].

Volume

The accessory glands supply their secretions in an ordered sequence to the ejaculate. The total volume of semen is therefore indicative of the functioning of the prostate, seminal vesicles and bulbourethral glands [8, 22]. Deviations from the lower reference value of 1.5 mL (fifth percentile, 95% CI, 1.4–1.7 mL) are therefore symptomatic of a glandular dysfunction [8, 9]. The initial volume of semen is an important parameter in an analysis as the concentration of spermatozoa and other cells in semen is based on the accurate determination of the volume [8]. The volume of a sample can be measured in two ways: firstly, by weighing the sample in the vessel in which it is collected and subtracting the pre-weighed weight of the vessel. This enables to calculate the volume from the sample weight, assuming the density of semen to be 1 g/mL [23, 24]. Secondly, it can be determined by reading the volume from a wide-mouthed graduated cylinder into which it was directly collected [8]. It is advised that the volume should not be determined by decanting the sample into a measuring cylinder or by aspirating it from the container into a pipette or syringe as volume lost can be between 0.3 and 0.9 mL [24, 25].

During the first 4 days following ejaculation, the volume of semen increases at a rate of 11.9%/day [26], and a 2–3 day abstinence period is therefore recommended by the WHO prior to a semen analysis. However, it must not be ruled out that a low volume of semen (hypospermia) can also indicate a pathological condition. A decrease in semen volume is observed in patients presenting with chronic bacterial prostatitis or suffering from retrograde ejaculation [27]. Retrograde ejaculation is referred to as partial or complete flow of ejaculate into the bladder, rather than an antegrade ejaculation through the urethra [28]. This can be due to structural damage to the neck of the bladder or functional impairment of the nerves and neurotransmitters at the bladder neck. Congenital absence of the vas deferens or obstruction of the ejaculatory ducts can also result in a low volume of semen [28]. Seminal fluid volume and thus the semen sample can also decrease with age [29]. Incomplete collection of the semen sample might be another simple explanation for a low semen volume. On the other hand, a high volume of semen, hypervolumeric, can be indicative of an inflammation of the accessory sex glands and is often coupled with poor semen quality [8, 11].

pH

Secretions from the accessory sex glands interact to dictate the pH level of semen. Semen is multi-glandular in origin with the acidic prostatic and alkaline seminal vesicle secretions combining to produce an alkaline fluid with a high pH ranging from approximately 7.2 to 8.0. Hence, abnormal pH levels in a semen analysis can signify glandular dysfunction [30, 31]. The pH is typically assessed with pH paper. In azoospermic patients, a pH value lower than 7.0 can be indicative of bilateral congenital absence of the vas deferens or obstruction of the ejaculatory ducts [8, 32, 33]. A pH with a raised alkaline level of greater than 7.8 can be indicative of dysfunctional seminal vesicles [1].

Microscopic Evaluation

On completion of the macroscopic evaluation, the sample can be microscopically evaluated to determine the number of sperm and non-sperm cellular elements as well as the nature of the spermatozoa (i.e. vitality, motility and morphology—see Table 24.1). A phase contrast microscope is recommended for all examinations of unstained preparations of fresh semen, while a brightfield (×100) oil-immersion objective is required for assessment of morphology.

In order for successful and reproducible microscopic evaluations, it is paramount that representative sampling must occur. This can be achieved by thorough mixing of the sample in the original container by aspirating it ten times into a wide-bore pipette without creating air bubble before aliquots are taken for assessment.

During routine microscopic evaluation, non-specific aggregation of spermatozoa (i.e. immotile sperm to each other or motile sperm to mucus strands, non-sperm cells' or debris) can be observed. Agglutination of spermatozoa (i.e. motile spermatozoa sticking to each other) should also be noted as it can be suggestive of anti-sperm antibodies and therefore impinge on motility and concentration assessment [34].

Motility

Motility is an important semen parameter in predicting subfertility as it is indicative of a decrease in the functional competence of spermatozoa [35] and is directly related to the quality of the spermatozoa [1]. Motility can be considered as a physiological variable as it is indicative of the spermatogenesis process [11]. The most recent WHO manual categorizes sperm motility according to a grading system: progressive motility (PR; spermatozoa moving actively, either linearly or in a large circle, regardless of speed), non-progressive motility (NP; all other patterns of motility with an absence of progression) and immotile (IM; no movement) [8]. Motility is typically assessed by a visual determination of a wet-mount slide (20 µm deep) under phase contrast optics at ×200 or ×400 magnification. After the sample has stopped drifting, approximately 200 spermatozoa should be scored [8]. It is also recommended to use an eyepiece reticle with grid to limit the area and allow for the same area of the slide to be assessed. The procedure can be performed at either room temperature or 37°C. CASA is currently also becoming very popular as an objective method of assessing sperm motility. Various factors can affect sperm motility, e.g. oxidative stress, genital infections, accessory sex gland dysfunction and varicocele which can affect motility negatively [1] and can ultimately lead to the impairment of fertility.

The latest lower reference limits for motility (PR + NP) is 40% (fifth percentile, 95% CI 38–42), and for PR is 32% (fifth percentile, 95% CI 31–34) as was determined in fertile men whose partners had a TTP of 12 months or less [9].

Concentration

The concentration or density of a semen sample is the oldest parameter reported to be investigated during a semen analysis [1, 36]. The concentration of semen depends on a variety of factors: the volume of the testes, the period of sexual abstinence prior to ejaculation and the size of epididymal sperm reserve as well as the extent of ductal patency [9]. Sperm concentration is reported in sperm/millilitre (mL) and determined preferably with a 100-µm-deep haemocytometer. The lower limit reference value for the concentration of sperm in a normal semen sample is 15×10^6 mL (fifth percentile, 95% CI $12–16 \times 10^6$) while that for the total number of spermatozoa per ejaculate is given at 39×10^6 (fifth percentile, 95% CI $33–46 \times 10^6$) [8, 9]. A low concentration as seen in oligozoospermic samples may be indicative of a short period of abstinence as well as incomplete collection of the sample [11]. Certain medical conditions can also impact on the total number of sperm produced, such as diabetes mellitus, cryptorchidism and varicocele [11]. Sperm concentration and sperm number per ejaculate have been shown to be predictors of conception [37, 38] as well as TTP and pregnancy rates [39, 40].

Morphology

A morphological examination provides vital information on the quality of the sperm in a sample. Morphology has been considered to be an essential parameter when establishing the fertility status of a patient [41–43] and can be an important variable in deciding which form of ART will be employed in subfertile patients [11]. During the maturation of spermatozoa, the morphogenetic process can result in imperfections and anomalies which can be seen in a routine semen analysis [42]. It must be considered that several factors can influence the spermatogenesis process such as chemical and environmental factors which could result in anomalies in the morphology of spermatozoa [42]. Therefore, morphologically abnormal spermatozoa in a sample could be indicative of these variables.

Due to the variability in morphology of human spermatozoa, assessment thereof is difficult. Defining the appearance of potentially fertilizing (morphologically normal) spermatozoa was done by examining spermatozoa recovered from post-coital endocervical mucus and the surface of the zona pellucida [41, 44, 45].

The two approaches used to measure sperm morphology to date were the previous WHO guidelines and the Tygerberg strict criteria. The Tygerberg strict criteria were developed on the basis of the morphological assessment of the sperm, especially the acrosomal region [1]. The basis of the criteria is that the morphological appearance, as a result of the size of the acrosome, is a reflection of the physiological and fertilizing capacity of the spermatozoa being graded. A threshold of 14% normal forms was the original reference value for the strict criteria. However, this value has been revised over the past years.

Once a semen smear has air-dried, the slide is stained with the recommended Papanicolaou, Shorr or Diff-Quick staining methods and mounted with a cover slip. For the visualization of the structural features of the spermatozoa, a ×100 oil-immersion brightfield objective and at least a ×10 eyepiece must be used [8]. Currently, the WHO manual classifies the morphology of sperm based on a simple abnormal/normal system as well as the optional test of determining the structural location of the abnormalities. The assessment of the percentage of morphologically normal spermatozoa that are regarded as having fertilizing potential is particularly beneficial in the prediction of a possible pregnancy [8]. The analysis of the parameter that is considered "normal" can therefore be considered to be the spermatozoa with "optimal fertilizing capability" [42]. A threshold of 4% (fifth percentile, 95% CI 3–4) normal forms is the lower reference value as calculated by Cooper [9] and accepted by the WHO [8]. This reference limit is only valid if the classification technique as described in the WHO manual is followed.

By strictly applying certain criteria of sperm morphology, several studies have established relationships between the percentage of normal forms and various fertility end points such as TTP and successful in vitro as well as natural fertilization rates [41–43, 46–51].

Sperm Vitality

Assessment of vitality, sometimes referred to as viability, indicates the percentage of alive and dead spermatozoa in a sample and is indicative of abnormalities in any of the genital organs [1]. Assessment of the vitality of spermatozoa is recommended if the motility of a sample is less than 10% [11]. Vitality is affected by numerous variables such as abnormal spermatogenesis and vesicular and prostatic fluids [1].

The principle of the test is based on the exclusion of dye by the sperm membrane. In living cells, the membrane remains intact and therefore excludes the dye from penetrating. However, in dead sperm, the membrane's integrity has been compromised, and hence cellular staining by the dye occurs [1]. Sperm vitality should be assessed as soon as possible after liquefaction of the semen sample and within 1 h after ejaculation to minimize environmental effects on vitality. The most common staining method used for vitality testing is the one-step eosin-nigrosin staining technique as described in the WHO manual [8]. The resultant investigation under brightfield optics will show sperm with dark pink heads (dead) and white heads (alive and membrane intact). The hypo-osmotic swelling (HOS) test may be used alternatively to dye exclusion [52]. This method is specifically useful at choosing sperm for intracytoplasmic sperm injection (ICSI) when staining of sperm must be avoided. This method is also based on intactness of cell membranes. Spermatozoa with intact membranes swell within 5 min when placed in a hypo-osmotic medium as indicated by curling of the tails while dead cells show no change. The lower reference limit for vitality is 58% (fifth centile, 95% CI 55–63).

Non-sperm Cellular Elements

Leukocytes are the most commonly observed cells in a semen sample besides spermatozoa [11]. The detection and quantification of leukocytes in semen is not considered part of a routine semen analysis and has little prognostic value in a spermiogram [53]. However, it is useful in a diagnostic sense as it can determine whether uncharacteristic semen parameters are a direct result of the presence of leukocytes [1]. The presence of leukocytes that exceed the WHO reference value of more than 10^6/mL is indicative of a genital tract infection, and the condition is termed leukocytospermia [9]. Certain methodologies for the identification of white blood cells in semen are controversial such as the Papanicolaou and Giemsa stains. This is due to difficulty in discriminating between leukocytes and other cells present in the semen [1]. The peroxidase stain and immunocytochemistry are the two tests that are most commonly employed when testing for leukocytospermia. Red blood cells are also found in a semen analysis, and in high concentrations, they can be indicative of infection and inflammation or possible ductal obstruction [11].

Biochemical Evaluation

The conventional semen analysis is the foundation of determining male factor infertility. However, with the advancement in the understanding of spermatozoa, various in vitro tests have arisen to assess the functional competence of spermatozoa beyond the basic spermiogram [54]. Examples of these tests that are not routinely performed in the traditional semen analysis include sperm–zona interaction, acrosome reaction and the measurement of ROS (reactive oxygen species) production. Their results can be particularly useful in determining the fertilizing ability of spermatozoa beyond the information provided by the basic sperm parameters [54]. These tests are expensive and not commonly performed and are therefore used rather in a research setting than in fertility clinics [11].

Applications to IVF/ART

The results of a semen analysis are the primary step in the assessment of a males' reproductive capacity and is essential in selecting patients for medical intervention such as IVF or ICSI treatment [12, 46]. Therefore, it is essential that the procedures are standardized and carried out precisely to achieve accurate results for the clinician's diagnosis [6].

ICSI has revolutionized the treatment of male infertility as it allows for sperm that would otherwise be incapable of penetrating the ovum to reach the cytoplasm and fertilize the oocyte [46]. This has led to many clinicians undermining the importance of the traditional semen analysis. However, despite the introduction of ICSI in ART treatment, the analysis of semen is still key as it forms the basis of decision-making on the therapeutic options to be taken when dealing with a couple experiencing difficulty in achieving a successful pregnancy [6, 12].

Conclusion

The traditional semen analysis is the established cornerstone of assessing male fertility, and the diagnostic management depends on a sequential, multi-step approach [43]. Recognized reference values for normality are essential due to the relationship between sperm quality and fertility [53]. The information provided by a semen analysis is the least invasive and most cost-effective assessment of a male's fertility status [7]. Despite the introduction of alternative techniques such as computer-assisted sperm analysis and the advancement of assisted conception, the prediction of fertilization in vitro is still crucial [10].

References

1. Andrade-Rocha FT. Physical analysis of ejaculate to evaluate the secretory activity of the seminal vesicles and prostate. Clin Chem Lab Med. 2005;43(11):1203–10.
2. Jequier AM. Is quality assurance in semen analysis still really necessary? A clinician's viewpoint. Hum Reprod. 2005;20(8):2039–42.
3. Jequier AM. Edward Martin (1859-1938). The founding father of modern clinical andrology. Int J Androl. 1991;14(1):1–10.
4. La Vignera S, Calogero AE, Condorelli R, Garrone F, Vicari E. Spermiogram: techniques, interpretation, and prognostic value of results. Minerva Endocrinol. 2007;32(2):115–26.

5. Alvarez C, Castilla JA, Martinez L, Ramirez JP, Vergara F, Gaforio JJ. Biological variation of seminal parameters in healthy subjects. Hum Reprod. 2003;18(10):2082–8.
6. Lewis SE. Is sperm evaluation useful in predicting human fertility? Reproduction. 2007;134(1):31–40.
7. Chong AP, Walters CA, Weinrieb SA. The neglected laboratory test. The semen analysis. J Androl. 1983;4(4):280–2.
8. WHO. WHO laboratory manual for the examination and processing of human semen. 5th ed. Geneva: WHO; 2010.
9. Cooper TG, Noonan E, von Eckardstein S, et al. World Health Organization reference values for human semen characteristics. Hum Reprod Update. 2010;16(3):231–45.
10. Sukcharoen N, Keith J, Irvine DS, Aitken RJ. Prediction of the in-vitro fertilization (IVF) potential of human spermatozoa using sperm function tests: the effect of the delay between testing and IVF. Hum Reprod. 1996;11(5):1030–4.
11. Agarwal A, Sabanegh ES, Bragais FM. Laboratory assessment of male infertility–a guide for the urologist. US Urology. 2009;4(1):70–3.
12. Joffe M. Semen quality analysis and the idea of normal fertility. Asian J Androl. 2004;12(1):79–82.
13. Zavos PM, Goodpasture JC. Clinical improvements of specific seminal deficiencies via intercourse with a seminal collection device versus masturbation. Fertil Steril. 1989;51(1):190–3.
14. Pound N, Javed MH, Ruberto C, Shaikh MA, Del Valle AP. Duration of sexual arousal predicts semen parameters for masturbatory ejaculates. Physiol Behav. 2002;76(4–5):685–9.
15. Cooper TG, Keck C, Oberdieck U, Nieschlag E. Effects of multiple ejaculations after extended periods of sexual abstinence on total, motile and normal sperm numbers, as well as accessory gland secretions, from healthy normal and oligozoospermic men. Hum Reprod. 1993;8(8):1251–8.
16. De Jonge C, LaFromboise M, Bosmans E, Ombelet W, Cox A, Nijs M. Influence of the abstinence period on human sperm quality. Fertil Steril. 2004;82(1):57–65.
17. Bjorndahl L, Kvist U. Sequence of ejaculation affects the spermatozoon as a carrier and its message. Reprod Biomed Online. 2003;7(4):440–8.
18. Cooper TG, Barfield JP, Yeung CH. Changes in osmolality during liquefaction of human semen. Int J Androl. 2005;28(1):58–60.
19. Lwaleed BA, Greenfield R, Stewart A, Birch B, Cooper AJ. Seminal clotting and fibrinolytic balance: a possible physiological role in the male reproductive system. Thromb Haemost. 2004;92(4):752–66.
20. Elzanaty S, Malm J, Giwercman A. Visco-elasticity of seminal fluid in relation to the epididymal and accessory sex gland function and its impact on sperm motility. Int J Androl. 2004;27(2):94–100.
21. Gonzales GF, Kortebani G, Mazzolli AB. Hyperviscosity and hypofunction of the seminal vesicles. Arch Androl. 1993;30(1):63–8.
22. Nieschlag E, Behre H, editors, Nieschlag S, Assist editor. Andrology. Male reproductive health and dysfunction. Berlin: Springer; 2000.
23. Auger J, Kunstmann JM, Czyglik F, Jouannet P. Decline in semen quality among fertile men in Paris during the past 20 years. N Engl J Med. 1995;332(5):281–5.
24. Cooper TG, Brazil C, Swan SH, Overstreet JW. Ejaculate volume is seriously underestimated when semen is pipetted or decanted into cylinders from the collection vessel. J Androl. 2007;28(1):1–4.
25. Brazil C, Swan SH, Drobnis EZ, et al. Standardized methods for semen evaluation in a multicenter research study. J Androl. 2004;25(4):635–44.
26. Carlsen E, Petersen JH, Andersson AM, Skakkebaek NE. Effects of ejaculatory frequency and season on variations in semen quality. Fertil Steril. 2004;82(2):358–66.
27. Robbins SL, Kumar V. Basic pathology. 4th ed. Philadelphia: W.B Saunders; 1987.
28. Roberts M, Jarvi K. Steps in the investigation and management of low semen volume in the infertile man. Can Urol Assoc J. 2009;3(6):479–85.

29. Ng KK, Donat R, Chan L, Lalak A, Di Pierro I, Handelsman DJ. Sperm output of older men. Hum Reprod. 2004;19(8):1811–5.
30. Sherwood L. Human physiology from cells to systems. 7th ed. Belmont: Brooks/Cole; 2007.
31. Fritjofsson A, Kvist U, Ronquist G. Anatomy of the prostate. Aspects of the secretory function in relation to lobar structure. Scand J Urol Nephrol Suppl. 1988;107:5–13.
32. de la Taille A, Rigot JM, Mahe P, et al. Correlation of genitourinary abnormalities, spermiogram and CFTR genotype in patients with bilateral agenesis of the vas deferens. Prog Urol. 1998;8(3):370–6.
33. Weiske WH, Salzler N, Schroeder-Printzen I, Weidner W. Clinical findings in congenital absence of the vasa deferentia. Andrologia. 2000;32(1):13–8.
34. Rose NR. Techniques for the detection of iso- and auto-antibodies to human spermatozoa. Clin Exp Immunol. 1976;23:4.
35. Gunalp S, Onculoglu C, Gurgan T, Kruger TF, Lombard CJ. A study of semen parameters with emphasis on sperm morphology in a fertile population: an attempt to develop clinical thresholds. Hum Reprod. 2001;16(1):110–4.
36. Macomber D, Sanders MD. The spermatozoa count: its value in the diagnosis, prognosis and concentration in fertile and infertile men. N Engl J Med. 1929;200:3.
37. Bonde JP, Ernst E, Jensen TK, et al. Relation between semen quality and fertility: a population-based study of 430 first-pregnancy planners. Lancet. 1998;352(9135):1172–7.
38. Larsen L, Scheike T, Jensen TK, et al. Computer-assisted semen analysis parameters as predictors for fertility of men from the general population. The Danish First Pregnancy Planner Study Team. Hum Reprod. 2000;15(7):1562–7.
39. Slama R, Eustache F, Ducot B, et al. Time to pregnancy and semen parameters: a cross-sectional study among fertile couples from four European cities. Hum Reprod. 2002;17(2):503–15.
40. Zinaman MJ, Brown CC, Selevan SG, Clegg ED. Semen quality and human fertility: a prospective study with healthy couples. J Androl. 2000;21(1):145–53.
41. Menkveld R, Stander FS, Kotze TJ, Kruger TF, van Zyl JA. The evaluation of morphological characteristics of human spermatozoa according to stricter criteria. Hum Reprod. 1990;5(5):586–92.
42. Auger J. Assessing human sperm morphology: top models, underdogs or biometrics? Asian J Androl. 2001;12(1):36–46.
43. Franken DR, Franken CJ, de la Guerre H, de Villiers A. Normal sperm morphology and chromatin packaging: comparison between aniline blue and chromomycin A3 staining. Andrologia. 1999;31(6):361–6.
44. Fredricsson B, Bjork G. Morphology of postcoital spermatozoa in the cervical secretion and its clinical significance. Fertil Steril. 1977;28(8):841–5.
45. Menkveld R, Franken DR, Kruger TF, Oehninger S, Hodgen GD. Sperm selection capacity of the human zona pellucida. Mol Reprod Dev. 1991;30(4):346–52.
46. Liu DY, Baker HW. Evaluation and assessment of semen for IVF/ICSI. Asian J Androl. 2002;4(4):281–5.
47. Coetzee K, Kruge TF, Lombard CJ. Predictive value of normal sperm morphology: a structured literature review. Hum Reprod Update. 1998;4(1):73–82.
48. Menkveld R, Wong WY, Lombard CJ, et al. Semen parameters, including WHO and strict criteria morphology, in a fertile and subfertile population: an effort towards standardization of in-vivo thresholds. Hum Reprod. 2001;16(6):1165–71.
49. Van Waart J, Kruger TF, Lombard CJ, Ombelet W. Predictive value of normal sperm morphology in intrauterine insemination (IUI): a structured literature review. Hum Reprod Update. 2001;7(5):495–500.
50. Garrett C, Liu DY, Clarke GN, Rushford DD, Baker HW. Automated semen analysis: 'zona pellucida preferred' sperm morphometry and straight-line velocity are related to pregnancy rate in subfertile couples. Hum Reprod. 2003;18(8):1643–9.

51. Liu DY, Baker HW. Disordered zona pellucida-induced acrosome reaction and failure of in vitro fertilization in patients with unexplained infertility. Fertil Steril. 2003;79(1):74–80.
52. Jeyendran RS, Van der Ven HH, Perez-Pelaez M, Crabo BG, Zaneveld LJ. Development of an assay to assess the functional integrity of the human sperm membrane and its relationship to other semen characteristics. J Reprod Fertil. 1984;70(1):219–28.
53. Ombelet W, Bosmans E, Janssen M, et al. Semen parameters in a fertile versus subfertile population: a need for change in the interpretation of semen testing. Hum Reprod. 1997;12(5):987–93.
54. Aitken RJ. Sperm function tests and fertility. Int J Androl. 2006;29(1):69–75; discussion 105–8.

Chapter 5
Sperm Assessment: Novel Approaches and Their Indicative Value

De Yi Liu, Harold Bourne, Claire Garrett, Gary N. Clarke, Shlomi Barak, and H.W. Gordon Baker

With the advance of assisted reproductive technology, there have been a number of attempts to develop new methods for the assessment of sperm over those of standard semen analysis (sperm number, motility and morphology), in the hope that they may improve the clinician's ability to manage and predict successful outcomes of treatment. In this chapter, we review a range of these tests, mainly those we have some experience with and discuss other possibilities for the future. The tests discussed can be performed in patients with sperm concentrations above 2×10^6/mL or total sperm count above 5×10^6 per ejaculate. We will not discuss assessment of sperm obtained surgically from the genital tract, patients with severe oligospermia (sperm concentration less than 2×10^6/mL), zero sperm motility, total teratozoospermia where all sperm have the same defect such as an absent heads, sperm autoimmunity and gonadotropin deficiency or suppression.

D.Y. Liu, PhD (✉) • S. Barak, MD • H.W.G. Baker, MD, PhD, FRACP
Melbourne IVF and Department of Obstetrics and Gynecology, Royal Women's Hospital, University of Melbourne, Suite 10/320 Victoria Parade, East Melbourne, VIC 3002, Australia
e-mail: deyliu.liu@mivf.com.au; Shlomi.barak@mivf.com.au; g.baker@unimelb.edu.au

H. Bourne, M Rep Sci
Reproductive Services/Melbourne IVF, The Royal Women's Hospital, Suite10/320 Victoria Parade, East Melbourne, VIC 3002, Australia
e-mail: Harold.bourne@mivf.com.au

C. Garrett
Melbourne IVF and Department of Obstetrics and Gynecology, Royal Women's Hospital, University of Melbourne, Suite 10/320 Victoria Parade, East Melbourne, VIC 3002, Australia
Reproductive Services/Melbourne IVF, The Royal Women's Hospital, Melbourne, VIC 3002, Australia
e-mail: Claire.garrett@mivf.com.au

G.N. Clarke, DSc
Andrology Unit and Department of Obstetrics and Gynaecology, The Royal Women's Hospital, University of Melbourne, 321 Cardigan Street, Carlton, VIC 3053, Australia
e-mail: Gary.clarke@thewomens.org.au

Before the introduction of ICSI, we conducted a number of studies of the relationship between various sperm tests and the outcomes of standard IVF. Couples with a range of semen abnormalities were included. Excess sperm prepared for insemination were tested and the results examined to determine their association with fertilization rate. Logistic regression analysis was used to show which groups of test results were independently significantly related to the fertilization rate. Although most sperm test results had some relationship with the fertilization rate, many were closely correlated, and when entered into the regression model, only a few remained significant. This approach allowed us to determine which sperm characteristics were most important for fertilization. There was a strong relationship between fertilization rate and sperm morphology assessed with the strict approach and some other factors such as DNA normality assessed with acridine orange florescence, automated sperm motility particularly straight line velocity (VSL) and the ability of sperm to bind to and penetrate the zona pellucida (studies summarized in [1, 2]).

The sperm–zona pellucida interaction results were most significantly associated with fertilization rates, and this led us to develop tests of sperm function using human oocytes which had failed to fertilize or were unsuitable for insemination or injection. Results of these tests confirmed that defective sperm–zona pellucida interaction is a major cause of failure of fertilization with standard IVF [3–8]. We provide details of the methods as any group associated with a clinical IVF programme could perform these tests.

Sperm Motility and Morphology

Several tests related to standard semen analysis measures of motility and morphology have been developed, but as yet none has an established place in patient management.

Hypoosmotic Swelling Test

Some investigators promoted hypoosmotic swelling as a predictor of IVF results, but we found results of this test were not significant when other sperm measures were taken into account [1].

DNA Normality

DNA or chromatin normality can be assessed by a variety of techniques including TUNEL and comet assays, but simpler methods involving sperm head decondensation and staining with dyes produce correlated results. We found little relationship between sperm head decondensation or aniline blue staining and fertilization rates, but acridine orange fluorescence assessed by microscopy was significantly related independent of sperm morphology and sperm–zona pellucida binding [1]. Subsequently, we investigated the use of the flow cytometry method involving acid denaturation of sperm and found that the increase in sperm with red fluorescence (the DNA fragmentation index, DFI) was inversely correlated with fertilization rates with standard IVF, but not with those of intracytoplasmic sperm injection. DFI was correlated with sperm motility, viability and morphology [9]. We showed the zona pellucida selectively binds sperm with normal acridine orange staining [10]. Meta-analysis of the results of the DFI test indicates that it is not a great advance over standard semen analysis. Also, claims that DFI results predict poor outcomes with implantation and subsequent pregnancy loss are unconvincing [11].

Sperm Movement Characteristics

We found several motility measurements assessed by computer-assisted semen analysis (CASA) were related to fertilization rates with standard IVF, particularly VSL [12]. Also, VSL and automated sperm morphology %Z (see below) together were the only independently significant semen characteristics related to natural conception rates in subfertile couples [13]. We believe there is potential for VSL to be included as a clinically useful semen analysis characteristic, but further large studies are required for confirmation.

Automated Sperm Morphology

Early studies showed that among the standard semen variables, sperm morphology was the strongest predictor of fertilization rates with IVF. We found that morphology was critical for sperm binding to the zona pellucida and that the population of sperm bound to the zona pellucida had higher normal morphology than those in the insemination medium [14–17]. We developed an automated method for computer image analysis of sperm morphometry and used the characteristics of sperm that most differentiated those bound to the zona pellucida from those in the insemination medium to develop a measure of sperm with zona binding capacity (%Z) as an overall assessment of sperm morphometry [13, 18]. Sperm morphometry should greatly improve the predictive value of semen analysis. Currently sperm morphology is assessed subjectively, and there are extreme variations between laboratories that are obvious in external quality assurance results. This should be improved by automation, but all current commercial CASA systems with sperm morphology modules may not give results comparable with those of manual methods or provide a measure equivalent to %Z.

Sperm Function Tests

Developing sperm function tests that would accurately predict fertility and the results of IVF has been an active interest of several groups for some time, but no test has become widely used because it either failed to live up to its promise or the assay is difficult, largely due to limited supply of human material for the tests and the unavailability of substitutes. For example, recombinant human zona proteins have been found inactive or inconsistently active [19].

Hamster Oocyte Penetration Test

Acrosome-reacted human sperm fuse with the oolemma of zona-free hamster oocytes and undergo nuclear decondensation in the ooplasm. This test is useful for research purposes [20]. Although promoted early as a human sperm function test that would predict the ability of sperm to fertilize in vitro, this was found not to be the case [21]. As discussed below with sperm defects, the main mechanism of interference with fertilization is reduced ability of sperm to bind to the zona pellucida or undergo the acrosome reaction on the zona pellucida. Defects of sperm–oolemma binding are uncommon [2]. Searches for oocytes from other species that could be used for testing human sperm binding and penetration or genetic modification of animal zona proteins that would allow human sperm interaction have been unsuccessful.

Human Sperm–Oocyte Interaction

We developed methods for testing stages of human fertilization using human oocytes that failed to fertilize in clinical IVF (Fig. 5.1). These tests improve evaluation of sperm function and have resulted in our identification of two defects of sperm–zona pellucida interaction: (1) low ability of the sperm to bind to the oocyte, called defective sperm–zona pellucida binding (DSZPB), and (2) failure of the acrosome reaction, called disordered zona pellucida-induced acrosome reaction (DZPIAR). Our reviews provide summaries of the results of applying these tests to study the signal transduction and effector pathways of the acrosome reaction and also describe extensions such as using different fluorescent dyes to stain test and control sperm [1, 2]. The method we currently use can measure both sperm–zona pellucida binding and the zona pellucida-induced acrosome reaction in the same test (Fig. 5.2).

5 Sperm Assessment: Novel Approaches and Their Indicative Value

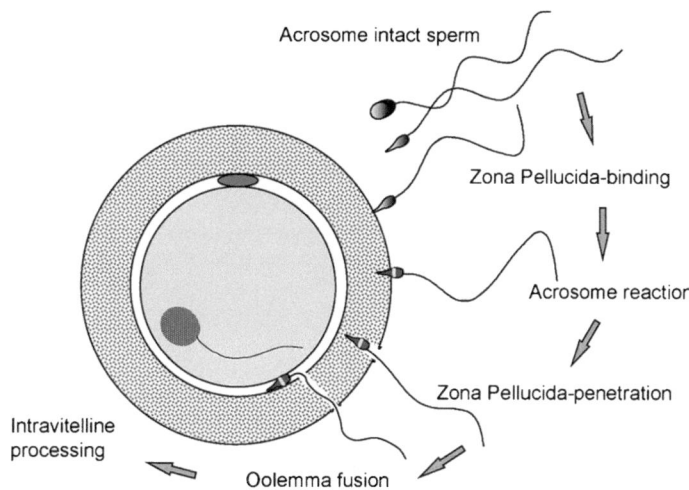

Fig. 5.1 Diagram of human sperm–oocyte interaction. Motile sperm swim through medium and cumulus oophorus (not shown) to attach to the surface of the zona pellucida. The acrosome reaction is stimulated, and the plasma and outer acrosomal membranes are shed as the sperm penetrates the zona pellucida. In the perivitelline space, the sperm plasma membrane persisting over the equatorial segment fuses with the oolemma, then the sperm is engulfed into the vitellus, and the sperm head decondenses

Oocytes that have failed to fertilize with standard IVF and immature oocytes (GV or MI) unsuitable for ICSI are used. The zona pellucida of these oocytes has similar biological activity as those of normal mature oocytes to bind sperm and induce the acrosome reaction [2]. The oocytes are used fresh or after storage in 1 M ammonium sulphate. Salt-stored oocytes are washed and incubated for 2 h with 2×10^6 motile sperm in 1 mL human tubal fluid medium with groups of four oocytes. Unbound sperm are removed by washing oocytes with a wide-bore pipette and sperm tightly bound to the surface of the zona pellucida are counted. Where there is normal sperm–zona pellucida binding, sperm bound to the surface of each zona pellucida are then removed by repeated aspiration of the oocyte with a narrow-bore pipette (120 µm, slightly smaller than the oocyte) with a small volume of medium placed on a slide and stained with fluorescein-labelled *Pisum sativum* agglutinin (Fig. 5.2). Two hundred sperm are counted for each test. Sperm penetrating the zona pellucida are counted, and the motility of sperm in the medium and the spontaneous acrosome reaction are also assessed at the end of the incubation period. The technician performs the counts blind to the condition of the patient. Assay reproducibility has been studied for the same sperm samples exposed to oocytes obtained from different IVF patients and for repeated ejaculates on different days from the same DZPIAR patients and normal men. For both, the variation in results is low (SD <10% [8]). Fresh and salt-stored oocytes give the same results, as do oocytes with or without

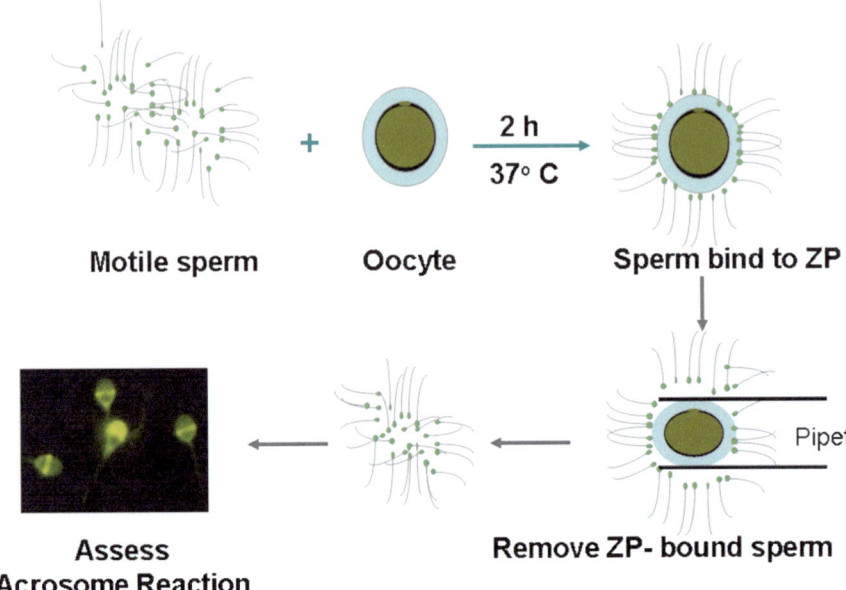

Fig. 5.2 Flow diagram of human sperm–oocyte interaction tests. Motile sperm are incubated with oocytes and sperm tightly bound to the zona pellucida counted after washing the oocytes to dislodge loosely adherent sperm. Sperm bound to the zona pellucida are removed by pipetting the oocyte with a pipette of diameter slightly smaller than that of the oocyte. Sperm penetrating the zona pellucida remain and are counted. The dislodged zona-bound sperm can be further assessed, for example, with fluorescein-labelled *Pisum sativum* agglutinin for acrosome status. Illustrated are one sperm with intact acrosome showing uniform florescence of the anterior half to two-thirds of the head and three acrosome-reacted sperm showing a florescent band in the equatorial region

sperm penetrating the zona pellucida from previous IVF. Under the conditions of the test, fertile men have >100 sperm tightly bound to each zona pellucida, and an average of ≤40 bound sperm/zona pellucida is defined as low. Using human tubal fluid medium plus 7–10% human serum, an average of 48% of zona pellucida-bound sperm undergoes the acrosome reaction, and a result of <16% is defined as low. Different culture media may have different effects on the acrosome reaction, and thus, the normal reference values depend on the medium and protein supplement. Because we use oocytes discarded from IVF, we have performed extensive studies on the effect of oocyte variability on the results of these tests [2]. We use four oocytes for each sperm sample because occasional oocytes will not bind sperm. We confirm abnormal results by repeating the test on another semen sample.

Defective Sperm–Zona Pellucida Binding

Low sperm–zona pellucida binding can be classified into two types according to semen analysis results: DSZPB types I and II [2, 8]. Type 1 has abnormal semen analysis: oligozoospermia, asthenozoospermia, teratozoospermia or a combination.

About 80% of patients with DSZPB type I have defects of sperm head shape that are obvious in routine semen analysis and presumably account for the low sperm–zona pellucida binding. In contrast, DSZPB type II has normal semen analysis, and the diagnosis can only be made by testing sperm–zona pellucida binding using human oocytes. About 13% of infertile men with normal semen analysis results have DSZPB type II [2, 4, 8]. It is likely that DSZPB originates from abnormal spermatogenesis or sperm maturation.

Disordered Zona Pellucida-Induced Acrosome Reaction

We found a group of infertile men with consistently normal routine semen analysis and normal sperm–zona pellucida binding, but sperm did not penetrate the zona pellucida because of a low acrosome reaction on the zona pellucida. We first identified this condition in a group of patients with unexplained infertility and repeated zero or low fertilization rates (<30%) with standard IVF [6, 22]. Normally an average of 48% (range 20–98%) of sperm bound to the zona pellucida undergo the acrosome reaction during the 2-h incubation involved in the test [6]. In contrast, with DZPIAR, very low proportions (mean 6%, range 1–16%) of sperm undergo the acrosome reaction on the zona pellucida. Studies on the frequency of DZPIAR in patients with unexplained infertility indicate about 25% are affected [6, 22]. Interestingly we have found that the zona pellucida-induced acrosome reaction is correlated with sperm concentration in the ejaculate, and although the patients had by definition sperm concentrations greater than 20×10^6/mL, those between 20 and 60×10^6/mL had significantly lower zona pellucida-induced acrosome reaction. Low zona pellucida-induced acrosome reaction is also frequent in oligospermic (<20×10^6/mL) and severely teratospermic (normal sperm morphology <5%) men with normal sperm–zona pellucida binding [5, 7].

Human Sperm–Oolemma Binding

It is possible to remove the zona pellucida from the oocyte with dilute acid treatment and then use a similar approach to sperm–zona pellucida binding (Fig. 5.2) to study sperm binding to the oolemma. We found evidence that sperm needed to be acrosome-reacted before binding to the oolemma and that globospermic sperm would not bind. However, we found no other patients with a specific defect of sperm–oolemma binding, making this test of little clinical value [1, 23].

Tests Correlated with Sperm Function

As well as the strong relationship between normal morphology and sperm–zona pellucida binding, we have found that two markers of sperm capacitation, hyperactivated motility and protein tyrosine phosphorylation in sperm tails, are correlated with the zona pellucida-induced acrosome reaction and sperm–zona pellucida binding.

Hyperactivation and Sperm–Zona Pellucida-Induced Acrosome Reaction

The proportion of sperm which undergo hyperactivation in culture medium assessed by CASA (Hamilton Thorne sperm analyser) is highly correlated with the zona pellucida-induced acrosome reaction, but not with sperm–zona pellucida binding capacity [24].

Protein Tyrosine Phosphorylation and Sperm–Zona Pellucida Binding

Tyrosine phosphorylated proteins increase mainly in the principle piece of human sperm with capacitation. There is a significant correlation between human sperm–zona pellucida binding and tyrosine phosphorylation in human sperm detected with the monoclonal antibody PY20 labelled with fluorescein [25].

Thus, these simple tests of hyperactivation and protein tyrosine phosphorylation, which could be performed as an addition to routine semen analysis, may be useful to screen for defects of human sperm–zona pellucida interaction. However, large prospective studies are needed to confirm this.

Summary and Conclusions

A number of sperm tests of varying complexity have been reviewed. Standard semen analysis remains the most useful clinically but has limited relationship with results of IVF. Sperm morphology assessed by the strict method is valuable for predicting poor fertilization with standard IVF, but its subjectivity causes problems with some laboratories failing to find it useful. Objective methods involving automated computer image analysis are being developed. Methods for assessing human sperm–oocyte interaction have been described, and these can be used for diagnosis. Some methods such as hamster oocyte penetration tests have been discarded, and others such as sperm DNA testing are of uncertain value.

While none of the tests discussed here have become established as useful in clinical practice, we believe automated semen analysis particularly for morphometry has great potential. We use the human sperm–oocyte interaction tests in patients with idiopathic infertility to detect those who have DSZPB or disordered sperm–zona pellucida-induced acrosome reaction and direct these patients to ICSI to avoid IVF treatments with low or zero fertilization rates. We also use these tests for assessing patients with isolated marginal sperm morphology. Those with confirmed poor zona binding require ICSI, while those with normal sperm–oocyte interaction can be treated by standard IVF. Further studies are necessary to determine if hyperactivated motility and immunofluorescence staining of tyrosine phosphorylation in sperm tails would be useful screening tests for the defects of human sperm–oocyte interaction.

Because of the range of abnormalities of human sperm and the variability in test results from day to day within the same patient, it is unlikely that a single predictive test that can be applied once will be found. Clinical information about the couple, together with a panel of repeated sperm test results, will always be required for predicting male fertility.

References

1. Liu DY, Baker HWG. Tests of human sperm function and fertilization in vitro. Fertil Steril. 1992;58:465–83.
2. Liu DY, Garrett C, Baker HWG. Clinical application of sperm-oocyte interaction tests in in vitro fertilization—embryo transfer and intracytoplasmic sperm injection programs. Fertil Steril. 2004;82:1251–63.
3. Liu DY, Baker HWG. Defective sperm-zona pellucida interaction: a major cause of failure of fertilization in clinical in-vitro fertilization. Hum Reprod. 2000;15:702–8.
4. Liu DY, Clarke GN, Martic M, Garrett C, Baker HWG. Frequency of disordered zona pellucida (ZP)-induced acrosome reaction in infertile men with normal semen analysis and normal spermatozoa-ZP binding. Hum Reprod. 2001;16:1185–90.
5. Liu DY, Baker HWG. Frequency of defective sperm-zona pellucida interaction in severely teratozoospermic infertile men. Hum Reprod. 2003;18:802–7.
6. Liu DY, Baker HWG. Disordered zona pellucida-induced acrosome reaction and failure of in vitro fertilization in patients with unexplained infertility. Fertil Steril. 2003;79:74–80.
7. Liu DY, Baker HWG. High frequency of defective sperm-zona pellucida interaction in oligozoospermic infertile men. Hum Reprod. 2004;19:228–33.
8. Liu DY, Liu ML, Garrett C, Baker HWG. Comparison of the frequency of defective sperm-zona pellucida (ZP) binding and the ZP-induced acrosome reaction between subfertile men with normal and abnormal semen. Hum Reprod. 2007;22:1878–84.
9. Apedaile AE, Garrett C, LD Y, Clarke GN, Johnston SA, Baker HWG. Flow cytometry and microscopic acridine orange test: relationship with standard semen analysis. Reprod Biomed Online. 2004;8:398–407.
10. Liu DY, Baker HW. Human sperm bound to the zona pellucida have normal nuclear chromatin as assessed by acridine orange fluorescence. Hum Reprod. 2007;22:1597–602.
11. Collins JA, Barnhart KT, Schlegel PN. Do sperm DNA integrity tests predict pregnancy with in vitro fertilization? Fertil Steril. 2008;89:823–31.
12. Liu DY, Clarke GN, Baker HWG. Relationship between sperm motility assessed with the Hamilton-Thorn motility analyzer and fertilization rates in vitro. J Androl. 1991;12:231–9.
13. Garrett C, Liu DY, Clarke GN, Rushford DD, Baker HWG. Automated semen analysis: 'zona pellucida preferred' sperm morphometry and straight-line velocity are related to pregnancy rate in subfertile couples. Hum Reprod. 2003;18:1643–9.
14. Garrett C, Liu DY, Baker HWG. Comparison of human sperm morphometry assessment models based on zona pellucida selectivity. Soc Reprod Fertil Suppl. 2007;65:357–61.
15. Liu DY, Baker HWG. Morphology of spermatozoa bound to the zona pellucida of human oocytes that failed to fertilize in vitro. J Reprod Fertil. 1992;94:71–84.
16. Liu DY, Baker HWG. Acrosome status and morphology of human spermatozoa bound to the zona pellucida and oolemma determined using oocytes that failed to fertilize in vitro. Hum Reprod. 1994;9:673–9.

17. Liu DY, Garrett C, Baker HWG. Low proportions of sperm can bind to the zona pellucida of human oocytes. Hum Reprod. 2003;18:2382–9.
18. Garrett C, Baker HWG. New fully automated system for the morphometric analysis of human sperm heads. Fertil Steril. 1995;63:1306–17.
19. Martic M, Moses EK, Adams TE, et al. Recombinant human zona pellucida proteins ZP1, ZP2 and ZP3 co-expressed in a human cell line. Asian J Androl. 2004;6:3–13.
20. WHO. World Health Organization (WHO) Laboratory manual for the examination and processing of human semen. 5th ed. Cambridge: Cambridge University Press; 2010.
21. Zainul Rashid MR, Fishel SB, Thornton S, et al. The predictive value of the zona-free hamster egg penetration test in relation to in-vitro fertilization at various insemination concentrations. Hum Reprod. 1998;13:624–9.
22. Liu DY, Baker HWG. Disordered acrosome reaction of sperm bound to the zona pellucida: a newly discovered sperm defect with reduced sperm-zona pellucida penetration and reduced fertilization in vitro. Hum Reprod. 1994;9:1694–700.
23. Bourne H, Liu DY, Clarke GN, Baker HWG. Normal fertilization and embryo development by intracytoplasmic sperm injection of round-headed acrosomeless sperm. Fertil Steril. 1995;63:1329–32.
24. Liu DY, Liu ML, Clarke GN, Baker HWG. Hyperactivation of capacitated human sperm correlates with the zona pellucida-induced acrosome reaction of zona pellucida-bound sperm. Hum Reprod. 2007;22:2632–8.
25. Liu DY, Clarke GN, Baker HW. Tyrosine phosphorylation on capacitated human sperm tail detected by immunofluorescence correlates strongly with sperm-zona pellucida (ZP) binding but not with the ZP-induced acrosome reaction. Hum Reprod. 2006;21:1002–8.

Chapter 6
Intracytoplasmic Morphologically Selected Sperm Injection

P. Vanderzwalmen, Magnus Bach, Batsuren Baramsai, A. Neyer,
Delf Schwerda, Astrid Stecher, Barbara Wirleitner, Martin Zintz,
Bernard Lejeune, S. Vanderzwalmen, Nino Guy Cassuto,
Mathias Zech, and Nicolas H. Zech

Since the beginning of in vitro fertilization (IVF), improvement in the stimulation protocols, in methods and strategies to select the best oocytes and embryos, in embryo culture media and protocol and in optimal preparation of the luteal phase are the main purposes of several studies and reports. Interestingly, since the introduction of intracytoplasmic sperm injection (ICSI), little attention has been paid to the spermatozoa. What is more, after the introduction of ICSI, several studies [1–3] find no relationship between ICSI outcomes with abnormal or normal sperm morphology. Such observations were probably biased by the selection performed by the embryologist who tried to select the best "normal-looking" motile spermatozoa prior to ICSI, which does not always reflect the quality of the whole semen population.

The evaluation of sperm morphology as a routine diagnostic control seems to be a powerful indicator of man's fertilizing potential in vitro and in vivo. The basic morphological evaluation (spermocytogram) is based on the WHO (World Health Organization) criteria [4] or Kruger's strict criteria [5] on ejaculated sperm after fixation and staining at magnification of ×1,000. Other powerful techniques such as transmission or scanning electronic microscopy permit a more accurate observation of nuclear defects or tail abnormalities (presence or absence of dynein arms) of spermatozoa. But, we have to recognize that it is impossible to select living morphologically normal spermatozoa with all those techniques requiring a fixation—staining step.

At the present, it is mostly believed that the success rate of ICSI mainly depends on morphological aspects of injected spermatozoa. De Vos et al. [6] observed a

P. Vanderzwalmen, Bio-Eng. MSc (✉) • M. Bach, Dip-Biol • B. Baramsai, MD • A. Neyer, MSc
D. Schwerda, MSc • A. Stecher, MSc • B. Wirleitner, PhD • M. Zintz, PhD
M. Zech, MD • N.H. Zech, MD, PhD
IVF Laboratory, IVF Centers Prof. H. Zech, Bregenz, Austria
e-mail: pierrevdz@hotmail.com

B. Lejeune, MD PhD • S. Vanderzwalmen, BSc
IVF Laboratory, Centre Hospitalier Inter Régional Cavell (CHIREC), Bruxelles, Belgium

N.G. Cassuto, MD
ART Unit, Drouot Laboratory, Paris, France

negative correlation with fertilization rates, ongoing pregnancies and implantation rates after ICSI, with occurrence of spermatozoa exhibiting elongated, tapered or amorphous heads, broken necks or cytoplasmic droplets.

As consequence, a more critical selection process of spermatozoa seems necessary.

During the last decade, there has been a growing interest on the development of new techniques that improve the preparation of the semen sample such as electrophoresis [7] or magnetic-activated cell sorting (MACS) [8]. Other techniques based either on a biochemical assay (hyaluronan binding assay) [9] or on high-magnification microscopical examination [10] were introduced to permit a better selection of those spermatozoa that can support embryo development to the birth of a healthy baby.

In this chapter, we will focus on a technique that allows us to assess the morphology of motile spermatozoa in real time before intracytoplasmic oocyte injection. The outcome of nuclear defect such as vacuole will be discussed.

Real-Time Morphological Approach: MSOME

The introduction of a new concept called "motile sperm organelle morphology examination" (MSOME) permits to examine the fine nuclear morphology of motile spermatozoa in real time, at a magnification of ×1,000 using Nomarski differential interference contrast optics [10, 11].

Morphological assessment at magnification up to more than ×10,000 is obtained after increasing the magnification with a zoom and coupling the microscope with a high-definition digital video camera and a high-definition video monitor. At identical magnification, the use of Nomarski differential interference contrast optics lets us observe more precisely the general morphology of the spermatozoa and, in addition, minimal structural defects in the head, as compared with the conventional Hoffman modulation contrast.

MSOME in Combination with ICSI: IMSI

The MSOME approach in observing spermatozoa was then considered as an additional tool to ICSI and takes the name "intracytoplasmic morphologically selected sperm injection" (IMSI).

Morphological Normalcy of Spermatozoa Assessed by MSOME

Bartoov et al. [10, 11] define the morphological normalcy on motile sperm nucleus according to the shape and chromatin content. The shape has to be smooth, symmetric and oval with an average length and width limits estimated to 4.75 ± 0.28

and 3.28 ± 0.20 µm, respectively. The chromatin mass has to be homogeneous and contain no extrusions or invaginations with a maximum of one vacuole involving less than 4% of the nuclear area.

Regarding the acrosome and the post-acrosomal lamina, they were considered abnormal if absent, partial or vesiculated. An abaxial neck, with the presence of disorders or cytoplasmic droplets, was considered abnormal, as well as the presence of broken, short or double and coiled tail.

Spermatozoa Selection and Reproductive Outcomes

IMSI with Morphologically Normal Spermatozoa

Fascinating results, showing the importance of the sperm morphology, were published immediately after the introduction of IMSI.

Bartoov et al. [11] stressed that among the group of subcellular organelles (head, tail, midpiece) observed by MSOME, the morphological normalcy of the sperm nucleus could be a crucial characteristic associated with a positive ICSI outcome.

They provided a first answer by performing MSOME on a leftover fraction of motile spermatozoa of 100 random couples referred for ICSI treatment. Among the different morphological aspects of the spermatozoa, the normalcy of the sperm nucleus (shape and chromatin content) was significantly related with fertilization, and no clinical pregnancy was achieved when less than 20% of the spermatozoa exhibit morphological normal nuclei.

Several publications report that selection of spermatozoa exhibiting normal nuclear shapes is positively associated with IVF outcomes after day 3 embryo transfers in couples with previous and repeated implantation failures [12–15] and in patients with an elevated degree of DNA-fragmented spermatozoa [16].

In a comparative prospective study, Bartoov et al. [12] compared the outcome of 50 couples that underwent IMSI with a group of 50 ICSI candidates after at least two previous failures of implantation and a maternal age of less than 37 year. The rate of good-quality embryos on day 3 (45.2% vs. 31.0%), the implantation (27.9% vs. 9.5%) and pregnancy rates (26.4% vs. 15.3%) were significantly higher after MSOME selection followed by injection of a morphologically normal spermatozoa. Significantly lower abortion rates were observed after application of IMSI (9.0% vs. 33.0%).

Hazout et al. [16] perform a similar trial on 125 couples with previous failures of implantation and in addition with men exhibiting different levels of DNA fragmentation. Their study stressed the advantage of MSOME selection in terms of clinical pregnancy (2.4% vs. 37.6%) and implantation (0.8% vs. 20.3%) rates and this independent of the rate of DNA fragmentation.

In a recent study, Berkovitz et al. [14] reinforced the power of performing IMSI with morphologically normal spermatozoa in a group of patients with at least two previous failures of implantation. After comparing 80 ICSI trials with 80 matched IMSI trials, their conclusions corroborate their previous studies [12]: an increase in the rate of embryo quality on day 3 (25.7% vs. 38.7%), in the clinical pregnancy (25% vs. 60%) and implantation (9.4% vs. 31.3%) rates and a reduction in the abortion rate in the IMSI group.

IMSI with Morphologically Abnormal Spermatozoa

There is a great heterogeneity between all the semen samples. Thus, the frequency by which good spermatozoa can be selected varies greatly from one patient to the other. In some cases, only one part of the oocytes can be injected with morphologically normal spermatozoa. For other patients, as noticed already earlier by Berkovitz et al. [13, 14], in spite of having a more powerful selection method at hand, it is not always possible to find and select morphologically completely normal-appearing spermatozoa for injection, even after extensive search.

Establishment of a Sperm Classification Using the MSOME Approach

As described in the previous chapter, Bartoov et al. [11] defined the morphological normalcy of the sperm nucleus according to the shape and chromatin content.

In the circumstances where no normal spermatozoa can be found, the only alternative consists then to select those that are morphologically second best. This meticulous approach towards sperm selection with the Nomarski differential interference contrast optics allows us to identify vacuole(s) in the sperm head that are otherwise not evident to detect at ×400 magnification with Hoffman modulation contrast.

It is then essential to know from the second choice spermatozoa with vacuoles and/or abnormal shape which one we have to select. For this reason, it appears that the establishment of a classification of the spermatozoa according to different types of abnormalities was necessary to select the spermatozoa in a more tangible way.

In order to know exactly the impact of specific sperm defects on embryo development and further outcome, Vanderzwalmen et al. [17] and Cassuto et al. [18] established a classification. The final aim was to classify individually the spermatozoon before injection combined with single embryo culture to day 5. With such an approach, they were able to compare and search for a relation between embryo development and the morphology of injected spermatozoa.

Vanderzwalmen et al. [17] classified the spermatozoa into four groups according to the presence and size of vacuoles: grade I, normal shape and absence of vacuoles; grade II, maximum of two small vacuoles; grade III, more than two small vacuoles or at least one large vacuole; and grade IV, large vacuoles in conjunction with abnormal head shapes or other abnormalities at the level of the base.

Cassuto et al. [18] established a detailed classification scoring scale ranging between 6 and 0 points according to the normalcy of the head (2 points if normal), the symmetry of the base (1 point if normal) and the absence of vacuole (3 points if absent). Three classes of scoring were established as follows: class 1, high-quality spermatozoa with calculated score of 4–6; class 2, medium-quality spermatozoa with calculated score of 1–3; and class 3, low-quality spermatozoa with calculated score of 0.

Effect of Injecting Morphologically Abnormal Spermatozoa on Reproductive Outcomes

Spermatozoa with unclassified defects. The importance of selecting normal spermatozoa is reinforced when comparing the reproductive outcomes in terms of fertilization, embryo development, pregnancy and abortions rates when oocyte injections are done with morphologically normal sperms and spermatozoa exhibiting different defects.

Berkovitz et al. [13] compared the IMSI outcome in two groups of 38 patients in which oocytes were injected with normal sperm or with spermatozoa exhibiting nucleus defects. They reported low fertilization rates (50.3% vs. 71.3%), low percentage of top-quality embryos on day 3 (19.4% vs. 34.9%) and low pregnancy (18.4% vs. 52.6%) and implantation rates (5.9% vs. 25.0%) after IMSI with spermatozoa exhibiting a large panel of nuclear malformations in terms of shape, size and the presence of vacuoles. The reproductive outcomes from this study were confirmed in a second larger study from the same group [14] comparing the reproductive outcome in two groups of respectively 70 patients injected with morphologically normal spermatozoa or second quality spermatozoa exhibiting defects.

Nuclear vacuoles. One particular sperm malformation that is better detectable (i.e. more precisely and easily) with the Nomarski optics is/are vacuole(s). Already in the early 1990s, their presence has been negatively associated with natural male fertility potential [19, 20]. The potential relationship between large vacuoles and late embryonic developmental effects raises concerns.

A more specific analysis on the impact of sperm cells with normal nuclear shape but large vacuoles was first carried out by Berkovitz et al. [21] on two matched IMSI groups of 28 patients each. Spermatozoa with strictly defined normal nuclear shape but large vacuoles were selected for injection and compared to a control group that included normal nuclear shape spermatozoa lacking vacuoles.

No difference in the fertilization and early embryo development up to day 3 was reported. However, injection of spermatozoa with strictly normal nuclear shape but large vacuoles appeared to reduce significantly pregnancy outcomes (18% vs. 50%) and seemed to be associated with early abortions (80% vs. 7%).

In two successive studies, Vanderzwalmen et al. [17] and Cassuto et al. [18] reported that the existence of large vacuoles in the nuclei of spermatozoa dramatically reduces the proportion of good-quality blastocysts on day 5.

Vanderzwalmen et al. [17] reported that the outcome of embryo development in a group of 25 patients after sibling oocyte injections with the four different grades of spermatozoa showed no differences in the fertilization rates as well in the rates of top-quality embryos on day 3. However, the occurrence of blastocysts formation was 56.3 and 61.4% with grades I and II spermatozoa, respectively (no significant difference), compared to 5.1% with grade III and 0% with grade IV, respectively ($p < 0.001$).

In the same way, the rate of good-quality blastocysts was significantly reduced (2.9%) when all the oocytes in a group of eight patients were injected with grade III/IV spermatozoa, as compared to the use of only grade I/II spermatozoa (19.1%) ($p < 0.01$) in a group of 34 patients.

Cassuto et al. [18] reported a statistically significant decrease in the fertilization rate according to the classes of injected spermatozoa (84% with class 1, 73% with class 2, 61% with class 3). In addition, a statistically significant relationship was noted when the comparison was made between the rate of expanded blastocysts (15% with class 1, 9% with class 2, 0% with class 3).

The size and the number of sperm nuclear vacuoles, identified accurately under the Nomarski optics, negatively affected blastocyst development and reinforced previous studies suggesting the early and late paternal effects on initial embryonic development [22–25]. The presence of a late paternal effect impacts embryo development after the onset of paternal DNA content contribution to embryonic development, which starts around day 3 after fertilization [25] and may often lead to early abortions.

These findings corroborate studies by Barth and Oko [26] and Thundathil et al. [27], who report that in the bovine species, nuclear vacuoles do not decrease fertilization rates but rather increase the incidence of early embryo losses.

Indications for IMSI

One of the most frequent questions with regard to IMSI relates to its indications.

History of Previous Failure of Implantation and/or DNA Fragmentation

As already mentioned in the previous chapter, MSOME-ICSI can be seen as a useful tool for patients with previous failure of implantation or for patients with high levels of DNA fragmentation [12, 14, 16]. Those previous studies were substantiated with recent data presented by Antinori et al. [28] and Nadalini et al. [29]. Antinori et al. [28] conducted a prospective randomized trial to assess the potential advantages of the IMSI technique (227 couples) over the conventional ICSI procedure (219 couples) in the management of patients with severe oligoasthenoteratozoospermia, regardless of the number of previous failed ICSI attempts. By comparing the two groups, the overall IMSI technique resulted in statistically significantly higher implantation and pregnancy rates than those for ICSI (17.3% vs. 11.3%, and 39.2% vs. 26.5%, respectively) in cases of severe male infertility, while no statistical differences were reported for miscarriage rates. Their data showed that the sub-group with at least two previous failed ICSI attempts received the greatest advantage from the IMSI procedure in terms of clinical pregnancy rate (29.9% vs.

12.9%). On the other hand, among these latter sub-groups of patients, no significant differences in miscarriage rates were reported, even though the clinical outcome was clearly in favour of the IMSI procedure, with a remarkable 50% reduction (17.4% vs. 37.5%).

Nadalini et al. [29] compared the reproductive outcome of couples with a history of at least one previous failed ICSI attempts who underwent IMSI with spermatozoa free of any nuclear morphological malformations (20 couples) with 37 couples referred for conventional ICSI treatment in the same period of time. As a result, the IMSI clinical outcome seemed to improve significantly in terms of clinical pregnancy rates (40% vs. 16.21%), and a positive trend towards reduction of miscarriages and biochemical pregnancies was seen.

Interestingly, the sub-group with fragmented DNA showed a significantly higher clinical pregnancy rate with respect to the ICSI control group (66.67% vs. 16.21%, $p = 0.005$) [29]. They therefore suggested that sperm selection and oocyte microinjection based on high-power microscopy at $>\times 6,000$ appeared to significantly increase the pregnancy outcome of previous failed ICSI treatments, above all in patients with several degrees of sperm DNA fragmentation corroborating the data of Hazout et al. [16].

Absence of Blastocysts in Previous IVF Cycles

We may also advice IMSI in case of absence of blastocyst formation after conventional ICSI treatment.

Unexplained Infertility

In case of unexplained infertility, a MSOME observation of the semen has to be advised. Our preliminary results in conjunction with those of Dr. Cassuto show a higher rate of class 4 [18] or grade IV [17] spermatozoa in an unexplained infertility patient as compared to a group of patients with pure tubal problem (personal observations).

General ICSI Candidates

Also, in our opinion, the question that brings a lot of debate is why not to select directly spermatozoa with the MSOME approach before ICSI?

The MSOME technique has to be considered as an additional tool for ICSI, particularly since the probability of selecting a normal spermatozoon is higher using the MSOME approach, as compared to the conventional ICSI approach.

Are we sure that with our conventional ICSI microscope, we can detect in all cases abnormal spermatozoa? Even after extensive search for patients who attend their first treatment, the frequency of selecting spermatozoa of normal morphological appearance greatly varies according to semen samples. We observed that in almost 50% of the semen sample, if selection had been performed using the classic ICSI approach, the likelihood of selecting sperm with a nuclear vacuoles would have been very high [17].

Considering the above, the following questions remain to be answered regarding the indications for IMSI: should IMSI be performed on all ICSI candidates or only on a sub-group of patients?

It is now obvious that assessment of sperm morphology by Kruger's strict criteria is routinely used and widely accepted as the best predictor of male fertility potential, better than sperm concentration or motility, highlighting the concept that sperm morphology is the most important parameter in the semen analysis. Everybody believes in this concept because the spermocytogram is one of the basic routine examinations.

As a consequence, we have to do all we can to select the best spermatozoa. There are absolutely no indications to select bad-quality spermatozoa if good ones are present in the prepared semen sample. Are there still indications where improved sperm selection before fertilization is not necessary or low-magnification microscopy using Hoffman modulation contrast is more than enough? Probably none.

At present, there is a big debate on which patients IMSI instead of ICSI should be recommended. Is it possible to find a threshold of normal spermatozoa above which selection at ×400 under Hoffman modulation contrast is sufficient?

There is a great heterogeneity between all the semen samples so that the frequency by which good spermatozoa can be selected varies greatly from one patient to the other. As consequence, the fundamental question to elucidate concerns the probability with which a normal spermatozoon can be selected with classical ICSI method under ×400 magnification instead of using the Nomarski optics.

The establishment of classification criteria, based on an assessment system, seems a valuable approach to determine a threshold limit for making the right therapeutic decision to advise ICSI or IMSI to patients entering an infertility treatment programme. For this reason, a prior screening of semen samples by MSOME to detect the presence of vacuoles would be a reasonable approach. But we have to recognize that at the present time, there are no studies reporting a threshold of percentages of normal forms for either recommending ICSI or IMSI.

Limiting Factors to Perform IMSI

However, there are some limiting factors that render MSOME selection almost not possible at all. In case of severe oligoteratozoospermia, the rare spermatozoa that are found are selected for injection. Even if the semen exhibit 100% abnormal morphology, it is difficult to select the best "second choice" from the sperm population.

MSOME for Routine Laboratory Semen Analysis

In order to assess the usefulness of the evaluation of sperm morphology by MSOME, two studies were undertaken in a first instance by Bartoov et al. [11] who estimated the correlation between MSOME and the WHO routine method [4] and more recently by Oliveira et al. [30] who compared the MSOME evaluation with the Tygerberg classification criteria [31].

Both works conclude that the MSOME criteria appear to be much more restrictive, presenting significantly lower sperm normalcy percentages for the semen samples in comparison to those found after routine analysis by WHO criteria and the Tygerberg classification. In addition, MSOME represented a much stricter evaluation, since the use of Nomarski optics enabled the identification of vacuoles that could not be described with the same accuracy with the other methods.

These studies point towards a benefit in sperm morphology and quality evaluation by including MSOME among the criteria for routine laboratory semen analysis prior to ICSI or conventional IVF procedure. A previous MSOME spermocytogram revealing a high percentage of vacuoles may be judicious to propose directly IMSI as the best therapy for ICSI candidates (Figs. 6.1 and 6.2). Furthermore the additional information gained by MSOME may help to avoid fertilization failure in IVF cycles.

With the aim to define a predictive value of sperm normalcy using the MSOME on the outcome of combined IVF-ICSI, Wittemer et al. [32] undertook a study including 55 couples with previous failure of implantation after IUI treatments. In their next attempt, a combination of conventional IVF and ICSI was proposed for each couple. They conclude that below a threshold of 8% of morphological normal spermatozoa observed by MSOME, ICSI must be performed instead of conventional IVF in order to avoid the risk of fertilization failure.

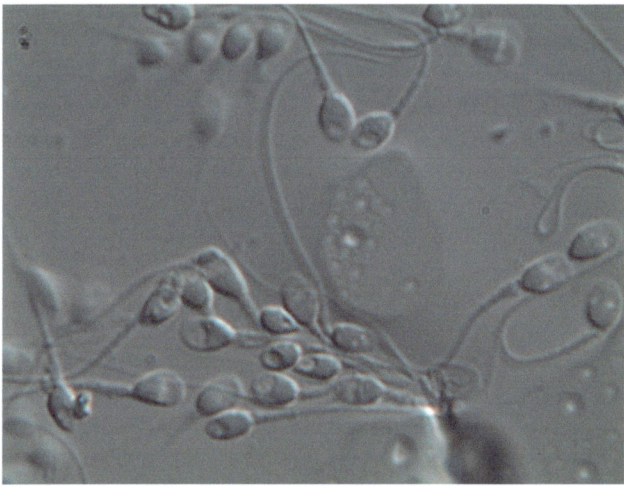

Fig. 6.1 Teratozoospermia semen observed by MSOME. DIC objective ×63 dry

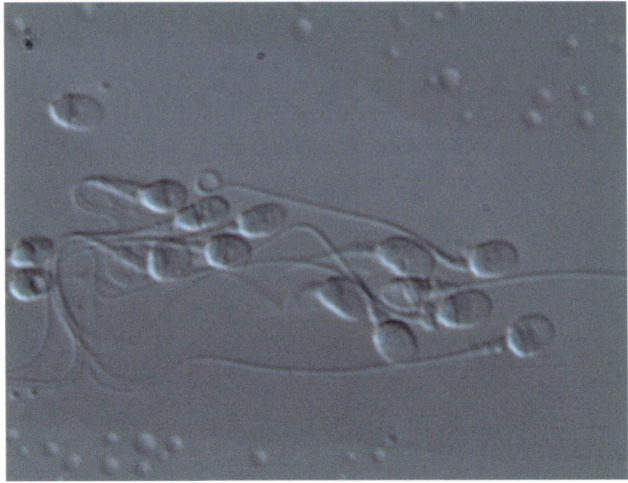

Fig. 6.2 Normal semen sample for conventional IVF observed by MSOME. DIC objective ×63 dry

The Importance of Selecting Morphologically Normal Sperm Without Vacuoles: A Phenomenon Raising a Lot of Questions

As described before, the main advantage of the MSOME technique is not only to select normal-shaped sperm but also to identify sperm which show special structural aberrations described as "vacuoles" in the sperm head. Although it seems to be well proven by the literature that the appearance of these structures is strongly related to reduced blastocyst outcome as well as pregnancy and implantation rates, we still do not know if there is a correlation between vacuoles and DNA damage.

Since it is more and more evident that vacuoles as well as DNA damage have a negative influence on the reproductive outcome, it would be valuable to comprehend if the presence of vacuole(s) in the sperm head is well correlated with DNA damage such as high degree of DNA fragmentation.

Effect of Vacuoles on Reproductive Outcome

In view of the evidence that nuclear defects negatively influence the outcome of embryo development, the argument that the oocyte itself supplies all the primary machinery for embryo development and that the sperm DNA only plays a secondary role probably has to be revised [33, 34]. Therefore, the pending question relates to the meaning of vacuoles, to their origin and, more importantly, to their possible negative effects they might have on the health of the offspring.

Effect of DNA Damage and Chromatin Disorganization on Reproductive Outcome

DNA damage in spermatozoa can affect both mitochondrial as well as nuclear DNA and can be induced by several mechanisms during the production of the spermatozoa (abortive apoptosis during meiosis, faulty chromatin remodelling during spermiogenesis) and/or mainly by oxidative stress during sperm transport through the seminiferous tubules and the epididymis or by endogenous caspases and endonucleases. Exogenous factors such as damage induced by radiotherapy and chemotherapy and by environmental toxicants can also induce DNA damage.

Several reports [35, 36] have shown that DNA damage is higher in the caudal epididymal and ejaculated sperm compared with testicular spermatozoa reinforcing the idea that during transport through the epididymis, levels of DNA fragmentation are higher.

We may consider DNA damage in three different forms: (1) fragmentation of the DNA in the form of single-stranded or double-stranded DNA strand breaks, (2) nuclear protein defects that may interfere with histone to protamine conversion and subsequent DNA compaction and (3) chromatin structural abnormalities causing altered tertiary chromatin configuration [36].

Such abnormalities of the paternal genome may affect blastocyst development [37–39] and pregnancy outcome [40, 41] after ICSI [42].

According to Hammadeh et al. [43], the integrity of the sperm chromatin may play the most important role, particularly in ICSI, in which most of the natural selection mechanisms are bypassed. In recent reports, Aitken [44] and Barratt et al. [45] report the possible negative influences of sperm DNA fragmentation both on pregnancy outcome and even on the next generation.

The argument that the oocyte supplies all the primary material (proteins and RNAs) and that the spermatozoa and their DNA only play a secondary role needs probably revision [33, 34]. A spermatozoon contains almost 3,000 different kinds of mRNA, some of which contain the code for proteins needed for early embryo development.

Is There a Correlation Between DNA Damage and the Presence of Vacuoles?

According to Berkovitz et al. [13], Cayli et al. [46] and Hazout et al. [16], vacuoles may reflect molecular defects responsible for anomalies of sperm chromatin packaging and abnormal chromatin remodelling during sperm maturation which, in turn, may render spermatozoa more vulnerable to DNA damage. According to Gopalkrishnan et al. [47], Hammadeh et al. [43] and Virro et al. [37], the integrity of the chromatin is related to the presence or absence of vacuoles in the head of spermatozoa, and loss of chromatin compaction renders the DNA more vulnerable to reactive oxygen species.

In order to substantiate these notions, recent studies [48–51] evaluated the integrity of the chromatin and the DNA fragmentation using the acridine orange staining procedure, aniline blue and the TUNNEL technique. All studies concluded that there is an obvious association between large vacuoles and high levels of denatured DNA. Garolla et al. [49] observed significantly better mitochondrial function, chromatin status and less aneuploidies in spermatozoa when nuclear vacuoles were lacking. For Franco et al. [48], there is an obvious association between large vacuoles and secondary as well as tertiary DNA structure damages in sperm nuclei: the association between high levels of denatured DNA in spermatozoa with large nuclear vacuoles suggests premature decondensation and desegregation of sperm chromatin fibres. The chromatin material of spermatozoa from patients with early pregnancy loss seems to be often either compact or partially compact and to have irregular nuclear borders with larger vacuoles. A regression analysis of 538 semen samples demonstrated that percentages of normal nuclear sperm and all spermatozoa with abnormalities of nuclear form at high magnification negatively correlated with percentages of DNA fragmentation. On the other hand, there was a positive correlation between percentages of spermatozoa with nuclear vacuoles and those with DNA fragmentation. Oliveira et al. [51] showed that both normal and abnormal nuclear forms appear to be equally vulnerable to DNA fragmentation as analysed under high magnification. The only sperm type that correlates with a high rate of DNA fragmentation is the category of sperm with >50% vacuolated nuclei, showing that selecting a spermatozoon based on morphology or motility is not a good criterion of DNA integrity.

Considering the thesis of reduced reproductive outcome due to DNA damage in sperm and the notion that such DNA damages are displayed by the formation of vacuoles which are accurately evaluated at high magnification by MSOME [30], we may suggest that the more sophisticated selection of spermatozoa using the MSOME approach will most probably substitute the classical ICSI sperm selection method within the next years.

When and Why Vacuoles Are Formed?

After analysing the influence of vacuoles on embryo development, another question to investigate concerns their origin.

A study by Peer et al. [52] demonstrated that after 2 h of incubation at 37°C in culture media, the incidence of spermatozoa with vacuolated nuclei was significantly higher compared to incubation at 21°C. They suggest that prolonged (≥ 2 h) sperm manipulations for assisted reproduction therapy should be performed at 21°C rather than 37°C.

Another hypothesis proposed by Kacem et al. [53] states that sperm nuclear vacuoles, as assessed by MSOME, are mostly associated with the presence of acrosomal material. Their data suggest that the vacuole-free spermatozoa that are microinjected during IMSI are mostly acrosome-reacted spermatozoa free of acrosomal enzymes, such as trypsin-like acrosin that may induce a harmful effect [54].

Several experiments were conducted in our centres in order to analyse if we could perceive the formation of vacuole in real time. We conducted a 24-h time-lapse recording approach, first on selected grade 1 spermatozoa incubated for 24 h at 37°C in culture media and in media containing different inducers of ROS (media in contact for 48 h with pool of plasma seminal containing high level of leucocytes or in media supplemented with different concentrations of H_2O_2). As compared to the control group, no changes in the morphology of the spermatozoa were observed. No vacuoles appeared. Even when the same experiment was conducted on spermatozoa with vacuoles, no changes in the size and shape of the spermatozoa after 24-h incubation at 37°C were observed (personal observation).

The same experiment was conducted with acrosome inducer (ionophore), but no change could be noticed. It is not fully understood at which time point in spermatogenesis vacuoles are formed and why they are such important indicators of sperm quality.

However, vacuoles seem to appear during the last maturation step of round spermatids. Could vacuoles be a selective mechanism of sperm to be removed in the natural selection process? We know that in sperm "incomplete apoptosis" is a common phenomenon [55]. Spermatozoa which do not pass the "quality control" due to, e.g. DNA defects or other aberration during spermatogenesis undergo the normal pathway towards apoptosis, but are not removed by phagocytes. Maybe the formation of vacuoles is a mechanism for abnormal spermatozoa to be attacked by ROS during storage and thereby being discarded.

Blastocyst Formation and Pregnancies with Vacuolated Spermatozoa: How Come?

Even though a negative impact of vacuoles is recognized, we still observe in some cases the formation of blastocysts followed by an ongoing pregnancy after IMSI with spermatozoa showing nuclear defects. How can we explain the ability of embryos to develop to the blastocysts stage and give rise to pregnancies after oocyte injection with spermatozoa exhibiting several small and/or large vacuoles?

It is no doubt that vacuoles have to be considered with attention. Several explanations such as the type and morphology of vacuoles, their location, the level of oxidative stress and repairing factors are still in suspend and may contribute in various ways or not at all to embryo development.

Type of Vacuoles

Spermatozoa contain heterogeneous vacuoles varying in number, size and content. To simplify this matter, we only refer to the term vacuole in any circumstance. But is vacuole the appropriate terminology? In a biological point of view, vacuoles are vesicles surrounded by a membrane. In the case of sperm vacuoles, what we call vacuoles represent more of a kind of depression in the nuclear part of the head. Some are deep, like a crater, or hollow. Watanabe et al. [56] reports that vacuoles are actually hollow whereby the plasma membrane falls into the nucleus, and Westbrook et al. [57] even speaks about nuclear crater formation in the sperm head. Toshimori [58] differentiates between large vacuoles with amorphous substances or membranous structures inside and small vacuolous patterns without any structures inside.

So the definition on its own is still an issue of controversial opinions and may explain why some spermatozoa can produce blastocysts and offsprings.

Location of Vacuoles

In a recent study, Hammoud et al. [59] analysed the rate of DNA fragmentation according to the position of the vacuoles on the sperm head. They report statistically higher degree of fragmentation if vacuoles are located in the posterior region. So it is also important that independently of the classification system, the location of the vacuole is taken into account.

Level of Endogenous and Exogenous ROS

The presence of vacuoles may reflect molecular defects responsible for abnormal chromatin remodelling during sperm maturation and might render sperm cells more vulnerable to DNA damage [46]. We may also postulate that when the oxidative stress during spermatogenesis and/or during sperm transport is below a critical level, the DNA and chromatin will not be affected. Above a critical level of ROS, genomic problems start to occur, thereby affecting the reproductive outcome.

DNA Damage-Repairing Factors

If we assume that a majority of nuclear defects reflected in vacuoles may be correlated with DNA integrity, we may have an optimistic view in the sense that this damage brought into the zygote by the fertilizing spermatozoon may be effectively repaired by oocyte factors [60, 61]. We may then postulate the possibility to obtain blastocysts that will further develop to a healthy baby even though the oocyte was injected with a spermatozoon carrying a large vacuole. This aspect is related to the tolerance of the oocytes towards DNA decays [60], especially if young and/or good-quality oocytes are capable of repairing and rescuing the DNA of poor-quality spermatozoa. As consequence, even if the fertilizing spermatozoon carries DNA damage in its genome, the oocyte could repair this damage, and, therefore, it would be of no consequence for embryo and foetal development.

However, we cannot determine whether the oocyte would be capable of repairing this damage. This mainly depends on the degree and the type of sperm DNA damage (single-stranded vs. double-stranded damage) [62]. Also, oocytes whose DNA repair mechanisms are not functional (ageing oocytes—in vitro culture conditions) or that have been damaged by endogenous (e.g. free radicals) or exogenous (e.g. radiation, environmental toxicants) factors might not be able to repair this damage.

Long-Term Safety

There remain concerns about the long-term safety of injecting spermatozoa carrying vacuoles. It is already well accepted that spermatozoa from older and/or infertile men have a higher level of imprinting disorders [62, 63]. The approach of selecting normal-appearing spermatozoa helps the oocytes in the DNA repair operations. However, when the DNA repair capacity in the oocyte is over passed, incomplete or mismatched, DNA repair mechanisms may lead to mutations. Under these circumstances, the damage may either remain unrepaired or be aberrantly repaired, creating DNA mutations. We have to be cautious, especially in the light of Aitken's work [44] on the possible negative effects of sperm DNA fragmentation in the next generation. Depending on the level of sperm nuclear DNA fragmentation, oocytes may partially repair fragmented DNA, producing blastocysts able to implant and produce live offspring. However, the incomplete repair may lead to long-term pathologies. The data of Fernández-Gonzalez et al. [64] in the mice model indicate that the use of DNA-fragmented spermatozoa in ICSI can generate effects that only emerge in later life, such as aberrant growth, premature ageing, abnormal behaviour and tumours from the mesenchymal lineage.

Up to now, there have not been sufficient numbers of children born after ICSI to draw any firm conclusions about the long-term safety of this procedure. However, it is important to emphasize that animal data are absolutely unequivocal on this point and clearly indicate that DNA damage in the male germ line is potentially damaging for the embryo and offspring [65]. According to a recent paper [66], sperm nucleus morphological normalcy, assessed at high magnification, could decrease the prevalence of major foetal malformations in ICSI children.

Therefore, how should we treat patients carrying 100% large vacuoles in their sperm samples? If such observation correlates with a positive DNA fragmentation test, antioxidant therapy may be proposed several months before the IVF treatment. But at the present, none of the studies report a significant benefit of specific antioxidant molecules therapy.

Knowing the potential risk of injecting abnormal spermatozoa, shall we continue the attempt with the patient's sperm or propose a testicular biopsy before proposing the option of a sperm donor if possible? As previously stated, reports have shown that sperm DNA damage is significantly lower in the seminiferous tubules compared with the cauda epididymis [67, 68] or ejaculated sperm [35]. Moreover, the use of testicular sperm in couples with repeated pregnancy failure in ART and high sperm DNA fragmentation in semen resulted in a significant increase in pregnancy rates in these couples.

Technical Aspect

For routine application and also to render the technique more user friendly, observations at ×1,000 magnification might suffice to select the right spermatozoa.

Some are reluctant to apply this new approach of selecting spermatozoa before ICSI. It is generally advocated that besides being time-consuming, IMSI is also expensive. The minimal requirement to observe and select spermatozoa using the MSOME criteria in a routine way consists to place the sperm suspension in a glass bottom dish and perform the observation under an inverted microscope equipped with Nomarski differential interference contrast optics with 63 and ×100 objective.

The adjunct of a vario-zoom, the amplification of the microscopic image with high-definition digital video camera, the video monitor as well as the computer software are not a priority to perform the observation and selection in a first instance.

Observation of moving spermatozoa at high magnification on the screen is difficult due to a more restricted field of observation.

The use of high magnification (>×6,000) in conjunction with digital image capture system permits to analyse spermatozoa in details. For example, MSOME spermocytogram can be done after capturing and storing several pictures of the prepared semen sample for later sperm morphological analysing.

Even though intracytoplasmic microinjection based on MSOME is a more time-consuming procedure, this should not be an argument not to start to perform IMSI. In order not to induce adverse affects to the oocyte quality, the IMSI procedure has to be envisaged in a way that the oocytes stay for a short time out of the incubator.

For both procedures, all the manipulations (observation, selection and injection) are done in glass bottom dishes. The first option consists to select the spermatozoa using the Nomarski microscope and perform the oocyte injection on a classical ICSI microscope.

A suspension of prepared spermatozoa is deposited in a drop of PVP. Morphologically motile spermatozoa are selected with an ICSI pipette and placed in a small drop of culture media. After collecting spermatozoa—if possible, 1.5× the amount of oocyte to inject—the dish is placed back in the incubator for temperature recovery. After this period of incubation (~15 to 30 min), the oocytes are placed in HEPES culture media, and ICSI is performed on a conventional Hoffman microscope. The advantage of this approach is that the IMSI microscope is not occupied for a too long period and that the oocytes finally stay out of the incubator only for the injection step.

When the purpose of the study is to follow the spermatozoa individually at very high magnification (observation on the screen at >×6,000 magnification), a maximum of two oocytes are placed in the dish. With this technique, a minimum of two dishes are prepared. This technique is easy to perform if dry objectives are used so that we have no problem with oil when we change the dish.

Conclusions

IMSI is now a reality in ART practice but still with a lot of question marks regarding (1) the terminology of vacuoles, their classification, their location on the sperm head, and their origin and meaning, (2) the application of IMSI instead of IVF in cases of unexplained infertility, (3) the age of the woman; is IMSI necessary in younger women with good-quality oocytes where cytoplasmic factors might be able to repair sperm nuclear defects? and (4) the technical aspect. We have to be aware that this technique is demanding and has to be performed in the best working conditions not to impair the oocyte quality.

The introduction of IMSI has the advantage that embryologists realize that more attention has to be paid during sperm selection even in case of classical ICSI. The application of IMSI leads to more and better quality blastocysts and, as consequence, it increases the chance to select the proper embryo for transfer with high implantation potential. Even though there is no real proof in the human species on the abnormal outcome generated by spermatozoa carrying vacuoles, a higher and better-resolution technique has to be added as an additional tool for ICSI knowing the possible consequence of sperm DNA damage for offsprings.

Furthermore, the effect of using MSOME approach to select spermatozoa manifests itself when it is performed in combination with day 5 embryo culture of all fertilized oocytes.

References

1. Svalander P, Jakobsson AH, Forsberg AS, et al. The outcome of intracytoplasmic sperm injection is unrelated to "strict criteria" sperm morphology. Hum Reprod. 1996;11:1019–22.
2. Mansour RT, Aboulghar MA, Serour GI, et al. The effect of sperm parameters on the outcome of intracytoplasmic sperm injection. Fertil Steril. 1995;64:982–6.
3. Nagy ZP, Liu J, Joris H, et al. The result of intracytoplasmic sperm injection is not related to any of the three basic sperm parameters. Hum Reprod. 1995;10:1123–9.
4. WHO. WHO laboratory manual for the examination of human semen and semen–cervical mucus interactions. Cambridge: Cambridge University Press; 1999.
5. Kruger TF, Acosta AA, Simmons KF, et al. Predictive value of abnormal sperm morphology in in vitro fertilization. Fertil Steril. 1988;49:112–7.
6. De Vos A, Van De Velde H, Joris H, et al. Influence of individual sperm morphology on fertilization, embryo morphology, and pregnancy outcome of intracytoplasmic sperm injection. Fertil Steril. 2003;79:42–8.
7. Ainsworth C, Nixon B, Jansen RP, et al. First recorded pregnancy and normal birth after ICSI using electrophoretically isolated spermatozoa. Hum Reprod. 2007;22:197–200.
8. Said TM, Grunewald S, Paasch U, et al. Advantage of combining magnetic cell separation with sperm preparation techniques. Reprod Biomed Online. 2005;10:740–6.

9. Huszar G, Jakab A, Sakkas D, et al. Fertility testing and ICSI sperm selection by hyaluronic acid binding: clinical and genetic aspects. Reprod Biomed Online. 2007;14:650–63.
10. Bartoov B, Berkovitz A, Eltes F. Selection of spermatozoa with normal nuclei to improve the pregnancy rate with intracytoplasmic sperm injection. N Engl J Med. 2001;345:1067–8.
11. Bartoov B, Berkovitz A, Eltes F. Selection of spermatozoa with normal nuclei to improve the pregnancy rate with intracytoplasmic sperm injection. N Engl J Med. 2001;345:1067–8.
12. Bartoov B, Berkovitz A, Eltes F, et al. Pregnancy rates are higher with intracytoplasmic morphologically selected sperm injection than with conventional intracytoplasmic injection. Fertil Steril. 2003;80:1413–9.
13. Berkovitz A, Eltes F, Yaari S, et al. The morphological normalcy of the sperm nucleus and pregnancy rate of intracytoplasmic injection with morphologically selected sperm. Hum Reprod. 2005;20:185–90.
14. Berkovitz A, Eltes F, Lederman H, et al. How to improve IVF-ICSI outcome by sperm injection? Reprod Biomed Online. 2006;12:634–8.
15. Junca AM, Cohen-Bacrie P, Hazout A. Improvement of fertilisation and pregnancy rate after intracytoplasmic fine morphology selected sperm injection. Fertil Steril. 2004;82 Suppl 2: S173.
16. Hazout A, Dumomt-Hassant M, Junca AM, et al. High-magnification ICSI overcomes paternal effect resistant to conventional ICSI. Reprod Biomed Online. 2006;12:19–25.
17. Vanderzwalmen P, Hiemer A, Rubner P, et al. Blastocyst development after sperm selection at high magnification is associated with size and number of nuclear vacuoles. Reprod Biomed Online. 2008;17:617–27.
18. Cassuto N, Bouret D, Plouchart J, et al. A new real-time morphology classification for human spermatozoa: a link for fertilization and improved embryo quality. Fertil Steril. 2009;92:1616–25.
19. Bartoov B, Eltes F, Pansky M, et al. Improved diagnosis of male fertility potential via a combination of quantitative ultramorphology and routine semen analyses. Hum Reprod. 1994;9:2069–75.
20. Mundy AJ, Ryder TA, Edmonds DK. A quantitative study of sperm head ultrastructure in subfertile males with excess sperm precursors. Fertil Steril. 1994;61:751–4.
21. Berkovitz A, Eltes F, Ellenbogen A, et al. Does the presence of nuclear vacuoles in human sperm selected for ICSI affect pregnancy outcome? Hum Reprod. 2006;21:1787–90.
22. Vanderzwalmen P, Bertin-Segal G, Geerts L, et al. Sperm morphology and IVF pregnancy rate: comparison between Percoll gradient centrifugation and swim-up procedures. Hum Reprod. 1991;6:581–8.
23. Shoukir Y, Chardonnens D, Campana A, et al. Blastocyst development from supernumerary embryos after intracytoplasmic sperm injection: a paternal influence. Hum Reprod. 1998;13: 1632–7.
24. Tesarik J, Greco E, Mendoza C. Late but not early paternal effect on human embryo development is related to sperm DNA fragmentation. Hum Reprod. 2004;19:611–5.
25. Tesarik J. Paternal effects on cell division in the preimplantation embryo. Reprod Biomed Online. 2005;10:370–5.
26. Barth AD, Oko RJ. Defects of the sperm head. In: Barth AD, Oko RJ, editors. Abnormal morphology of bovine spermatozoa. Ames: IS Iowa State University Press; 1988. p. 130–92.
27. Thundathil J, Palasz A, Barth A, et al. Fertilization characteristics and in vitro embryo production with bovine sperm containing multiple vacuoles. Mol Reprod Dev. 1998;50:328–33.
28. Antinori M, Licata E, Dani G, et al. Intracytoplasmic morphologically selected sperm injection: a prospective randomized trial. Reprod Biomed Online. 2008;16:835–41.
29. Nadalini M, Tarozzi N, Distratis V, et al. Impact of intracytoplasmic morphologically selected sperm injection on assisted reproduction outcome. Reprod Biomed Online. 2009;19:45–55.
30. Oliveira JB, Massaro FC, Mauri AL, et al. Motile sperm organelle morphology examination is stricter than Tygerberg criteria. Reprod Biomed Online. 2009;18:320–6.
31. Menkveld R, Stander FS, Kotze TJ, et al. The evaluation of morphological characteristics of human spermatozoa according to stricter criteria. Hum Reprod. 1990;5:586–92.

32. Wittemer C, Pujol A, Boughali H, et al. The impact of high-magnification evaluation of sperm on ART outcome. Hum Reprod. 2006;22 Suppl 1:i59–60.
33. Lalancette C, Miller D, Li Y, et al. Paternal contributions: new functional insights for spermatozoal RNA. J Cell Biochem. 2008;6:633–42.
34. Dadoune JP. Spermatozoal RNAs: what about their functions? Microsc Res Tech. 2009;72: 536–51.
35. Greco E, Scarselli F, Iacobelli M, et al. Efficient treatment of infertility due to sperm DNA damage by ICSI with testicular spermatozoa. Hum Reprod. 2005;20:226–30.
36. Sakkas D, Juan G, Alvarez JG. Sperm DNA fragmentation: mechanisms of origin, impact on reproductive outcome, and analysis. Fertil Steril. 2010;93(4):1027–36.
37. Virro MR, Larson-Cook KL, Evenson DP. Sperm chromatin structure assay (SCSA) parameters are related to fertilization, blastocyst development, and ongoing pregnancy in in vitro fertilization and intracytoplasmic sperm injection cycles. Fertil Steril. 2004;81:1289–95.
38. Seli E, Gardner DK, Schoolcraft WB, et al. Extent of nuclear damage in ejaculated spermatozoa impacts on blastocyst development after in vitro fertilization. Fertil Steril. 2004;82: 378–83.
39. Muriel L, Garrido N, Fernandez JL, et al. Value of the sperm deoxyribonucleic acid fragmentation level, as measured by the sperm chromatin dispersion test, in the outcome of in vitro fertilization and intracytoplasmic sperm injection. Fertil Steril. 2006;85:371–83.
40. Nasr-Esfahani MH, Salehi M, Razavi S, et al. Effect of sperm DNA damage and sperm protamine deficiency on fertilization and embryo development post-ICSI. Reprod Biomed Online. 2005;11:198–205.
41. Larson K, DeJonge C, Barnes A, et al. Relationship of assisted reproductive technique (ART) outcomes with sperm chromatin integrity and maturity as measured by the sperm chromatin structure assay (SCSA). Hum Reprod. 2000;15:1717–22.
42. Jones G, Trounson A, Lolatgis N, et al. Factors affecting the success of human blastocyst development and pregnancy following in vitro fertilization and embryo transfer. Fertil Steril. 1998;70:1022–9.
43. Hammadeh M, Nkemayim D, Georg T, et al. Sperm morphology and chromatin condensation before and after semen processing. Arch Androl. 2000;44:221–6.
44. Aitken R. Origins and consequences of DNA damage in male germ cells. Reprod Biomed Online. 2007;14:727–33.
45. Barratt C, Aitken J, Björndahl L, et al. Sperm DNA: organisation, protection and vulnerability: from basic science to clinical applications—a position report. Hum Reprod. 2010;25:824–38.
46. Cayli S, Jakab A, Ovari L, et al. Biochemical markers of sperm function: male fertility and sperm selection for ICSI. Reprod Biomed Online. 2003;7:462–8.
47. Gopalkrishnan K, Padwal V, Meherji PK, et al. Poor quality of sperm as it affects repeated early pregnancy loss. Arch Androl. 2000;45:111–7.
48. Franco JG, Baruffi RL, Mauri AL, et al. Significance of large nuclear vacuoles in human spermatozoa: implications for ICSI. Reprod Biomed Online. 2008;17:42–5.
49. Garolla A, Fortini D, Menegazzo M, et al. High power magnification microscopy and functional status analysis of sperm in the evaluation and selection before ICSI. Reprod Biomed Online. 2008;17:610–6.
50. Baborova P, Uher P, Stecher A. Correlation between morphological semen parameters and sperm nuclear DNA damage: focus on the nuclear vacuoles and patient with environmental stress. J Reproduktionsmed Endokrinol. 2008;5:289–90.
51. Oliveira J, Massaro F, Baruffi R, et al. Correlation between semen analysis by motile sperm organelle morphology examination and sperm DNA damage. Fertil Steril. 2010;94(5): 1937–40.
52. Peer S, Eltes F, Berkovitz A, et al. Is fine morphology of the human sperm nuclei affected by in vitro incubation at 37 degrees C? Fertil Steril. 2007;88:1589–94.
53. Kacem O, Sifer C, Barraud-Lange V, et al. Sperm nuclear vacuoles, as assessed by motile sperm organellar morphological examination, are mostly of acrosomal origin. Reprod Biomed Online. 2010;20:132–7.

54. Morozumi K, Yanagimachi R. Incorporation of the acrosome into the oocyte during intracytoplasmic sperm injection could be potentially hazardous to embryo development. Proc Natl Acad Sci U S A. 2005;102:14209–14.
55. Gandini L, Lombardo F, Paoli D, et al. Study of apoptotic DNA fragmentation in human spermatozoa. Hum Reprod. 2000;15:830–9.
56. Watanabe S, Tanaka A, Fujii S, Mizunuma H, et al. No relationship between chromosome aberrations and vacuole-like structures on human sperm head. Hum Reprod. 2009;24:i96–9.
57. Westbrook A, Diekman A, Klotz K, et al. Spermatid-specific expression of the novel X-linked gene product SPAN-X localized to the nucleus of human spermatozoa. Biol Reprod. 2000; 63:469–81.
58. Toshimori K. In: Toshimori K, editors. In: Dynamics of the Mammalian Sperm Head: Modifications and Maturation Events From Spermatogenesis to Egg Activation. In Advances in Anatomy, Embryology and Cell Biology. Dynamics of the mammalian sperm head, dynamics of the sperm nucleus; 2009. p. 43–51. Kindle Edition.
59. Hammoud I, Albert M, Bergere M, et al. Can IMSI (X6000) be more efficient than ICSI to select spermatozoa without nuclear fragmentation? Hum Reprod. 2009;24:i214–7.
60. Menezo Y, Russo G, Tosti E, et al. Expression profile of genes coding for DNA repair in human oocytes using pangenomic microarrays, with a special focus on ROS linked decays. J Assist Reprod Genet. 2007;24:513–20.
61. Brandriff B, Pedersen RA. Repair of the ultraviolet-irradiated male genome in fertilized mouse eggs. Science. 1981;211:1431–3.
62. Kobayashi H, Sato A, Otsu E, et al. Aberrant DNA methylation of imprinted loci in sperm from oligospermic patients. Hum Mol Genet. 2007;16:2542–51.
63. Marques CJ, Costa P, Vaz B, Carvalho F, et al. Abnormal methylation of imprinted genes in human sperm is associated with oligozoospermia. Mol Hum Reprod. 2008;14:67–74.
64. Fernández-Gonzalez R, Nuno Moreira P, Perez-Crespo M, et al. Long term effects of mouse intracytoplasmic sperm injection with DNA-fragmented sperm on health and behavior of adult offspring. Biol Reprod. 2008;78:761–72.
65. Lewis S, Aitken R. DNA damage to spermatozoa has impacts on fertilization and pregnancy. Cell Tissue Res. 2005;322:33–41.
66. Berkovitz A, Eltes F, Paul M, et al. The chance of having a healthy normal child following intracytoplasmic morphologically-selected sperm injection (IMSI) treatment is higher compared to conventional IVF-ICSI treatment. Fertil Steril. 2007;88:S20.
67. Suganuma R, Yanagimachi R, Meistrich ML. Decline in fertility of mouse sperm with abnormal chromatin during epididymal passage as revealed by ICSI. Hum Reprod. 2005;20: 3101–8.
68. Steele EK, McClure N, Maxwell RJ, Lewis SE. A comparison of DNA damage in testicular and proximal epididymal spermatozoa in obstructive azoospermia. Mol Hum Reprod. 1999;5:831–5.

Chapter 7
Sperm Testing and ICSI Selection by Hyaluronic Acid Binding: The Hyaluronic Acid-Coated Glass Slide and Petri Dish in the Andrology and IVF Laboratories

Gabor Huszar

Overview of Sperm Biomarkers

Infertility has been commonly defined as failure to conceive following 12 months of regular intercourse. In the 2008 national US statistics, 35% of the IVF-ET cycles reported in the United States were diagnosed with male factor infertility either as a single (17%) or combined (18%) diagnosis.

Semen analysis is routinely used to evaluate the male partner of the infertile couple. Although widely used normal semen measures have been published by the WHO, the current normal parameters for sperm concentration, motility, and morphology fail to meet rigorous clinical, technical, and statistical standards [1]. With the advent of ICSI [2], it is imperative to provide solid scientific base for the characterization of sperm that are enabled to fertilize and provide paternal contribution. The ongoing research, focusing on biochemical markers of sperm function [3], have taken high prominence, as the pathology in male factor infertility patients, who require ICSI treatment, is likely to be of high complexity.

In the past 2 decades, the Huszar laboratory made major advances upon the biochemical markers of human sperm maturity and function [4–6]. In this chapter, an overview is presented, including clinical application of the biochemical markers, the cell biology of sperm maturity and genetic integrity, the lack of relationship between sperm shape and chromosomal aneuploidies, sperm hyaluronic acid (HA) binding, the application of sperm-HA binding score in the Andrology laboratory, and preferential selection for ICSI spermatozoa that fully completed cellular development.

In the early phase of sperm studies, we were searching for an objective biochemical parameter that may predict sperm fertility, independently from the

G. Huszar, MD (✉)
Department of Obstetrics, Gynecology, and Reproductive Sciences, Male Fertility Program and Sperm Physiology Laboratory, Yale University School of Medicine, 333 Cedar Street, New Haven, CT 06510, USA
e-mail: gabor.huszar@yale.edu

classical semen parameters. In assessments of B-type creatine kinase (CK), we found significantly higher sperm CK content in men with diminished fertility [4, 7, 8]. One of the first recognized markers was cytoplasmic retention which was measured by the excess cytoplasm in sperm; biochemically this observation translated to an increased sperm creatine phosphokinase (CK) activity [8]. The variations of CK activity in semen samples have been well documented, as well as the fact that sperm recovered from pellets of density gradient centrifugation had substantially lower CK content [9]. A logistic regression analysis of 180 couples with oligozoospermic husbands, treated with intrauterine insemination (IUI), indicated that the increased levels of CK activity in these oligozoospermic, men predicted a lower likelihood for pregnancy [8, 10]. The CK-immunostaining patterns indicated that the high sperm CK activity was a direct consequence of increased cytoplasmic protein and CK concentrations in individual spermatozoa [11]. This suggested a sperm developmental defect in terminal spermiogenesis when the surplus cytoplasm is normally extruded from elongating spermatid [12, 13].

We have also found another sperm protein with ATP content in mature sperm [14]. This protein was later characterized as the 70-kDa testis-expressed HspA2 chaperone [15]. Thus, the proportional concentrations of CK and HspA2 (or HspA2 ratio) reflect the representation of fully developed and dysmature spermatozoa in semen samples [14]. In three studies (approximately 500 men), there were similarly close correlations between sperm CK activities and HspA2 ratios ($r = -0.69, -0.71$, and -0.76; $p < 0.001$; $N = 159, 134$, and 194) [14, 16, 17]. The proportion of mature and immature sperm, whether the men were normozoospermic or oligozoospermic, showed a day-to-day and man-to-man variation in semen samples [15]. Indeed, in a study of couples treated with IUI, a logistic regression analysis indicated that sperm CK activity did, but sperm concentrations did not, provide a predictive attribute for pregnancies to occur [10].

In further studies of sperm-hemizona (halved unfertilized human oocytes) complexes, all zona pellucida-bound sperm were clear-headed without cytoplasmic retention. Thus, immature sperm with retained cytoplasm and low expression of HspA2 were deficient in the zona-binding site [9]. We hypothesized that during normal spermiogenesis, a plasma membrane remodeling step occurs. In a blinded study, focusing upon β1, 2,-galactosyltransferase (present exclusively in the sperm plasma membrane), the cytoplasmic content of CK or HspA2, and the membrane density of β1-, 2-galactosyltransferase were closely related (both $r > -0.8$ and >0.8, respectively, with $p < 0.001$) [18]. Thus, during normal spermiogenesis and plasma membrane remodeling, along with formation of the zona pellucida-binding site, and as found later, the formation of the hyaluronic acid (HA)-binding site also occurs, which is the basis for the HA-mediated fertility testing and ICSI sperm selection in men.

Male Fertility and Semen Parameters

Contemporary studies, directed to the relationship between semen attributes and male infertility, focus on the experience with IUI which, from the perspective of sperm-zona pellucida interaction, is similar to that of natural conception. There are two major IUI studies on the relationship between semen parameters and fertility. One is a major collaborative effort conducted at seven sites utilizing approximately 1,600 couples [19]. The other work summarizes the data of 26 IUI publications encompassing over 30,000 cycles in 14,000 couples [20]. The authors of both studies concluded that assessment of single sperm attributes, even strict sperm morphology, is of limited predictive value. These data confirm our findings regarding the predictive value of biochemical markers with no contributions by sperm concentrations or motility [10].

With respect to IVF-ICSI data, several investigators attempted both IVF and ICSI in the same cycle on sibling oocytes [21–24]. In the van der Westerlaken study using 106 couples (1,518 oocytes), 28 of the couples were treated with ICSI, while 78 couples were treated with both IVF and ICSI. Two couples failed to fertilize in both IVF and ICSI, while the 26 women who were treated only with ICSI showed a 57% fertilization rate (182 oocytes). In the remaining 78 patients, 528 oocytes were treated with conventional IVF yielding a 51% fertilization rate, and 858 oocytes were treated with ICSI resulting in a 56% fertilization rate. The pregnancy rates similarly fail to show differences, as the transfer rates were 54% for IVF and 48% for ICSI.

It seems that above a threshold motile sperm density, no semen parameters are identified that would predict whether IVF or ICSI is more beneficial toward for a particular couple. The data of sperm-HA binding and ICSI with HA-selected sperm support that the sperm-HA binding assay contributes to an objective assessment of sperm function and male fertility and thus optimize the mode of fertility treatment. ICSI selected with hyaluronic acid binding (the PICSI dish) is increasingly efficient in the below 60%, low sperm-HA binding score level (high incidence of dysmature sperm). The ability to measure the proportion of sperm that are able to bind to the zona pellucida greatly enhances the benefits of semen analysis. In addition, considering sperm concentration, motility, and morphology, our understanding regarding the pathogenesis of male infertility is improved. Indeed, the sperm-HA binding assay is more on target compared to the so far most advanced approach, the sperm-hemizona assay, as the HA slides are of uniform quality as opposed to the functional variations among unfertilized human oocytes.

Spermiogenetic Events and Sperm Fertilizing Function

From the perspective of male gamete evolvement. It is important that synthesis of the HSP70 family of chaperone proteins (HspA2 in men) is regulated developmentally and that they contribute to the maintenance of the synaptonemal complex and to the meiotic function during spermatocyte development [25–28]. With respect to human sperm, our laboratory was the first to demonstrate the two-wave expression of HspA2 (Fig. 7.1), first in spermatocytes as a meiotic component within the synaptonemal complex and second in elongating spermatids during terminal spermiogenesis [15]. Further, in human and stallion studies, we found that all CK and

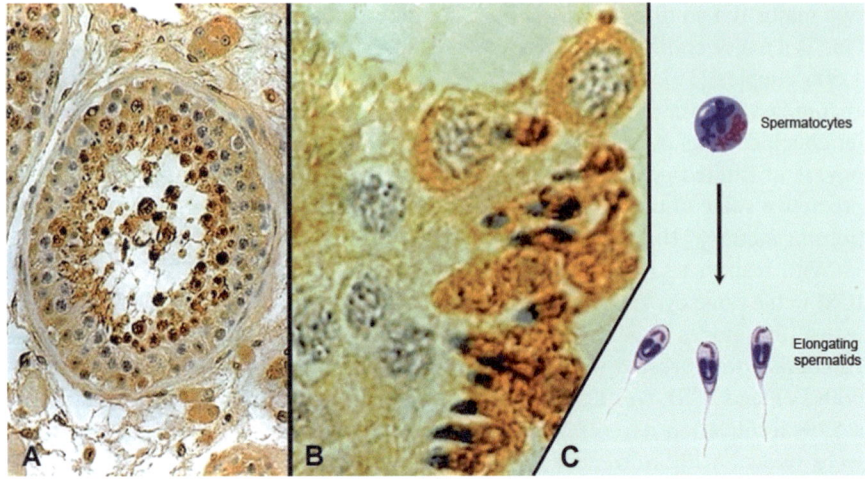

Fig. 7.1 Human testicular biopsy tissue immunostained with heat shock protein HspA2 antiserum. (**a**) Illustrates the structure of the seminiferous tubuli and the staining pattern of the adluminal area. HspA2 expression begins in meiotic spermatocytes, and there is a second wave of expression in elongating spermatids (**b, c**) (from Huszar et al. [3], with permission)

HspA2-related maturational events are completed in sperm cells prior to reaching the caput epididymis [29].

In considering the potential diagnostic value of the sperm-HA binding assay, it should be noted that the relationship between male fertility and the conventional semen parameters is inconsistent. In addition to the clinical utility of sperm CK activity [10], expression levels of the sperm HspA2 chaperone protein were also tested in blinded studies of in vitro fertilization couples. In one blinded study, we assigned 84 husbands from the Jones Institute and Yale, based only on their sperm CK-HspA2 levels (while their semen parameters or reproductive histories were unknown), into "high likelihood" (>10% HspA2) and "low likelihood" (<10% HspA2) for fertility subgroups [16]. All pregnancies were found in the "high-likelihood" group. An additional benefit of the HspA2 levels was apparent: 9 of the 22 "low-likelihood" men were normozoospermic but had sperm dysmaturity. Thus, the HspA2 level provides a diagnostic utility for unexplained male infertility (infertile men with normal semen [16]). Recently, the utility of HspA2 levels was reexamined in 194 couples treated with IVF at Yale. The ROC analysis showed a 100% predictive value for failure to achieve pregnancy in the range of <10.4% HspA2 threshold. As in the 1992 study, 9 of the 15 men with <10% HspA2 ratio (18 of the 37 men (45%) in the two studies) and pregnancy failure were normozoospermic; thus, their diminished fertility would be unsuspected [30]. In summary, the expression levels of HspA2 correlate well with sperm cellular development and IVF success.

Sperm Structure and Function: Nuclear and Cytoplasmic Biochemical Markers

The recognition that HspA2 reflects the meiotic process, as well as the cytoplasmic and nuclear downstream events of cellular development in spermatozoa, was a key advance [3, 15,112]. The spermatid phase is a dividing point between normally developing and diminished maturity sperm. In elongating spermatids with a substantial upregulation of HspA2, *normal sperm development* occurs with the orderly extrusion of cytoplasm and simultaneous plasma membrane remodeling, yielding a spermatozoon with normal head morphology and fully formed binding sites for the zona pellucida and hyaluronic acid (Fig. 7.2).

In contrast, spermatids with low HspA2 expression (sperm dysmaturity) show increased cytoplasmic retention and higher frequencies of chromosomal aneuploidies due to synaptonemal complex defects, as well as DNA chain breaks as a result of inadequate delivery of DNA repair enzymes. The latter is likely due to diminished

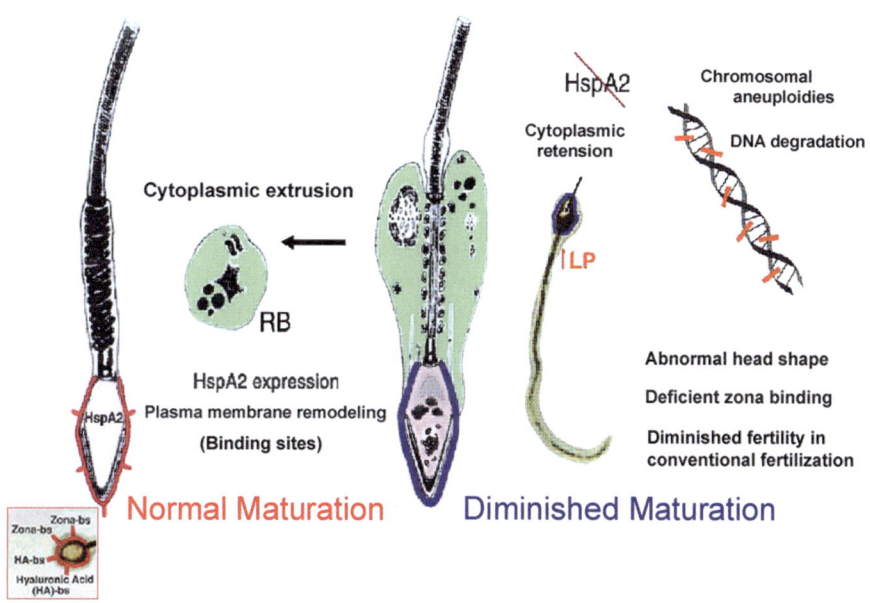

Fig. 7.2 A model of normal development and dysmaturation of human spermatozoa. In normal sperm maturation (*left*), elongating spermatids undergo cytoplasmic extrusion (represented by the loss of the residual body, RB) and plasma membrane remodeling, leading to the formation of the zona pellucida and hyaluronic acid-binding sites (bs) (change from *blue* membrane to *red* membrane with the stubs). Dysmature spermatozoa have low heat shock protein HspA2 expression, which may causes meiotic defects and chromosomal aneuploidies. Also, in dysmature sperm, there is a higher retention of CK and other cytoplasmic enzymes, increased levels of lipid peroxidation (LP) and consequential DNA fragmentation, abnormal sperm morphology, and deficiency in the zona and hyaluronic acid-binding sites (from Huszar et al. [3], with permission)

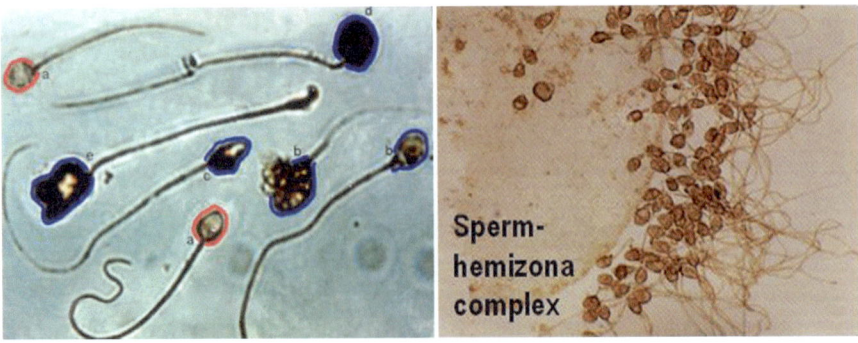

Fig. 7.3 Zona pellucida binding of normally developed and dysmature human spermatozoa. *Left*: Normally developed and dysmature sperm (cytoplasmic retention and abnormal morphology are highlighted with creatine kinase immunostaining) in dysmature spermatozoa. Also, the plasma membrane remodeling is illustrated by the *red* and *blue* colors, respectively. *Right*: Sperm-hemizona complexes immunostained with creatine kinase antiserum. Please note that only the clear sperm without cytoplasmic retention and normal morphology are able to bind to the zona pellucida (from Huszar et al. [46], with permission)

HspA2 chaperone activity [25, 26]. These dysmature sperm are characterized by cytoplasmic retention, abnormal head morphology, increased levels of reactive oxygen species, and consequential DNA fragmentation. Further, due to the incomplete spermiogenetic process, the plasma membrane remodeling and the formation of the zona pellucida and hyaluronic acid-binding sites fail to occur. Thus, dysmature sperm are unable to bind to the zona pellucida or fertilize via natural or IVF conception, only by ICSI. Conversely, none of the hemizona-bound spermatozoa have cytoplasmic retention (Fig. 7.3). The likely reason why such sperm do not demise prior to ejaculation is the presence of antiapoptotic protein Bclx2 in the surviving germ cells [9, 31].

Sperm Head Shape and Sperm Genetic Integrity: Shape or Dimensional Properties Do Not Facilitate the Selection of Haploid Sperm for ICSI

The potential relationship between abnormal sperm morphology and chromosomal aberrations has been of long-term interest [32, 33]. Earlier data supporting this association were based on the frequencies of abnormally shaped or aneuploid sperm in semen samples, but not within the same sperm. Examination of the same individual sperm for both shape and aneuploidies has become possible when the data from the Huszar laboratory established that sperm preserve their shape after undergoing the decondensation and denaturation steps that are a prerequisite of FISH analysis [34]. Based on this finding, we studied the potential role of shape attributes in ICSI sperm selection [35].

First, using objective shape measurements, by the Metamorph computer-assisted program, 1,286 individual sperm were evaluated from 15 men: 900 haploid cells, utilizing three-color FISH for chromosomes 17, X, and Y and two-color FISH for the 10 and 11 chromosomes, and all the disomic and diploid sperm images that were found in the samples (368 cells). Second, we sorted the 900 nonaneuploid sperm and classified into three groups as "small head," "intermediate head," and "large head." Third, we sorted the 256 aneuploid and 130 diploid sperm according to the head-size parameter ranges established in the nonaneuploid sperm group and determined the frequencies of disomies and diploidies within the "small," "intermediate," and "large" groups.

Aneuploidies and diploidies were present within all three categories. The proportions of the 256 disomic sperm in the small, intermediate, and large sperm head category groups were 66 (27 ± 2%), 56 (23 ± 1%), and 133 (50 ± 2%), respectively. Similarly, the mean number of diploidies in the three sperm head categories were 3.0 ± 1, 8.0 ± 1, and 89.0 ± 2%, respectively. Interestingly, approximately 27% of sperm with disomy and 3% with diploidy of the 386 nonhaploid sperm were among the 300 sperm were within the "small" and "normal" dimensions.

In another analysis of the 1,286 images, we examined sperm shape according to their characteristics as symmetrical ($N = 367$), asymmetrical ($N = 368$), irregular ($N = 504$), and amorphous ($N = 47$). Disomic and diploid sperm were present in all four groups with an increasing frequency of 18, 18, 41, and 98%, respectively [35]. Finally, according to the Kruger strict morphology method as normal and abnormal, the proportion of sperm with normal morphology in the symmetrical, asymmetrical, irregular, and amorphous groups was 26, 3, 1, and 0%, respectively. There were aneuploid sperm even within the Kruger normal group.

Thus, it is evident that visual shape assessment, i.e., choosing the "best-looking" sperm, is an unreliable method for ICSI selection of haploid spermatozoa [35, 36]. This inconsistent relationship between sperm chromosomal aberrations and sperm shape seems to be in contrast with the ICSI sperm selection approach based on enhanced microscopic imaging. However, there were no studies yet on sperm chromosomal aneuploidies, persistent histones, or DNA chain integrity in sperm selected by the high magnification imaging approach [37, 38].

Testing of Sperm Development by Hyaluronic Acid-Binding in the Andrology and IVF Laboratories

Concurrently with the studies on sperm development we investigated the effects of hyaluronic acid (HA) or hyaluronan on human sperm function. HA-containing medium increased sperm velocity, retention of long-term motility and viability with an immediate increase in sperm tail cross-beat frequency, and sperm velocity upon HA exposure [39, 40]. When these sperm were exposed to media lacking HA, the motility and velocity properties returned to those of the control sperm. Thus, the HA effects appear to be receptor-mediated [41–43]. In line with this idea, dysmature sperm with cytoplasmic retention, and thus retarded plasma membrane remodeling, were not stimulated by HA [39, 40].

Fully developed spermatozoa may selectively bind to solid-state HA. Indeed, sperm bound to HA were oriented head first, as with sperm-zona pellucida binding. This finding is in agreement with the HA binding pattern in monkey sperm [41, 44]. Also, in line with previous hemizona binding experiments, sperm bound to HA exhibited a uniform shape conforming to normal cells of the Kruger classification which is based on the zona pellucida-bound spermatozoa [35, 45–47]. Further attributes of HA-bound mature spermatozoa indicated that HA-selected sperm are viable. Nonviable sperm do not bind and may be removed from the HA slide with gentle washing (Fig. 7.4). HA-bound sperm are also devoid of cytoplasmic retention, persistent histones, DNA fragmentation, and the apoptotic marker caspase 3 (Fig. 7.5). Indeed, in a recent study, we demonstrated that each spermatozoa bound to the HA spot of the sperm selection PICSI dish exhibits green fluorescence (Fig. 7.6) with the acridine orange reagent (represent the lack of DNA chain degradation in the HA-bound sperm fraction) [48]. These properties are very important because nuclear and cytoplasmic sperm dysmaturity, particularly the presence of DNA fragmentation, is known to adversely affect the paternal contribution of sperm to the zygote [4, 13, 31, 34, 49–54].

The comparable sperm selection properties of zona pellucida and HA were further confirmed in a collaborative study between the Huszar and Kruger laboratories. In 37 of the 63 samples with <14% Kruger normal (teratozoospermic) score, the HA-bound sperm vs. semen sperm fractions showed an approximately fourfold enrichment in Kruger normal spermatozoa. The likelihood ratio was 3.04× (95% confidence limits: 1.9–4.7× considering the three blinded investigators). This enrichment is comparable

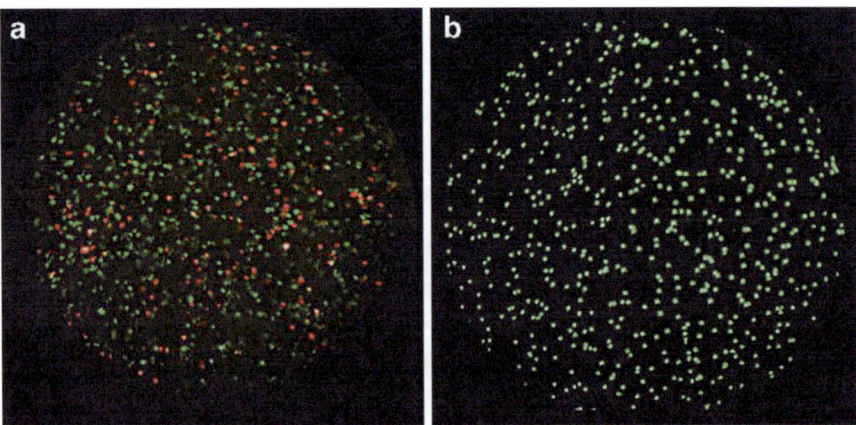

Fig. 7.4 Sperm viability and hyaluronic acid (HA) binding. (**a**) A drop of semen treated with a combination of Cyber green and propidium iodide, respectively, in order to highlight viable (*green*) and nonviable (*red*) spermatozoa. (**b**) HA-bound spermatozoa are gently rinsed and stained with the same combination of dyes. Only the viable green spermatozoa remain bound to the HA slide (from Huszar et al. [52], with permission)

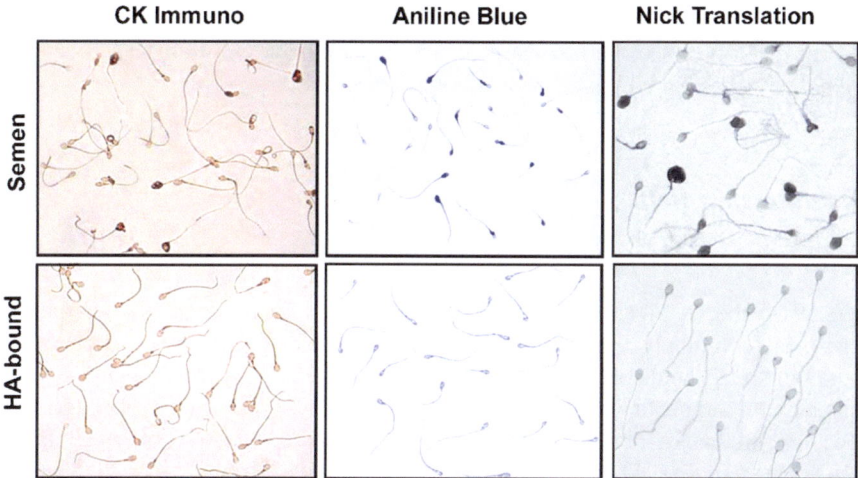

Fig. 7.5 Hyaluronic acid (HA)-bound mature spermatozoa do not contain cytoplasmic retention (creatine kinase [CK] immunostaining), persistent histones (aniline blue staining), or DNA fragmentation (detected by DNA-nick translation; Sati et al. [53]). *Upper*: Spermatozoa, including dysmature cells, from whole semen showing various degrees of staining. *Lower*: The HA-bound sperm stained with the respective cytoplasmic and nuclear biochemical markers. HA-bound normally developed spermatozoa show patterns clear from the biochemical markers of dysmaturity (cytoplasmic retention, persistent histones, DNA fragmentation)

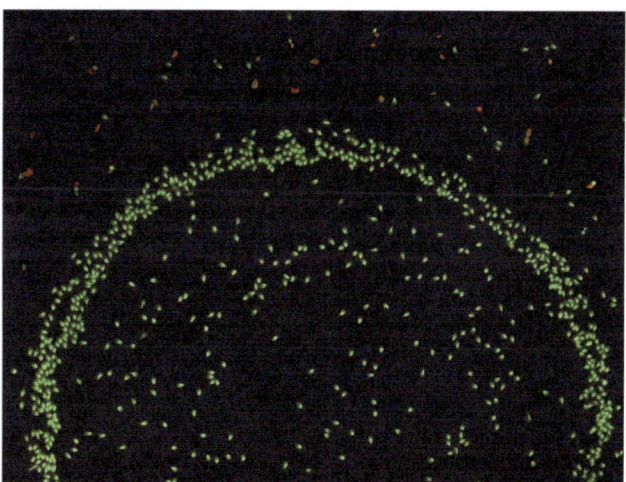

Fig. 7.6 PICSI dish picture. Acridine orange-stained sperm in the area of the HA-selection spot and in the outside control area of the HA spot-modified Petri dish (PICSI dish). Please note the almost exclusive presence of sperm with *green acridine orange* fluorescence (represent sperm with no DNA fragmentation) within the HA-selected sperm fraction. In the outside control area, the original semen is shown before HA selection with about 40% sperm with *red acridine orange* staining (sperm with fragmented DNA). The higher density of sperm around the perimeter of the HA spot is due to an HA ridge, which is caused by the application tool for placing the HA spot (48, with permission)

to the 3.9× improvement reported by Kruger in the zona pellucida bound vs. semen sperm [55–57]. Since sperm-zona pellucida binding is the penultimate fertilization step, sperm-HA binding is very important evidence.

Relationship Between Sperm Binding to Hemizonae and Hyaluronic Acid

We tested the validity of the idea that the HA-binding and zona-binding sites in sperm are commonly regulated via plasma membrane remodeling in a comparative study of sperm-hemizona binding and sperm-HA binding scores in aliquots of the same sperm sample in 60 men [18, 46, 52, 58]. By using bisected unfertilized human oocytes and the HA-binding slides, there was a close correlation between the binding scores to either HA or hemizona ($r = 0.73$, $p < 0.001$, $N = 54$) [59]. Thus, if the zona-binding properties of sperm were low or high, it was followed by a similar pattern by the HA-binding properties. Indeed, we suggest that the correlation is not closer because of the undefined sperm-binding ability of unfertilized oocytes, a factor which is more variable than the properties of the uniformly manufactured HA-coated binding slide.

A Semen Chamber Device for the Sperm-HA Binding Assay

Based on the fact that mature sperm selectively bind to solid-state HA, we have developed the sperm-HA binding assay, both as a clinical Andrology test and as a method for selection of mature sperm for ICSI. Sperm binding occurs within 8–10 min. The time-lapse photography highlights the pattern of motile sperm and arrested motile sperm (see examples in Fig. 7.7). The assessment of HA binding is based on the proportions of bound sperm with increased tail cross-beat frequency vs. the unbound swimming sperm that do not "perceive" the HA. Nonmotile sperm without tail movement are not considered [52]. In line with the inverse relationship between the spermiogenetic events of arrested cytoplasmic extrusion (increased CK retention), and sperm plasma membrane remodeling (formation of the HA-binding sites), there was a close correlation between sperm CK activity and HA binding ($r = -0.78$, $p < 0.001$, $N = 56$).

Because the clinical utility of sperm CK activity and HspA2 levels were already established in IUI and IVF studies [10, 16, 30], we formulated a general idea regarding the expected clinical application of the sperm-HA binding score. We considered three binding zones in 56 men: (1) *≥80% binding* (excellent binding, $N = 32$). In these men, the sperm CK activity was 0.18 ± 0.02 CK IU/10^8 sperm (normal range <0.25); thus, there was no male factor infertility or need for intervention. (2) *Binding between 60 and 80%* (intermediate binding, $N = 14$). In this group, the sperm CK activity was elevated to 0.50 ± 0.06 CK IU/10^8 sperm. These couples

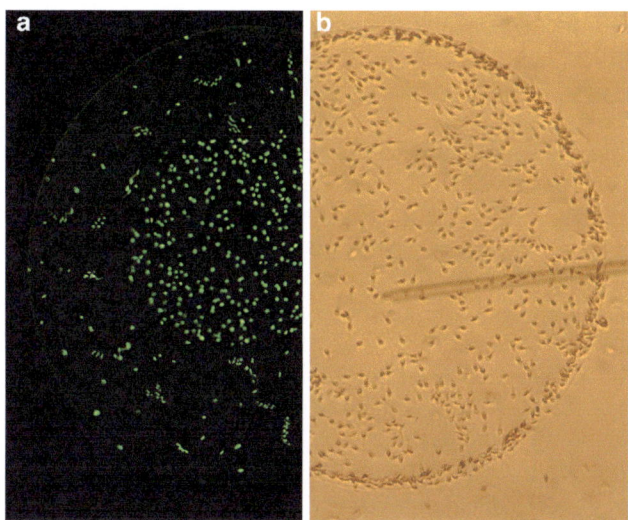

Fig. 7.7 Time-lapse photography of spermatozoa stained with Cyber green stain. *Left*: Semen drop placed on a glass slide. Please observe the progress of moving free spermatozoa. *Right*: A drop of the same semen observed on hyaluronic acid-coated slide. Most sperm (the normally developed ones) are bound by the sperm head (remodeled plasma membrane) to the hyaluronic acid and exhibit vigorous tail beating. Some dysmature sperm (no membrane remodeling) still swim freely and do not perceive the hyaluronic acid coating as they lack the hyaluronic acid receptors

may benefit from IUI. (3) *Binding* ≤60% (diminished binding, $N = 10$). In this group, the CK activity was a high 2.8 ± 0.1 CK IU/10^8 sperm (tenfold higher than the normal sperm CK activity range), indicating a high level of sperm cells with cytoplasmic retention. These men should be retested, and if the diminished binding is confirmed, these couples may be best treated with ICSI after HA sperm selection. These application guidelines are being confirmed with prospective studies and clinical experience [86–88]. As with the other biochemical markers, HA binding was largely independent from sperm concentrations. Among men within the <20 million sperm/ml concentration range ($N = 18$ of 56 men), we identified three excellent, seven intermediate, and eight diminished HA binders [60].

Considerations in Men with Excessive Semen ROS Production

Sperm preparation for assisted reproduction in men with high seminal ROS may improve sperm quality if media containing antioxidants such as reduced glutathione or catalase/EDTA [61–63]. Such approach may improve the quality of gametes used by protecting the spermatozoa from high oxidative stress.

Another approach available is the hyaluronic acid-mediated sperm selection. The rationale for this approach is as follows: (a) A close correlation has been shown between ROS production and cytoplasmic retention which represent gamete dysmaturity [9]. Thus, it is expected that dysmature sperm, which produce and\or have been affected by ROS, would have a high amount of DNA degradation and due to the arrested spermiogenesis, would not bind to hyaluronic acid. (b) Sperm selection by HA binding is also helpful as hyaluronic acid-bound sperm is also devoid of excess persistent histones, DNA fragmentation, and the apoptotic process. Thus, sperm selection by deselection of dysmature spermatozoa, and positive selection of normally developed spermatozoa with low or no ROS production, is an appropriate and practical solution [3].

Another advancement is the utilization of sperm extracted from the testes (TESE sperm). It is established that sperm originating in the adluminal area are protected from oxidative attack, whereas most ROS-initiated DNA fragmentation occurs during epididymal storage [64]. A number of reports indicate that sperm DNA damage is significantly lower in the seminiferous tubules compared to the cauda epididymis or ejaculated sperm [64, 65]. The use of TESE sperm in couples with repeated pregnancy failure in ART, and high sperm DNA fragmentation in semen, resulted in a significant increase in pregnancy rates [66]. Thus, use of sperm with very low levels of sperm DNA fragmentation reduces the burden of sperm DNA repair by the zygote. With respect to sperm in the seminiferous tubuli and in the epididymis, the usefulness of the TESE approach is limited to the location of the testicular origin, i.e., whether sperm extracted from the testes would originate in the seminiferous tubuli, in which the spermatozoa was already released from the adluminal compartment after all aspects of the sperm cellular maturation has been completed [29]. No ICSI selection may be performed with the PICSI dish in TESE sperm, due to the lack of progressive motility in these testes-extracted spermatozoa.

The Key Role of Sperm Chromatin Maturation

The formation of fully developed spermatozoa is a unique process involving a series of steps in both the nuclear and cytoplasmic compartments including histone-transition protein-protamine replacement [67]. A greater than tenfold compaction of sperm DNA is achieved during the final phases of spermatogenesis when the normally occurring histone that is bound to DNA is almost completely replaced by protamines.

Earlier studies showed an association between male infertility and diminished histone-transition protein-protamine exchange in sperm, and this may be detected by aniline blue staining of the excess persistent lysine-rich histones [68–72, 75]. Accordingly, based on the variations in sperm maturity, staining intensity was light, intermediate, and dark tone and represent sperm with mature, moderately immature, and severely immature developmental status, respectively [53]. It is clear that sperm chromatin is essential for sperm function and subsequent embryonic development because defects in sperm chromatin are linked to natural reproductive failures, such as spontaneous abortion as well as assisted reproductive failure [73–75].

The relationship between persistent histones and DNA degradation was highlighted in a recent report from the Huszar labroatory. In sperm with dark aniline blue staining, representing extensive levels of persistent histones, there was a lack of signal for fluorescence in situ hybridization (FISH) chromosome-probe binding [75]. Thus, deficiency in sperm chromatin development, improper DNA folding, and fragmented DNA chains caused diminished FISH probe binding, as there were limited number of long DNA sequences that facilitate the binding of FISH probes.

Regarding the interrelationship between sperm dysmaturity and persistent histones, a report by the Huszar group indicates that diminished sperm fertility and reduced paternal contribution of sperm to the embryo may not originate only in the arrested histone-protamine remodeling, but along with the persistent histones, there are other associated factors of dysmaturity in the same spermatozoa [53]. In these studies, a double-staining method was developed: First, sperm are stained with aniline blue for probing persistent histones. Second, after recording the aniline blue-stained sperm fields, and a subsequent destaining step, the same sperm are probed for cytoplasmic retention with creatine kinase immunostaining, for the apoptotic process with caspase 3 immunostaining, for DNA chain fragmentation with in situ DNA-nick translation, and for sperm shape [53].

The evaluation of the same sperm after the first and the subsequent probes convincingly showed an approximately 75% agreement between the aniline blue staining patterns whether light (no probe presence), intermediate (some probe detection), and dark staining (heavy probe presence) and of the various other biochemical probes, such as cytoplasmic retention, DNA degradation, caspase 3 apoptotic marker, or Kruger normal/abnormal sperm shape. This indicated that indeed, there is a relationship between the attributes of arrested development or dysmaturity within the same sperm. Also, the experiments demonstrated that the nuclear and cytoplasmic, as well as the early and late events of spermatogenesis and spermiogenesis, are related. Thus, sperm with persistent histones and arrested chromatin remodeling, and failing to initiate proper DNA folding in the nucleus, are also characterized by dysmaturity and diminished sperm function [53].

Does Sperm-HA Binding Test Predict High DNA Integrity: Studies with Two Different Approaches

In previous studies [4, 52] with the methods of in situ DNA-nick translation, it was demonstrated that HA-bound spermatozoa are viable; exhibit lack of cytoplasmic retention, persistent histones, and apoptotic probes; and also show high DNA chain integrity. Another recent paper, on acridine orange staining of HA-bound spermatozoa, a reagent which provides green fluorescence for DNA with high chain integrity and orange fluorescence for damaged DNA, Liu and Baker reported that the zona pellucida-bound sperm has mostly green fluorescence [76]. In the Huszar laboratory, the acridine orange assay was performed with sperm bound to the HA spot of the PICSI dish, a device which is used for ICSI sperm selection in IVF laboratories.

The data indicated, using the very high quality Polysciences Inc. acridine orange, that literally, 100% of the hundreds of HA-bound sperm were of green fluorescence (Fig. 7.7). Thus, whether we probe DNA integrity with nick translation or acridine orange reagent, the DNA of HA-bound sperm had high integrity [3, 48]. This experiment using the classic acridine orange assay supported that HA-mediated sperm selection, by the PICSI dish, is an optimal tool for ICSI sperm selection.

Furthermore, in a more refined experiment, semen aliquots were smeared on glass slides, and the sperm were fixed for the various markers. Another aliquot of the same semen was incubated on hyaluronic acid-coated slides. After the 15-min binding process, the unbound sperm were gently rinsed off, and the HA-bound fraction was fixed. In the semen sperm fraction, there were sperm with cytoplasmic retention, DNA degradation (detected in individual spermatozoa with DNA-nick translation), aberrant shape, and persistent histones with aniline blue staining, whereas in the HA-bound sperm fraction, there was no presence of sperm with any of the cytoplasmic, nuclear, or shape defects [3].

Aneuploidy Frequencies in the HA-Bound Spermatozoa

Regarding the HA-mediated ICSI sperm selection, in addition to the DNA integrity, there is now focus on the increase in chromosomal aneuploidies with the embryologist-selected sperm, as the aneuploidy frequencies are 3–4 times higher in the ICSI offspring. Pointing out the relationship between meiotic and late spermiogenetic events, it was shown that sperm with cytoplasmic retention defects and sperm dysmaturity also have increased frequencies of chromosomal aneuploidies with a significant correlation at the level of $r > 0.75, p < 0.001$ [77]. Thus, these data, along with the below discussed experiments by Jakab et al. with FISH studies of >20,000 spermatozoa [58], suggest that the filtering effect of the zona pellucida has been reconstructed and tested by hyaluronic acid binding. No matter how high the aneuploidy frequency was in the initial semen sperm fraction, in the sperm bound, and removed from HA, there was a 4–6× decline in disomy and diploidy frequencies to the 0.1–0.2% normal range, which is customary in babies conceived with natural conception or with conventional IVF (Fig. 7.8). Thus, the clinical use of HA-mediated sperm selection could ultimately solve the pertinent problem of ICSI with increased frequency of aneuploidies in the offspring when the ICSI is performed with embryologist-selected sperm from samples with high proportion of dysmature spermatozoa which can be detected by the score of the sperm-HA binding assay.

ICSI Sperm Selection by HA-Binding: FISH Analysis of Sperm in Semen and in the Respective HA-Selected Sperm Fractions

The increased rate of chromosomal aberrations and other potential consequences of using immature sperm for ICSI are of major concern [78–81]. Based on the presence of the HA receptors in mature, but not in dysmature sperm, coupled with a

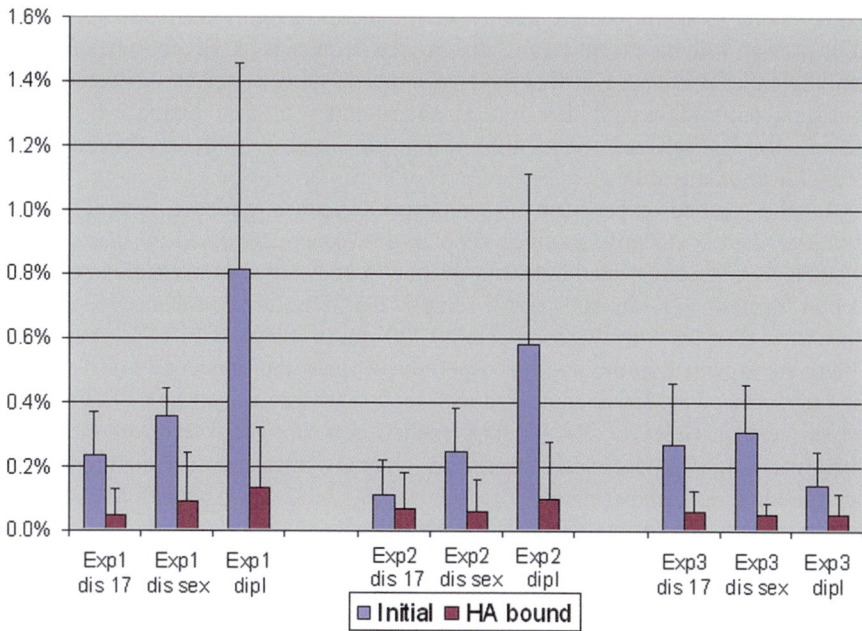

Fig. 7.8 Aneuploidy frequency results after the three experiments (experiments 1–3). *dis* disomy; *dis sex* sex chromosome disomy; *dipl* diploidy (from Jakab et al. [58], with permission)

respective device with an HA-coated surface, we expected that the method will facilitate the selection of single mature sperm with high DNA integrity and low frequencies of chromosomal aneuploidies for ICSI. As demonstrated (Fig. 7.6), the HA-selected mature sperm are devoid of cytoplasmic retention, persistent histones, and DNA fragmentation.

Regarding ICSI sperm selection, we have tested the efficiency of elimination of aneuploid and diploid sperm from the HA-bound population [58] in three experiments. The sperm selection studies utilized Falcon Petri dishes with HA spots for ICSI sperm selection, so-called PICSI dishes (Biocoat Inc., Fort Washington, PA).

A drop of washed sperm was placed close to the edge of the HA spot, and the sperm were allowed to spontaneously migrate. The mature sperm that had completed plasma membrane remodeling bound to the HA, while arrested maturity sperm with lower HA receptor concentrations moved freely over the HA (Fig. 7.8, left). The HA-bound sperm also exhibited vigorous beating with increased tail cross-beat frequency [39, 40, 52]. After 15 min, the HA-bound sperm were collected with the ICSI micropipette (Fig. 7.7, right), fixed with methanol-acetic acid, and subjected to FISH, using centromeric probes for the X, Y, and 17 chromosomes [58].

In the control semen fraction of 34 men we analyzed a mean of 4,770 sperm, or 162,210 sperm in all. In the HA-bound and micropipette collected sperm fractions, due to the burdens of the task, there were fewer sperm studied.

In the first experiment, 12 moderately oligozoospermic men (sperm concentration: $20.6 \pm 1.7 \times 10^6$/mL, motility: $52.1 \pm 2.5\%$, all data mean ± SEM) were examined based on 7,530 sperm (range: 224–1,142 per man). In the HA-selected sperm vs. initial semen with the exception of Y disomy, the frequencies of all other aneuploidies and diploidies declined: Fourfold for 17 disomy, 5.7-fold for sex chromosome disomies, and 6.2-fold for diploidies. Indeed, no matter how high the frequencies were in semen, the HA-selected sperm were within the range of normozoospermic men (Fig. 7.8, experiment 1).

In the second experiment (12 normozoospermic patients, sperm conc.: $121.3 \pm 21.4 \times 10^6$/mL, motility: $59.5 \pm 4.9\%$), we addressed the question of whether HA selection would cause a decline in chromosomal aberrations even in sperm fractions of normozoospermic samples that were further enhanced in mature sperm via gradient centrifugation about 9,720 sperm (range: 373–1,955 sperm per man). As expected, in the normozoospermic samples, the frequencies of disomies and diploidies were lower compared with those of oligozoospermic men (Fig. 7.8, experiment 2). However, HA binding resulted in a substantial selection effect, as there was a 4.3-fold decline in sex chromosome disomies and a 5.8-fold reduction in diploidies. As in experiment 1, the frequencies of individual aneuploidies or diploidies were in the very low 0.04–0.1% range.

In the third experiment, ten oligozoospermic men were studied (sperm concentration: $12.6 \pm 1.2 \times 10^6$/mL, motility: $49.3 \pm 4.0\%$) in a setting similar to IVF-ICSI laboratories where the embryologist collect the HA-bound sperm individually. In the *third experiment* of individually selected sperm, 24,420 sperm were evaluated. In this approach, which required marathon collection sessions, we studied a mean of 2,442 HA-selected sperm in each of the 10 men (range: 1,086–3,973). As Fig. 7.8, experiment 3 indicates, neither the frequencies of disomies nor the significant reduction in disomy frequencies in the HA-selected sperm differed from those produced in experiments 1 and 2.

Overall Results

In the HA-bound sperm vs. unselected sperm, the chromosomal disomy frequencies, with the three probes studied, were reduced to 0.16 from 0.52%, diploidy to 0.09 from 0.51%, and sex chromosome disomy to 0.05 from 0.27% (a 5.4-fold reduction vs. a 4–5-fold respective increase in ICSI offspring). No matter how high the aneuploidy frequencies in the semen sperm fractions were, the respective frequencies were within the narrow low 0.04–0.10% range per probed chromosome in HA-bound sperm, comparable to the range of normozoospermic fertile men. The fivefold decline in X, Y, and XY disomies is consistent with the increase in chromosomal aberrations in ICSI children conceived with visually selected sperm [80, 82].

Although the primary ICSI candidates are men with severe oligozoospermia (notwithstanding the fact that success-oriented IVF laboratories use ICSI almost exclusively, thus almost any couple may be exposed to the ICSI risks), it was necessary to use oligozoospermic and borderline oligozoospermic samples in order to collect sufficient numbers of spermatozoa to statistically validate the experimental results. However, because ICSI sperm selection reflects the maturity status and binding of single sperm, we believe that *HA-bound mature sperm* of a severely oligozoospermic man or of men with higher sperm density should not be different. If a sperm binds to HA, it will bind whether there are ten or thousands of mature or dysmaturity sperm in the drop. Thus, due to the polymorphic nature of sperm, similar to the zona pellucida binding, HA selections of mature sperm are likely to be independent from seminal sperm concentrations. This hypothesis is well supported by the sperm-HA binding studies, and by the three aneuploidy experiments, in which the aneuploidy frequencies in the HA-selected sperm fractions were similar and within a narrow, low, and normal range (Fig. 7.8).

Methods of HA-Mediated ICSI Sperm Selection Using PICSI Dishes

The methods of PICSI-mediated sperm selection maybe summarized as follows:

1. Sperm preparation is normally performed by using density gradient protocol (45 and 90% Isolate). A PICSI dish (modified Petri dish) has orienting lines, each ending with round HA-coated spot, in order to facilitate the approach to sperm selection. A 5–10 µL of washing media (modified human tubal fluid with 10% human serum albumin) is added to each ring at 37°C, under sterile conditions, and covered up with oil.
2. Thereafter, 1–5 µL of sperm suspension prepared in fertilization media (the suspension is ready for ICSI) should be placed into the media drop around the PICSI HA spot. (The volume of the sperm suspension will depend on the motile sperm concentration in the suspension; the lower the motile sperm concentration, the more sperm suspension media is needed).
3. The incubation with the PICSI dishes is carried out for 5–15 min at 34–36°C (Fig. 7.9). (The PICSI dish has some temperature-filtering effect; thus, alteration of the stage temperature should not be mandatory. During the observation time, one can clearly distinguish between spermatozoa which is normally developed, underwent the plasma membrane remodeling and bind to the HA spot, as well as they exhibit a higher tail cross-beat frequency or the dysmature spermatozoa that do not perceive the HA, and swims along).
4. Following the observation step, the PICSI dish is moved to the micromanipulation microscope. At this time, ICSI dishes should be ready to put the collected sperm from the PICSI dishes. Sperm should be collected using ICSI (microinjection) needle. In 5–15-min incubation time, there will be enough sperms attached to the HA spot. Using ICSI needle, 10–100 of attached sperm should be collected. The embryologist should prefer to pick up and collect sperm with the fastest tail cross beat frequency. This is important because of the sperm with faster tail cross-beat frequency have a more enhanced HA receptor density, indicating that the sperm membrane remodeling was more effective.
5. The sperm are collected from the PICSI HA spot with an ICSI needle and are ejected into a sperm ICSI washing media. This will be followed by the routine procedure of ICSI injection with the collected sperm.

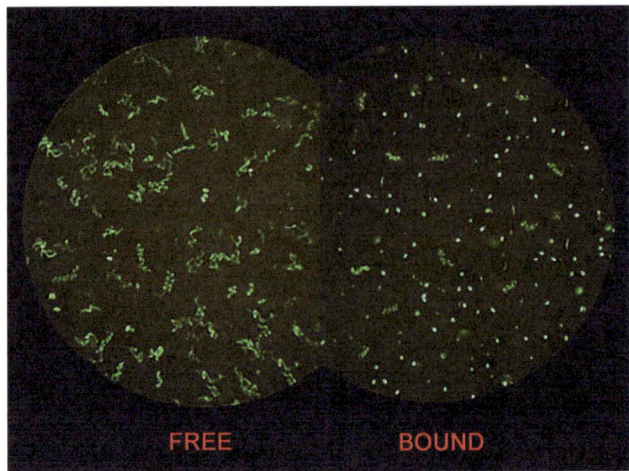

Fig. 7.9 Selection of mature spermatozoa for intracytoplasmic sperm injection (ICSI). (**a**) Time-lapse photography. Spermatozoa applied to the periphery of an HA spot. Normally developed spermatozoa bind to HA (*solid spots*) and maintain their tail-beating activity, whereas dysmature spermatozoa, lacking HA receptors, freely proceed over the HA coating. (**b**) After removal of the unbound spermatozoa by gentle rinsing, the normally developed, HA-bound, spermatozoa are selected with the ICSI pipette (from Huszar et al. [3], with permission)

IVF-ICSI Data with HA-Mediated Sperm Selection

There are now several laboratories that have initiated use of HA-mediated sperm selection. It is important that none of the groups that practice the HA sperm selection reported any adverse effect on fertilization or embryo development. In one 2005 ESHRE presentation, data on 18 pregnancies were reported. Comparing ICSI results with *visually selected ICSI sperm* ($N = 84$) vs. *HA-selected ICSI sperm* ($N = 18$): fertilization rates: 69.7% vs. 67.0%; good grade embryos: 56.6% vs. 51.7%; pregnancy rates: 45.3% vs. 33%; miscarriage rates: 7% vs. 0%; take-home baby rates: 46.5% vs. 39.0% [83].

Another related 2006 study was performed by the Brussel group on 20 unselected couples treated with ICSI in which at least eight MII oocytes were recovered. The sibling oocytes were injected either with HA-selected or with visually selected spermatozoa ($N = 146$ and 145). The fertilization rates (72.9 and 66.9%), oocyte degeneration rates (9.6 and 13.8%), rate of embryo cleavage (cell numbers), embryo quality, embryo transfer, and embryo cryopreservation rates were all similar. The authors suggest that in addition to the sperm selection utility in ICSI, the use of HA-selected sperm may be useful in patients undergoing preimplantation genetic screening in which the chromosomal status of the embryos can be related to the sperm selection technique [84].

In another relevant publication [85] improvements with HA-selected sperm were reported in porcine IVF. Porcine embryos were produced by IVF, ICSI, and ICSI performed with HA-selected sperm. The HA-mediated sperm selection was superior to visual sperm selection in producing chromosomally normal embryos and increasing ICSI efficiency by reducing the early embryonic mortality and thus enhancing ICSI success rates.

A number of recent studies have indicated that HA-bound sperm used in the ICSI procedure (the so-called physiological ICSI) may lead to increased implantation rates. In one such study, Parmegiani et al. [86] showed that in 293 couples treated with HA-ICSI vs. 86 couples treated with conventional ICSI (historical control group), all outcome measures of fertilization, embryo quality, implantation, and pregnancy were the same or improved in the HA-bound sperm group [86]. The implantation rate was increased from 10.3% in conventional ICSI to 17.1% in the HA group. The authors concluded that if multicenter randomized studies confirm the beneficial effects on ICSI outcome, HA could be considered as a routine choice for "physiologic" sperm selection prior to ICSI. A smaller clinical trial assessing the same technology by Worrilow et al. has also shown that clinical pregnancy rates are improved when using HA-selected sperm compared to conventional ICSI [87]. Furthermore, the sperm-HA binding score (the proportion of sperm that underwent plasma membrane remodeling in spermatogenesis and binds to hyaluronic acid) is an important diagnostic indicator. Men with <55% binding score would particularly benefit, as their ICSI success rates were improved (20–30% higher pregnancy rates) by using the HA-mediated sperm selection [87]. Thus, it is important that in IVF programs, the Andrology laboratory performs the sperm-HA binding test for the husbands of IVF-ICSI couples, based on the HA-binding score which provides the information on the proportion of sperm with attributes of dysmaturity, such as DNA fragmentation, chromosomal aneuploidies, persistent histones, cytoplasmic retention, and lack of HA-binding ability, consequential to dysmaturity. The IVF team triages the couples according to their HA-binding score in order to perform conventional IVF or ICSI. Another aspect of the markers of sperm development is the enhancement of sperm with normal morphology in the HA-bound sperm fraction. Studies in the Huszar laboratory indicated that there was a 2–3-fold enrichment of Tygerberg normal morphology sperm compared to the respective semen sperm fraction, which, interestingly, agreed with the finding of the Tygerberg group with respect to the enrichment of normal morphology sperm in the zona pellucida bound vs. semen sperm fraction [56, 57].

In a more recent 2006 study of 26 patients (273 oocytes retrieved and 177 embryos created by ICSI), the fertilization rates with visually selected and HA-selected sperm were similar (66.6 and 61.1%). Among the 22 couples with embryo replacement, 8 couples received embryos fertilized with visually selected sperm, 7 couples received embryos with HA-selected sperm, and another 7 couples received embryos of both origins. The respective pregnancy rates were 25, 57.1, and 57.1% with significantly higher rates in the two groups that received HA-selected embryos. Regarding miscarriage rates, they were higher in the group that received visually selected embryos ($p = 0.013$) [88]. All of these data were confirmed by a recent larger multicenter study, comparing ICSI outcomes with eye-selected and HA-selected spermatozoa which was presented at recent meetings by Worrilow et al. [87–88]

Other ICSI Sperm Selection Methods

Sperm Selection by Sperm Charge Properties

The Aitken's group recently reported a novel *electrophoretic sperm isolation* device utilizing a separation strategy based on sperm size and electronegative charge. The suspensions generated by the electrophoretic separation technique contained motile, viable, and morphologically normal spermatozoa while exhibited low levels of DNA damage. Reportedly, the electrophoretic sperm isolation procedure is both time and cost-effective [89], and the first pregnancy using this method for a couple suffering from extensive sperm DNA damage was reported [90]. Further, in a clinical trial of IVF and ICSI fertilization with gradient prepared sperm and electrophretically prepared sperm, the resulys were compbarable with repect to fertilizarion rates, cleavage and embryu quality [113].

Intracytoplasmic Morphologically Selected Sperm Injection

In 2001, Bartoov et al. [91] reported the selection of spermatozoa with normal nuclei to improve the pregnancy rate with intracytoplasmic sperm injection. They further verified this technique by performing ICSI using morphologically normal sperm, strictly defined by high power light microscopy ($\times > 6,000$). Sixty-two couples, with at least two previous consequent pregnancy failures after ICSI, underwent a single ICSI trial preceded by morphological selection of spermatozoa with normal nuclei. Fifty of these couples were matched with couples who underwent a routine ICSI procedure at the same IVF center and exhibited the same number of previous ICSI failures. The matching study revealed that the pregnancy rate after modified ICSI was significantly higher than that of the routine ICSI procedure (66.0% vs. 30.0%).

More recently, Antinori et al. conducted a prospective randomized study to assess the advantages of intracytoplasmic morphologically selected sperm injection (IMSI) over the conventional ICSI procedure [92]. A total of 446 couples with 3 years of primary infertility, the woman aged 35 years or younger, without workup for female factor, and husbands of severe oligoasthenoteratozoospermia were randomized to eye-selected ICSI ($N = 219$; group 1) and IMSI ($N = 227$; group 2) treatment groups. The data showed that IMSI resulted in a higher clinical pregnancy rate (39.2% vs. 26.5%; $p = 0.004$) than ICSI.

The use of IMSI appears promising [93]. Some drawbacks are however present, in particular, the belief that it is a complicated technique that cannot be routinely performed [94–96]. As the high-magnification approach is increasingly used, more studies will be focused upon the selected sperm, their respective levels of cytoplasmic retention, persistent histones, DNA chain integrity, aneuploidy rates, tyrosine phosphorylation, or apoptotic markers should be performed in order to verify the safety with respect to the potential public health concerns.

Potential Benefits of the HA-Mediated Sperm Selection Method for the ICSI Offspring

The HA-mediated ICSI sperm selection, by introducing only mature spermatozoa, will maintain the genetic impact and paternal contribution of sperm to the zygote at the traditional evolutionary level. Thus, the HA method may alleviate the potential problems related to chromosomal aneuploidies and DNA chain fragmentation that presently cause concern due to ICSI fertilization with visually selected sperm that may be of arrested maturity [9, 31, 35, 49, 52–54, 78, 97]. The safety of HA-mediated sperm selection is supported by various lines of evidence. First, HA occurs normally in the female reproductive tract and in the cumulus oophorus. Thus, it is likely that HA is carried with the sperm into oocytes even during in vivo conception. In the case of ICSI, the removal of sperm from HA may cause a few HA molecules to attach to sperm or a fraction of μm^2 of sperm membrane from the area of the acrosomal cap (which is lost otherwise during the acrosomal reaction) to remain attached to the HA.

DNA damage is associated with a decline in pregnancy rates following natural conception, but it has also been linked to diminished success in assisted conception due to reduced rates of fertilization, disrupted development of the zygote, and early pregnancy loss [4, 50, 54, 98, 99]. This is an increasingly important factor because 3–6% of the populations in developed countries now utilize assisted conception for reproduction. Another, related, concern is raised by the relationship between paternal and maternal (in pregnancy) smoking and other associated oxidative damage to DNA in response to xenobiotics, pesticides, and environmental chemicals which may promote testicular cancer and childhood cancer [50, 100–102].

Arrested maturity, or dysmature sperm with DNA damage and arrested membrane remodeling, that is unable to fertilize in natural conception is likely be eliminated by HA-mediated ICSI sperm selection with potential improvements in various areas: (a) Following ICSI fertilization with visually selected sperm, there were increased rates of de novo numerical chromosomal aberrations and also cytogenetically detectable structural chromosomal aberrations. These are most likely due to increased rates of chromosomal aneuploidies, primarily sex chromosome disomies, in sperm of ICSI fathers [79–82, 103]. (b) With visually selected sperm and ICSI, there is a reportedly higher incidence of spontaneous abortions in the 18% range, compared to the 10% rate following normal conception [81]. (c) In a recent multicenter study from five European countries which focused upon 5-year-old singleton children, a potentially increased risk of birth defects was reported; the odds for malformations were 2.77 for ICSI vs. naturally conceived children ($N = 540$ and 538, respectively) [79]. (d) Men treated with ICSI also show a higher rate of chromosomal rearrangements, such as reciprocal and Robertsonian translocations. These rearrangements may be associated with oligozoospermia and infertility, as well as, via interchromosomal effects, disomies and diploidies. Thus, the HA-mediated sperm selection for ICSI may reduce the risk for the chromosomal aberrations for the offspring, if a man has a common origin of chromosomal rearrangements, numerical aberrations, and arrested sperm maturity [104–106].

(e) Regarding structural chromosomal abnormalities in ICSI-derived pregnancies after visual sperm selection, the incidence of abnormal karyotypes was examined via chorionic villus sampling and amniocentesis. In 1,586 subjects, there were 47 children (3%) with abnormal fetal karyotypes, and 25 of these (1.6%) were de novo. Regarding the role of sperm maturity, the frequency of structural chromosomal abnormalities was approximately tenfold higher (24/1,120 or 2.1% vs. 1/1,419 or 0.24%, $p = 0.006$) following ICSI fertilization by oligozoospermic and severely oligozoospermic men [107]. (f) In line with the idea of the Brussels group who see a potential for fertilization with HA-selected sperm for couples who plan to undergo preimplantation genetic diagnosis or preimplantation genetic haplotyping, fertilization with HA-selected mature sperm may delineate into the oocyte aneuploidies and chromosomal aberrations found in embryos. Data supporting this approach arising from recent studies [108, 109]. (g) Using HA-selected mature sperm may increase pregnancy success following ICSI by reduction of sperm-derived aneuploidies and defects of oocyte activation that lead to early embryo failure [110, 111].

Acknowledgments This research was supported by the NIH (HD-19505, HD-32902, OH-04061). The HA-related diagnostic and sperm selection devices were invented by Gabor Huszar, MD; the invention was assigned to Yale University who owns the patent. Yale University has licensed the invention to Biocoat Inc. Gabor Huszar is acting as a scientific advisor.

References

1. WHO. WHO laboratory manual for the examination of human semen and sperm-cervical mucus interaction. 4th ed. Cambridge: Cambridge University Press; 1999.
2. Palermo G, Joris H, Devroey P, Van Steirteghem AC. Pregnancies after intracytoplasmic injection of single spermatozoon into an oocyte. Lancet. 1992;340:17–8.
3. Huszar G, Jakab A, Sakkas D, Ozenci CC, Cayli S, Delpiano E, Ozkavukcu S. Fertility testing and ICSI sperm selection by hyaluronic acid binding: clinical and genetic aspects. Reprod Biomed Online. 2007;14:650–63.
4. Cayli S, Jakab A, Ovari L, Delpiano E, Celik-Ozenci C, Sakkas D, Ward D, Huszar G. Biochemical markers of sperm function: male fertility and sperm selection for ICSI. Reprod Biomed Online. 2003;7:462–8.
5. Huszar G, Jakab A, Celik-Ozenci C, Sati G. Hyaluronic acid binding by sperm: andrology evaluation of male infertility and sperm selection for ICSI. In: Oehninger S, Kruger T, editors. Male infertility: diagnosis and treatment. Oxford, UK: Informa Ltd; 2006.
6. Huszar G, Ozkavukcu S, Jakab A, Celik-Ozenci C, Sati GL, Cayli S. Hyaluronic acid binding ability of human sperm reflects cellular maturity and fertilizing potential: selection of sperm for intracytoplasmic sperm injection. Curr Opin Obstet Gynecol. 2006;18:260–7.
7. Huszar G, Corrales M, Vigue L. Correlation between sperm creatine phosphokinase activity and sperm concentrations in normospermic and oligospermic men. Gamete Res. 1988; 19:67–75.
8. Huszar G, Vigue L, Corrales M. Sperm creatine phosphokinase activity as a measure of sperm quality in normospermic, variable spermic, and oligospermic men. Biol Reprod. 1988;38:1061–6.
9. Huszar G, Vigue L. Correlation between the rate of lipid peroxidation and cellular maturity as measured by creatine kinase activity in human spermatozoa. J Androl. 1994;15:71–7.

10. Huszar G, Vigue L, Corrales M. Sperm creatine kinase activity in fertile and infertile oligospermic men. J Androl. 1990;11:40–6.
11. Huszar G, Vigue L. Incomplete development of human spermatozoa is associated with increased creatine phosphokinase concentration and abnormal head morphology. Mol Reprod Dev. 1993;34:292–8.
12. Clermont Y. The cycle of the seminiferous epithelium in man. Am J Anat. 1963;112:35–51.
13. Huszar G, Gordon E, Irvine D, Aitken R. Absence of DNA cleavage in mature human sperm selected by their surface membrane receptors. In: Annual meeting of the American Society for Reproduction Medicine. San Francisco, CA; 1998.
14. Huszar G, Vigue L. Spermatogenesis-related change in the synthesis of the creatine kinase B-type and M-type isoforms in human spermatozoa. Mol Reprod Dev. 1990;25:258–62.
15. Huszar G, Stone K, Dix D, Vigue L. Putative creatine kinase M-isoform in human sperm is identified as the 70-kilodalton heat shock protein HspA2. Biol Reprod. 2000;63:925–32.
16. Huszar G, Vigue L, Morphed M. Sperm creatine phosphokinase M-isoform ratios and fertilizing potential of men: a blinded study of 84 couples treated with in vitro fertilization. Fertil Steril. 1992;57:882–8.
17. Lalwani S, Sayme N, Vigue L, Corrales M, Huszar G. Biochemical markers of early and late spermatogenesis: relationship between the lactate dehydrogenase-X and creatine kinase-M isoform concentrations in human spermatozoa. Mol Reprod Dev. 1996;43:495–502.
18. Huszar G, Sbracia M, Vigue L, Miller DJ, Shur BD. Sperm plasma membrane remodeling during spermiogenetic maturation in men: relationship among plasma membrane beta 1,4-galactosyltransferase, cytoplasmic creatine phosphokinase, and creatine phosphokinase isoform ratios. Biol Reprod. 1997;56:1020–4.
19. Guzick DS, Overstreet JW, Factor-Litvak P, Brazil CK, Nakajima ST, Coutifaris C, Carson SA, Cisneros P, Steinkampf MP, Hill JA, Xu D, Vogel DL. Sperm morphology, motility, and concentration in fertile and infertile men. N Engl J Med. 2001;345:1388–93.
20. Ombelet W, Deblaere K, Bosmans E, Cox A, Jacobs P, Janssen M, Nijs M. Semen quality and intrauterine insemination. Reprod Biomed Online. 2003;7:485–92.
21. Nagy ZP, Janssenswillen C, Janssens R, De Vos A, Staessen C, Van de Velde H, Van Steirteghem AC. Timing of oocyte activation, pronucleus formation and cleavage in humans after intracytoplasmic sperm injection (ICSI) with testicular spermatozoa and after ICSI or in-vitro fertilization on sibling oocytes with ejaculated spermatozoa. Hum Reprod. 1998;13:1606–12.
22. Pisarska MD, Casson PR, Cisneros PL, Lamb DJ, Lipshultz LI, Buster JE, Carson SA. Fertilization after standard in vitro fertilization versus intracytoplasmic sperm injection in subfertile males using sibling oocytes. Fertil Steril. 1999;71:627–32.
23. Tournaye H, Verheyen G, Albano C, Camus M, Van Landuyt L, Devroey P, Van Steirteghem A. Intracytoplasmic sperm injection versus in vitro fertilization: a randomized controlled trial and a meta-analysis of the literature. Fertil Steril. 2002;78:1030–7.
24. van der Westerlaken L, Naaktgeboren N, Verburg H, Dieben S, Helmerhorst FM. Conventional in vitro fertilization versus intracytoplasmic sperm injection in patients with borderline semen: a randomized study using sibling oocytes. Fertil Steril. 2006;85:395–400.
25. Allen JW, Dix DJ, Collins BW, Merrick BA, He C, Selkirk JK, Poorman-Allen P, Dresser ME, Eddy EM. HSP70-2 is part of the synaptonemal complex in mouse and hamster spermatocytes. Chromosoma. 1996;104:414–21.
26. Eddy EM. Role of heat shock protein HSP70-2 in spermatogenesis. Rev Reprod. 1999;4:23–30.
27. Son WY, Hwang SH, Han CT, Lee JH, Kim S, Kim YC. Specific expression of heat shock protein HspA2 in human male germ cells. Mol Hum Reprod. 1999;5:1122–6.
28. Tsunekawa N, Matsumoto M, Tone S, Nishida T, Fujimoto H. The Hsp70 homolog gene, Hsc70t, is expressed under translational control during mouse spermiogenesis. Mol Reprod Dev. 1999;52:383–91.
29. Huszar G, Patrizio P, Vigue L, Willets M, Wilker C, Adhoot D, Johnson L. Cytoplasmic extrusion and the switch from creatine kinase B to M isoform are completed by the

commencement of epididymal transport in human and stallion spermatozoa. J Androl. 1998;19:11–20.
30. Ergur AR, Dokras A, Giraldo JL, Habana A, Kovanci E, Huszar G. Sperm maturity and treatment choice of in vitro fertilization (IVF) or intracytoplasmic sperm injection: diminished sperm HspA2 chaperone levels predict IVF failure. Fertil Steril. 2002;77:910–8.
31. Cayli S, Sakkas D, Vigue L, Demir R, Huszar G. Cellular maturity and apoptosis in human sperm: creatine kinase, caspase-3 and Bcl-XL levels in mature and diminished maturity sperm. Mol Hum Reprod. 2004;10:365–72.
32. Lee JD, Kamiguchi Y, Yanagimachi R. Analysis of chromosome constitution of human spermatozoa with normal and aberrant head morphologies after injection into mouse oocytes. Hum Reprod. 1996;11:1942–6.
33. Yakin K, Kahraman S. Certain forms of morphological anomalies of spermatozoa may reflect chromosomal aneuploidies. Hum Reprod. 2001;16:1779–80.
34. Celik-Ozenci C, Catalanotti J, Jakab A, Aksu C, Ward D, Bray-Ward P, Demir R, Huszar G. Human sperm maintain their shape following decondensation and denaturation for fluorescent in situ hybridization: shape analysis and objective morphometry. Biol Reprod. 2003;69:1347–55.
35. Celik-Ozenci C, Jakab A, Kovacs T, Catalanotti J, Demir R, Bray-Ward P, Ward D, Huszar G. Sperm selection for ICSI: shape properties do not predict the absence or presence of numerical chromosomal aberrations. Hum Reprod. 2004;19:2052–9.
36. Zavaczki Z, Celik-Ozenci C, Ovari L, Jakab A, Sati GL, Ward DC, Huszar G. Dimensional assessment of X-bearing and Y-bearing haploid and disomic human sperm with the use of fluorescence in situ hybridization and objective morphometry. Fertil Steril. 2006;85:121–7.
37. Bartoov B, Berkovitz A, Eltes F, Kogosowski A, Menezo Y, Barak Y. Real-time fine morphology of motile human sperm cells is associated with IVF-ICSI outcome. J Androl. 2002; 23:1–8.
38. Berkovitz A, Eltes F, Lederman H, Peer S, Ellenbogen A, Feldberg B, Bartoov B. How to improve IVF-ICSI outcome by sperm selection. Reprod Biomed Online. 2006;12:634–8.
39. Huszar G, Willetts M, Corrales M. Hyaluronic acid (sperm select) improves retention of sperm motility and velocity in normospermic and oligospermic specimens. Fertil Steril. 1990;54:1127–34.
40. Sbracia M, Grasso J, Sayme N, Stronk J, Huszar G. Hyaluronic acid substantially increases the retention of motility in cryopreserved/thawed human spermatozoa. Hum Reprod. 1997;12: 1949–54.
41. Cherr GN, Yudin AI, Li MW, Vines CA, Overstreet JW. Hyaluronic acid and the cumulus extracellular matrix induce increases in intracellular calcium in macaque sperm via the plasma membrane protein PH-20. Zygote. 1999;7:211–22.
42. Kornovski BS, McCoshen J, Kredentser J, Turley E. The regulation of sperm motility by a novel hyaluronan receptor. Fertil Steril. 1994;61:935–40.
43. Ranganathan S, Ganguly AK, Datta K. Evidence for presence of hyaluronan binding protein on spermatozoa and its possible involvement in sperm function. Mol Reprod Dev. 1994;38: 69–76.
44. Vines CA, Li MW, Deng X, Yudin AI, Cherr GN, Overstreet JW. Identification of a hyaluronic acid (HA) binding domain in the PH-20 protein that may function in cell signaling. Mol Reprod Dev. 2001;60:542–52.
45. Gergely A, Kovanci E, Senturk L, Cosmi E, Vigue L, Huszar G. Morphometric assessment of mature and diminished-maturity human spermatozoa: sperm regions that reflect differences in maturity. Hum Reprod. 1999;14:2007–14.
46. Huszar G, Vigue L, Oehninger S. Creatine kinase immunocytochemistry of human sperm-hemizona complexes: selective binding of sperm with mature creatine kinase-staining pattern. Fertil Steril. 1994;61:136–42.
47. Kruger TF, Menkveld R, Stander FS, Lombard CJ, Van der Merwe JP, van Zyl JA, Smith K. Sperm morphologic features as a prognostic factor in vitro fertilization. Fertil Steril. 1986; 46:1118–23.

48. Yagci A, Murk W, Stronk J, Huszar G. Spermatozoa bound to solid state hyaluronic acid show chromatin structure with high DNA chain integrity: an acridine orange fluorescence study. J Androl. 2010;31(6):566–72.
49. Aitken RJ, Baker MA, Sawyer D. Oxidative stress in the male germ line and its role in the etiology of male infertility and genetic disease. Reprod Biomed Online. 2003;7:65–70.
50. Aitken RJ, Koopman P, Lewis SE. Seeds of concern. Nature. 2004;432:48–52.
51. Aoki VW, Liu L, Jones KP, Hatasaka HH, Gibson M, Peterson CM, Carrell DT. Sperm protamine 1/protamine 2 ratios are related to in vitro fertilization pregnancy rates and predictive of fertilization ability. Fertil Steril. 2006;86:1408–15.
52. Huszar G, Ozenci CC, Cayli S, Zavaczki Z, Hansch E, Vigue L. Hyaluronic acid binding by human sperm indicates cellular maturity, viability, and unreacted acrosomal status. Fertil Steril. 2003;79 Suppl 3:1616–24.
53. Sati L, Ovari L, Bennett D, Simon SD, Demir R, Huszar G. Double probing of human spermatozoa for persistent histones, surplus cytoplasm, apoptosis and DNA fragmentation. Reprod Biomed Online. 2008;16:570–9.
54. Seli E, Sakkas D. Spermatozoal nuclear determinants of reproductive outcome: implications for ART. Hum Reprod Update. 2005;11:337–49.
55. Huszar G, Prinosilova P, Ozkavukcu S, Vigue L, Kruger T. Sperm bound to hyaluronic acid or to zona pellucida exhibit similar levels of improvement in Tygerberg strict morphology scores. In: ASRM annual meeting. New Orleans, LA; 2006.
56. Menkveld R, Franken DR, Kruger TF, Oehninger S, Hodgen GD. Sperm selection capacity of the human zona pellucida. Mol Reprod Dev. 1991;30:346–52.
57. Prinosilova P, Kruger T, Sati L, Ozkavukcu S, Vigue L, Kovanci E, Huszar G. Selectivity of hyaluronic acid binding for spermatozoa with normal Tygerberg strict morphology. Reprod Biomed Online. 2009;18:177–83.
58. Jakab A, Sakkas D, Delpiano E, Cayli S, Kovanci E, Ward D, Revelli A, Huszar G. Intracytoplasmic sperm injection: a novel selection method for sperm with normal frequency of chromosomal aneuploidies. Fertil Steril. 2005;84:1665–73.
59. Cayli S, Sakkas D, Celik-Ozenci C, Vigue L, Demir R, Huszar G. Hyaluronic acid binding is a test of human sperm maturity and function: correlation between the hyaluronic acid binding and hemizona binding tests. In: Annual Meeting of ESHRE. Madrid, Spain; 2003.
60. Huszar G, Celik-Ozenci C, Vigue L. Sperm maturity and fertility: testing by hyaluronic acid (HA) binding annual meeting of ESHRE. Austria: Vienna; 2002.
61. Chi HJ, Kim JH, Ryu CS, Lee JY, Park JS, Chung DY, Choi SY, Kim MH, Chun EK, Roh SI. Protective effect of antioxidant supplementation in sperm-preparation medium against oxidative stress in human spermatozoa. Hum Reprod. 2008;23:1023–8.
62. Donnelly ET, McClure N, Lewis SE. Glutathione and hypotaurine in vitro: effects on human sperm motility, DNA integrity and production of reactive oxygen species. Mutagenesis. 2000;15:61–8.
63. Griveau JF, Le Lannou D. Effects of antioxidants on human sperm preparation techniques. Int J Androl. 1994;17:225–31.
64. Steele EK, McClure N, Maxwell RJ, Lewis SE. A comparison of DNA damage in testicular and proximal epididymal spermatozoa in obstructive azoospermia. Mol Hum Reprod. 1999;5:831–5.
65. Suganuma R, Yanagimachi R, Meistrich ML. Decline in fertility of mouse sperm with abnormal chromatin during epididymal passage as revealed by ICSI. Hum Reprod. 2005;20:3101–8.
66. Greco E, Scarselli F, Iacobelli M, Rienzi L, Ubaldi F, Ferrero S, Franco G, Anniballo N, Mendoza C, Tesarik J. Efficient treatment of infertility due to sperm DNA damage by ICSI with testicular spermatozoa. Hum Reprod. 2005;20:226–30.
67. Ward WS, Coffey DS. DNA packaging and organization in mammalian spermatozoa: comparison with somatic cells. Biol Reprod. 1991;44:569–74.
68. Aoki VW, Moskovtsev SI, Willis J, Liu L, Mullen JB, Carrell DT. DNA integrity is compromised in protamine-deficient human sperm. J Androl. 2005;26:741–8.

69. Dadoune JP. The nuclear status of human sperm cells. Micron. 1995;26:323–45.
70. Filatov MV, Semenova EV, Vorob'eva OA, Leont'eva OA, Drobchenko EA. Relationship between abnormal sperm chromatin packing and IVF results. Mol Hum Reprod. 1999;5: 825–30.
71. Ramos L, van der Heijden GW, Derijck A, Berden JH, Kremer JA, van der Vlag J, de Boer P. Incomplete nuclear transformation of human spermatozoa in oligo-astheno-teratospermia: characterization by indirect immunofluorescence of chromatin and thiol status. Hum Reprod. 2008;23:259–70.
72. Steger K. Transcriptional and translational regulation of gene expression in haploid spermatids. Anat Embryol (Berl). 1999;199:471–87.
73. Bungum M, Humaidan P, Axmon A, Spano M, Bungum L, Erenpreiss J, Giwercman A. Sperm DNA integrity assessment in prediction of assisted reproduction technology outcome. Hum Reprod. 2007;22:174–9.
74. Carrell DT, Emery BR, Hammoud S. Altered protamine expression and diminished spermatogenesis: what is the link? Hum Reprod Update. 2007;13:313–27.
75. Ovari L, Sati L, Stronk J, Borsos A, Ward DC, Huszar G. Double probing individual human spermatozoa: aniline blue staining for persistent histones and fluorescence in situ hybridization for aneuploidies. Fertil Steril. 2010;93:2255–61.
76. Liu DY, Baker HW. Human sperm bound to the zona pellucida have normal nuclear chromatin as assessed by acridine orange fluorescence. Hum Reprod. 2007;22:1597–602.
77. Kovanci E, Kovacs T, Moretti E, Vigue L, Bray-Ward P, Ward DC, Huszar G. FISH assessment of aneuploidy frequencies in mature and immature human spermatozoa classified by the absence or presence of cytoplasmic retention. Hum Reprod. 2001;16:1209–17.
78. Barri PN, Vendrell JM, Martinez F, Coroleu B, Aran B, Veiga A. Influence of spermatogenic profile and meiotic abnormalities on reproductive outcome of infertile patients. Reprod Biomed Online. 2005;10:735–9.
79. Bonduelle M, Wennerholm UB, Loft A, Tarlatzis BC, Peters C, Henriet S, Mau C, Victorin-Cederquist A, Van Steirteghem A, Balaska A, Emberson JR, Sutcliffe AG. A multi-centre cohort study of the physical health of 5-year-old children conceived after intracytoplasmic sperm injection, in vitro fertilization and natural conception. Hum Reprod. 2005;20:413–9.
80. Simpson JL, Lamb DJ. Genetic effects of intracytoplasmic sperm injection. Semin Reprod Med. 2001;19:239–49.
81. Van Steirteghem A, Bonduelle M, Devroey P, Liebaers I. Follow-up of children born after ICSI. Hum Reprod Update. 2002;8:111–6.
82. Bonduelle M, Liebaers I, Deketelaere V, Derde MP, Camus M, Devroey P, Van Steirteghem A. Neonatal data on a cohort of 2889 infants born after ICSI (1991–1999) and of 2995 infants born after IVF (1983–1999). Hum Reprod. 2002;17:671–94.
83. Sanchez M, Aran B, Blanco J, Vidal F, Veiga A, Barri PN, Huszar G. Preliminary clinical and FISH results on hyaluronic acid sperm selection to improve ICSI. 21st annual meeting of European society for human reproduction and embryology (ESHRE), Copenhagen, Denmark, 2005. Hum Reprod. 2005;20 Suppl 1:556.
84. Janssens R, Verheyen G, Bocken G. Use of PICSI dishes for sperm selection in clinical ICSI practice: results of a pilot study. In: Annual meeting of the Belgian Society Reproductive Medicine. Brussels, Belgium; 2006.
85. Park CY, Uhm SJ, Song SJ, Kim KS, Hong SB, Chung KS, Park C, Lee HT. Increase of ICSI efficiency with hyaluronic acid binding sperm for low aneuploidy frequency in pig. Theriogenology. 2005;64:1158–69.
86. Parmegiani L, Cognigni GE, Ciampaglia W, Pocognoli P, Marchi F, Filicori M. Efficiency of hyaluronic acid (HA) sperm selection. J Assist Reprod Genet. 2010;27:13–6.
87. Worrilow K, Huynh H, Bower J, Peters A, Johnston J. The clinical impact associated with the use of PICSI derived embryos. In: Annual meeting of ASRM. Atlanta; 2009.
88. Worrilow KC, Huynh HT, Bower JB, Peters AJ, Johnston JB. The clinical impact associated with the use of PICSI TM-derived embryos. Fertil Steril. 2006;86(3 Suppl 1):S62.

89. Ainsworth C, Nixon B, Aitken RJ. Development of a novel electrophoretic system for the isolation of human spermatozoa. Hum Reprod. 2005;20:2261–70.
90. Ainsworth C, Nixon B, Jansen RP, Aitken RJ. First recorded pregnancy and normal birth after ICSI using electrophoretically isolated spermatozoa. Hum Reprod. 2007;22:197–200.
91. Bartoov B, Berkovitz A, Eltes F. Selection of spermatozoa with normal nuclei to improve the pregnancy rate with intracytoplasmic sperm injection. N Engl J Med. 2001;345:1067–8.
92. Antinori M, Licata E, Dani G, Cerusico F, Versaci C, d'Angelo D, Antinori S. Intracytoplasmic morphologically selected sperm injection: a prospective randomized trial. Reprod Biomed Online. 2008;16:835–41.
93. Nadalini M, Tarozzi N, Distratis V, Scaravelli G, Borini A. Impact of intracytoplasmic morphologically selected sperm injection on assisted reproduction outcome: a review. Reprod Biomed Online. 2009;19 Suppl 3:45–55.
94. Cohen-Bacrie P, Dumont M, Junca A, Belloc S, Hazout A. Indications for IMSA. J Gynecol Obstet Biol Reprod. 2007;36:S105–8.
95. Junca AM, Cohen-Bacrie P, Belloc S, Dumont M, Menezo Y. Teratozoospermia at the time of intracytoplasmic morphologically selected sperm injection (IMSI). Gynecol Obstet Fertil. 2009;37:552–7.
96. Mauri AL, Petersen CG, Oliveira JB, Massaro FC, Baruffi RL, Franco Jr JG. Comparison of day 2 embryo quality after conventional ICSI versus intracytoplasmic morphologically selected sperm injection (IMSI) using sibling oocytes. Eur J Obstet Gynecol Reprod Biol. 2010;150:42–6.
97. Lewis SE, Aitken RJ. DNA damage to spermatozoa has impacts on fertilization and pregnancy. Cell Tissue Res. 2005;322:33–41.
98. Borini A, Tarozzi N, Bizzaro D, Bonu MA, Fava L, Flamigni C, Coticchio G. Sperm DNA fragmentation: paternal effect on early post-implantation embryo development in ART. Hum Reprod. 2006;21:2876–81.
99. Lopes S, Sun JG, Jurisicova A, Meriano J, Casper RF. Sperm deoxyribonucleic acid fragmentation is increased in poor-quality semen samples and correlates with failed fertilization in intracytoplasmic sperm injection. Fertil Steril. 1998;69:528–32.
100. Pettersson A, Kaijser M, Richiardi L, Askling J, Ekbom A, Akre O. Women smoking and testicular cancer: one epidemic causing another? Int J Cancer. 2004;109:941–4.
101. Robaire B, Hales BF. Advances in male mediated developmental toxicity. New York: Kluwer/Plenum; 2003.
102. Sorahan T, Prior P, Lancashire RJ, Faux SP, Hulten MA, Peck IM, Stewart AM. Childhood cancer and parental use of tobacco: deaths from 1971 to 1976. Br J Cancer. 1997;76:1525–31.
103. Lam R, Ma S, Robinson WP, Chan T, Yuen BH. Cytogenetic investigation of fetuses and infants conceived through intracytoplasmic sperm injection. Fertil Steril. 2001;76:1272–5.
104. Anton E, Blanco J, Egozcue J, Vidal F. Sperm FISH studies in seven male carriers of Robertsonian translocation t(13;14)(q10;q10). Hum Reprod. 2004;19:1345–51.
105. Morel F, Roux C, Bresson JL. Disomy frequency estimated by multicolour fluorescence in situ hybridization, degree of nuclear maturity and teratozoospermia in human spermatozoa. Reproduction. 2001;121:783–9.
106. Ogawa S, Araki S, Araki Y, Ohno M, Sato I. Chromosome analysis of human spermatozoa from an oligoasthenozoospermic carrier for a 13;14 Robertsonian translocation by their injection into mouse oocytes. Hum Reprod. 2000;15:1136–9.
107. Schreurs A, Legius E, Meuleman C, Fryns JP, D'Hooghe TM. Increased frequency of chromosomal abnormalities in female partners of couples undergoing in vitro fertilization or intracytoplasmic sperm injection. Fertil Steril. 2000;74:94–6.
108. Chatzimeletiou K, Taylor J, Marks K, Grudzinskas JG, Handyside AH. Paternal inheritance of a 16qh-polymorphism in a patient with repeated IVF failure. Reprod Biomed Online. 2006;13:864–7.
109. Renwick PJ, Trussler J, Ostad-Saffari E, Fassihi H, Black C, Braude P, Ogilvie CM, Abbs S. Proof of principle and first cases using preimplantation genetic haplotyping—a paradigm shift for embryo diagnosis. Reprod Biomed Online. 2006;13:110–9.

110. Baltaci V, Satiroglu H, Kabukcu C, Unsal E, Aydinuraz B, Uner O, Aktas Y, Cetinkaya E, Turhan F, Aktan A. Relationship between embryo quality and aneuploidies. Reprod Biomed Online. 2006;12:77–82.
111. Menezo YJ. Paternal and maternal factors in preimplantation embryogenesis: interaction with the biochemical environment. Reprod Biomed Online. 2006;12:616–21.
112. Miller D, Brough S, al-Harbi O. Characterization and cellular distribution of human spermatozoal heat shock proteins. Hum Reprod. 1992;7(5):637–45.
113. Fleming SD, Ilad RS, Griffin AM, Wu Y, Ong KJ, Smith HC et al. Prospective controlled trial of an electrophoretic method of sperm preparation for assisted reproduction: comparison with density gradient centrifugation. Human Reprod. 2008;23: 2646–51.

Chapter 8
Electrophoretic Sperm Separation

Steven Fleming and John Aitken

Principles of Electrophoresis

Electrophoresis is a term used to define the motion of a particle within a liquid medium, the electrolyte, in response to a spatially uniform electric field. This electrokinetic phenomenon occurs as a result of the particles displaying a net positive or negative surface charge against which an external electric field can exert an electrostatic force. In fact, a surface charge may not even be necessary for electrokinesis, as it is theoretically possible that even neutral particles could migrate in response to an electric field by virtue of the molecular structure of water at their interface. This concept relates to the so-called double layer theory, whereby a diffuse layer of ions having the same but opposite charge to the particle surface screens them from the surrounding medium. Consequently, the electric field exerts an electrostatic force on the ions within the diffuse layer in the opposite direction to that exerted upon the particles, resulting in viscous stress, termed the electrophoretic retardation force. This hydrodynamic friction applied to the particles depends also upon the viscosity of the liquid medium in which they are dispersed, ultimately determining their electrophoretic mobility. Hence, it is necessary to carefully consider the molecular weight and charge of the particles relative to the conductivity and viscosity of the electrolyte to achieve the electrophoretic mobility required.

S. Fleming, BSc (Hons), MSc, PhD
Assisted Conception Australia, Greenslopes Private Hospital, Newdegate Street, Greenslopes, Brisbane, QLD 4120, Australia

J. Aitken, PhD, ScD, FRSE (✉)
ARC Centre of Excellence in Biotechnology and Development, University of Newcastle, Callaghan, Newcastle, NSW 2308, Australia
e-mail: John.aitken@newcastle.edu.au

Electrophoretic Properties of Spermatozoa

Normal, mature spermatozoa carry a net negative charge that is imparted by the sperm glycocalyx, which is rich in sialic acid residues [1, 2]. One of these residues, called CD52, is a highly sialated glycosylphosphatidylinositol (GPI)-anchored protein that is acquired during epididymal transit and located on the sperm plasmalemma [3–5]. During spermatogenesis, there is a massive cell-cell transfer of GPI-anchored CD52 that occurs at the sperm surface, the magnitude of which may be dependent upon the negative charge associated with the sperm plasmalemma [6]. Therefore, the presence of a negative charge may reflect normal spermatogenesis, especially since CD52 expression appears to be significantly correlated with capacitation and normal sperm morphology [5]. Consequently, this differential negative charge imparted by the sperm plasmalemma has been exploited as a means for sperm separation using either simple electrostatic [7, 8] or sophisticated electrophoretic techniques [9–11].

Development of Electrophoretic Technology for Sperm Sorting

The life separations company, NuSep, has been concerned with the development of bioseparations products for the past 30 years. In collaboration with Prof. John Aitken at the University of Newcastle, NuSep further developed their laboratory protein separations instrument, the ProteomeSep MF110, to create a prototype instrument designed for sperm separation, called the cell sorter 10 (CS10; Fig. 8.1). The CS10 was based upon preparative isolation by membrane electrophoresis (PrIME) technology, a patented technique that is capable of purifying most macromolecules from complex biological samples. The principle of this mode of separation was developed from the hypothesis that the CS10 preferentially selects cells on the basis of charge differences between human spermatozoa due to the differential presence of sialated proteins on the sperm plasmalemma [9]. A subsidiary commercial entity of NuSep, called SpermGen, is developing the CS10 into a regulatory compliant production unit, known as the SpermSep CS10.

The CS10 applies an electric potential via platinum-coated titanium mesh electrodes to move spermatozoa across a 5-μm polycarbonate separation membrane, the pore size of which allows the passage of morphologically normal spermatozoa while restricting larger cells within semen, such as immature germ cells and leukocytes (Figs. 8.2 and 8.3). Spermatozoa, which are negatively charged when suspended in a physiological buffer, are attracted towards the positive electrode, or anode. Consequently, spermatozoa not possessing a normal negative charge have less electrophoretic mobility and do not manage to pass through the separation membrane during the relatively short period (5 min) of electrophoresis. The exploitation of this concept has been found to yield a high percentage of morphologically normal, motile spermatozoa with intact DNA following electrophoretic sperm separation [9].

8 Electrophoretic Sperm Separation

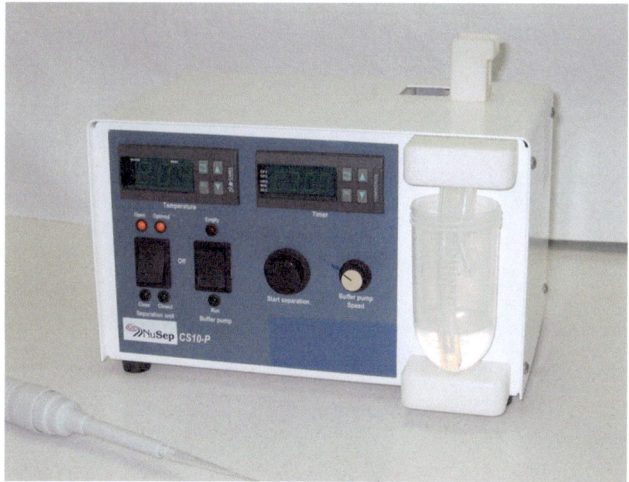

Fig. 8.1 The prototype CS10 instrument

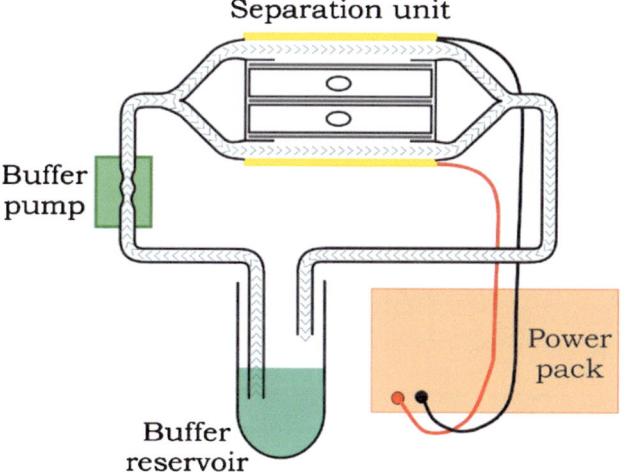

Fig. 8.2 Diagrammatic representation of the CS10 design

Equipment Setup and Separation Parameters

Separation Cartridges and Sample Handling

The separation cartridge of the prototype CS10 is a self-assembled device that has either a symmetric or an asymmetric format. In the asymmetric design, the inoculation or loading chamber has a volume of 2 mL and a collection or separation

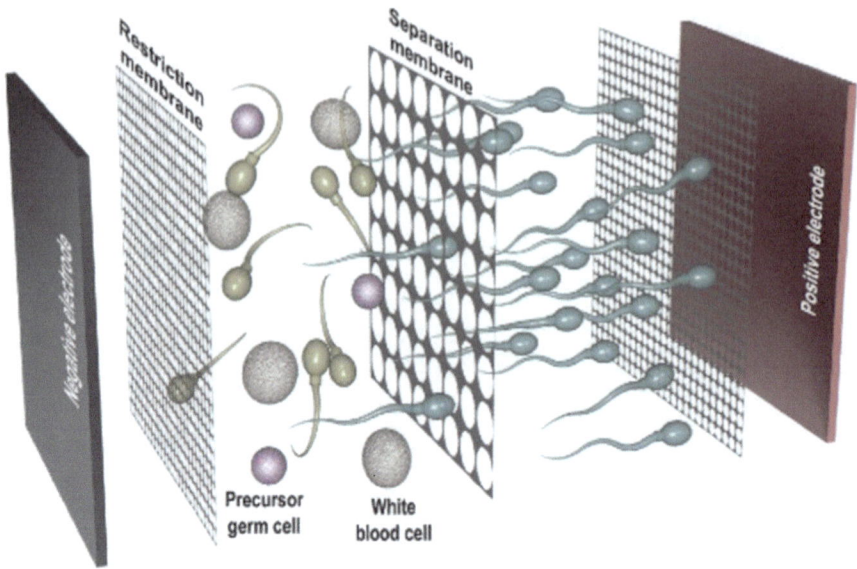

Fig. 8.3 Schematic diagram showing sperm electrophoretic mobility

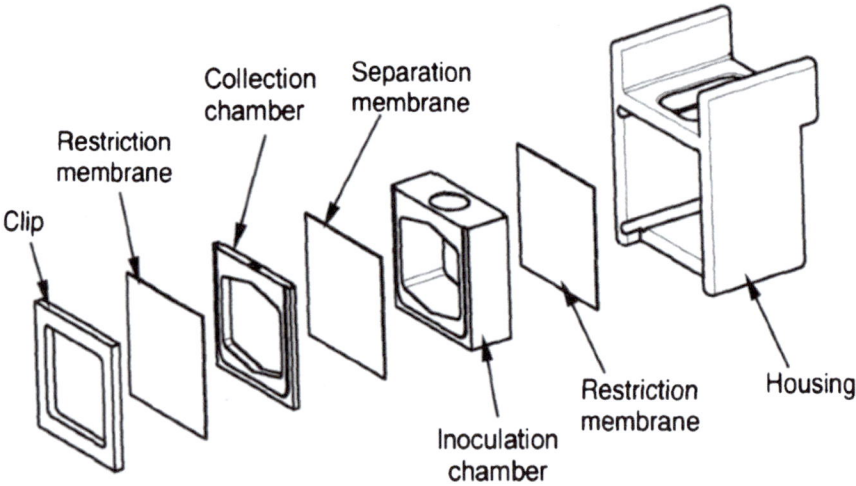

Fig. 8.4 Exploded diagram of the asymmetric separation cartridge

chamber volume of 400 µL (Fig. 8.4). Conveniently, 400 µL is also the estimated mean volume of the human uterine cavity and is, therefore, often the volume of sperm preparation inserted during intrauterine insemination (IUI) procedures. Consequently, the potential exists for electrophoretic sperm separation to be followed immediately by IUI of the entire volume of the sperm preparation retrieved, providing that the prostaglandins present within seminal plasma have been removed or reduced to clinically insignificant levels. However, for the purposes of in vitro fertilisation (IVF) and intracytoplasmic sperm injection (ICSI), the spermatozoa could be used directly, provided that they are separated into an appropriate medium within the separation chamber. The component parts of the separation cartridge can be autoclaved to ensure sterility. A 5-μm polycarbonate membrane, with an active membrane area of 20 × 15 mm, separates the loading and separation chambers which are bounded by polyacrylamide restriction membranes with a pore size of 15 kDa that prevent cross-contamination between the semen sample and electrophoresis buffer, while permitting free transit of electrolytes (Figs. 8.3 and 8.4).

The separation cartridge is inserted into the cartridge housing on top of the SpermSep CS10 (Fig. 8.1), the housing being designed to ensure the cartridge can only be inserted in the correct orientation. Once the separation unit sealing mechanism is activated, the cartridge components are made watertight by the machine sealing pressure applied by the SpermSep CS10. Semen samples are simply pipetted into the loading chamber of the cartridge using a sterile, nontoxic, disposable plastic pipette, left for 5 min to equilibrate, then subjected to electrophoresis. Once separated, the sperm preparation is aspirated from the separation chamber of the cartridge using an elongated, sterile, nontoxic, disposable micropipette tip, as typically used in standard gel electrophoresis.

Electrophoresis Buffers and Temperature Settings

The electrophoresis buffer contains 10 mM HEPES, 30 mM NaCl and 0.2 mM sucrose, having an osmolarity of 310 mOsm.kg^{-1} and a pH of 7.4, following adjustment using 2 M KOH. It is filter-sterilised prior to use with a 0.22-μm filter (Millipore Corp., Bedford, MA, USA). In order to provide a physiological medium in which to maintain sperm viability, 400 μL of electrophoresis buffer is placed into the separation chamber prior to running a sperm separation. A sterile, disposable buffer reservoir is filled with 80 mL electrophoresis buffer and placed into the reservoir housing on the front of the SpermSep CS10 (Fig. 8.1). In order to prevent overheating during operation of the instrument, the buffer is maintained at 25°C and is circulated round the instrument by means of a buffer pump (Fig. 8.2). In order to complete the electrical circuit, the buffer pump is run for at least 1 min prior to performing any sperm separations.

Current and Voltage Settings

The input power specifications of the SpermSep CS10 are 115–240 V at 50–60 Hz. Electrophoresis is achieved via a constant current of 75 mA at a variable voltage of 18–21 V applied over a 5-min period. No electrical potential is applied until the separation run is initiated.

Cleaning of Equipment

At the conclusion of each sperm separation, any electrophoresis buffer remaining in the buffer reservoir is replaced with sterile, distilled water, and the buffer pump is actuated to rinse the buffer lines. If no more separations are to be performed that day, the water is replaced with a 0.1 M NaOH cleaning solution, and the buffer pump is run for 30 s to circulate it through the lines of the SpermSep CS10, and the cleaning solution is left in place overnight. The following morning, the cleaning solution is thoroughly rinsed out with a minimum of three washes of sterile, distilled water.

Method Validation

Initial validation of the SpermSep CS10 system was performed using semen samples from normozoospermic sperm donors and a separation cartridge with a symmetrical design, the loading and separation chambers both having a capacity of 400 µL [9].

Sample Recovery and Purity

The mean sample concentration loaded into the system was $52 \pm 5.2 \times 10^6$ mL^{-1}. During an initial 5-min equilibration period, the starting concentration of spermatozoa in the separation chamber was $1.67 \pm 0.58 \times 10^6$ mL^{-1} (3.2% recovery), presumably as a consequence of the inherent motility of spermatozoa. Following just 30 s of electrophoresis, the sperm concentration increased to $3.55 \pm 0.42 \times 10^6$ mL^{-1} (6.8% recovery), reaching a peak concentration of $22.31 \pm 5.85 \times 10^6$ mL^{-1} (42.9% recovery) after 15 min. The purity of the electrophoretically separated sperm preparations was extremely high, with contamination by round cells proving undetectable using phase-contrast microscopy [9].

Sperm Vitality and Motility

Sperm vitality, assessed using the eosin dye (0.05% eosin in phosphate buffered saline) exclusion test, was $83 \pm 1.5\%$ in the original semen samples prior to electrophoresis. The percentage of viable spermatozoa in the electrophoretically separated sperm preparations was found to be consistent with that of the original samples, and there was no significant change in vitality observed over the entire period (15 min) of electrophoresis [9].

Sperm motility, assessed using computer-assisted semen analysis (CASA), was $72 \pm 2.1\%$ in the original semen samples prior to electrophoresis. Similar to sperm vitality, percentage sperm motility was found to be consistent with that of the original samples and not significantly affected by the duration of electrophoresis, though a slight reduction was observed after 15 min [9]. Similarly, kinematic analysis by CASA demonstrated that the duration of electrophoresis had no significant effect upon the quality of sperm motility observed.

Sperm Morphology and DNA Integrity

The percentage of normal spermatozoa observed following staining by a modification of the Papanicolaou method [12] and assessed using the sperm deformity index (SDI) [13] was significantly increased ($P < 0.001$) by electrophoresis [9]. A higher percentage of morphologically normal spermatozoa within the separated sperm preparation was observed regardless of the duration of electrophoresis, with no significant variation between different time periods. Furthermore, SDI values for the separated spermatozoa were significantly below ($P < 0.001$) the threshold SDI value of 0.93 for all electrophoretic time-points, indicating their normal fertilisation potential [13].

DNA damage, assessed using the terminal deoxynucleotidyl transferase-mediated deoxyuridine triphosphate nick-end labelling (TUNEL) assay, was significantly reduced ($P < 0.05$) in the sperm preparation separated by electrophoresis [9]. This reduction was only observed at all time-points up to 10 min of electrophoresis, beyond which there was no significant difference in the percentage of DNA-damaged spermatozoa.

Clinical Applications

The first successful clinical application of electrophoretic sperm separation was published as a case report following ICSI [10]. This provided proof of principle that electrophoresis could be used to prepare spermatozoa for use in assisted reproduction. However, since ICSI had been used to fertilise the oocytes in this instance, it was still unknown whether electrophoresis might compromise aspects of sperm function necessary for normal fertilisation. This uncertainty was resolved following a prospective, split-sample, split-cohort controlled clinical trial, involving patients having both ICSI and IVF, with sperm prepared either by standard density gradient centrifugation (DGC) or by electrophoresis [11]. The design of this trial ensured that any differences in gamete quality between semen samples and cohorts of oocytes were controlled for. Approximately 400 oocytes were inseminated by either DGC or electrophoretically prepared spermatozoa, resulting in comparable rates of fertilisation (63.6 vs. 62.4%, respectively), cleavage (88.5 vs. 99.0%, respectively) and embryo quality (26.1 vs. 27.4% top grade embryos, respectively), regardless of whether ICSI or IVF was employed as the method of insemination [11].

Furthermore, six pregnancies resulted from the use of electrophoretically prepared spermatozoa, two of them from patients receiving ICSI and four from patients receiving IVF [11].

Previous work has demonstrated that spermatozoa can be efficiently isolated from a variety of sources [10]. Separation of frozen-thawed, cryostored semen ($39.6 \pm 11.1 \times 10^6$ mL^{-1}) resulted in 27% recovery of separated spermatozoa ($10.8 \pm 3.8 \times 10^6$ mL^{-1}) after just 5 min electrophoresis [10]. These sperm preparations were devoid of detectable contaminating cells, the separated spermatozoa displaying significantly greater viability ($P < 0.01$), motility ($P < 0.05$) and normal morphology ($P < 0.001$) than the cryostored semen [10]. Therefore, electrophoresis may prove an advantageous method for preparing cryostored semen, especially since it has recently been shown that such material is particularly vulnerable to oxidative stress and subsequent DNA damage during processing by standard DGC [14–16].

A particularly promising potential application of electrophoretic sperm separation is the isolation of spermatozoa exhibiting low levels of sperm DNA damage from more complex mixtures of cells such as those found in surgically recovered aspirates and biopsies of the epididymis and testis. Testicular biopsy material, containing a range of mature and immature spermatozoa, has been shown to rapidly yield cells with greater residual motility, vitality and normal morphology than those in the original biopsy following electrophoretic sperm preparation [10]. Importantly, the recovery of spermatozoa from the biopsy material was good ($28.4 \pm 7.1\%$).

Closing Remarks

Combined, the basic scientific and clinical data suggest that electrophoretic sperm separation is particularly suitable for those patients requiring ICSI or IVF where the cause of infertility is due to poor sperm morphology and/or significantly damaged sperm DNA. Though electrophoresis has previously been demonstrated to be detrimental to sperm motility in a free-flow electrophoretic system [17], such impacts on sperm quality do not appear to be a problem with the SpermSep CS10. The latter would therefore seem to offer some promise as a fast, efficient method for isolating spermatozoa exhibiting low levels of DNA damage for assisted conception applications, ranging from IUI to ICSI [11].

References

1. Kallajoki M, Virtanen I, Suominen J. Surface glycoproteins of human spermatozoa. J Cell Sci. 1986;82:11–22.
2. Calzada L, Salazar EL, Pedron N. Presence and chemical composition of glycoproteic layer on human spermatozoa. Arch Androl. 1994;33:87–92.
3. Schroter S, Kirchhoff C, Yeung CH, Cooper T, Meyer B. Purification and structural analysis of sperm CD52, a GPI-anchored membrane protein. Adv Exp Med Biol. 1997;424:233–4.

4. Kirchhoff C, Schroter S. New insights into the origin, structure and role of CD52: a major component of the mammalian sperm glycocalyx. Cells Tissues Organs. 2001;168:93–104.
5. Giuliani V, Pandolfi C, Santucci R, Pelliccione F, Macerola B, Focarelli R, Rosati F, Della Giovampaola C, Francavilla F, Francavilla S. Expression of gp20, a human sperm antigen of epididymal origin, is reduced in spermatozoa from subfertile men. Mol Reprod Dev. 2004;69:235–40.
6. Schroter S, Derr P, Conradt HS, Nimtz M, Hale G, Kirchhoff C. Male-specific modification of human CD52. J Biol Chem. 1999;274:29862–73.
7. Chan PJ, Jacobson JD, Corselli JU, Patton WC. A simple zeta method for sperm selection based on membrane charge. Fertil Steril. 2006;85:481–6.
8. Kam TL, Jacobson JD, Patton WC, Corselli JU, Chan PJ. Retention of membrane charge attributes by cryopreserved-thawed sperm and zeta selection. J Assist Reprod Genet. 2007;24:429–34.
9. Ainsworth C, Nixon B, Aitken RJ. Development of a novel electrophoretic system for the isolation of human spermatozoa. Hum Reprod. 2005;20:2261–70.
10. Ainsworth C, Nixon B, Jansen RP, Aitken RJ. First recorded pregnancy and normal birth after ICSI using electrophoretically isolated spermatozoa. Hum Reprod. 2007;22:197–200.
11. Fleming SD, Ilad RS, Griffin AM, Wu Y, Ong KJ, Smith HC, Aitken RJ. Prospective controlled trial of an electrophoretic method of sperm preparation for assisted reproduction: comparison with density gradient centrifugation. Hum Reprod. 2008;23:2646–51.
12. Panidis D, Matalliotakis I, Papathanasiou K, Roussos C, Koumantakis E. The sperm deformity and the sperm multiple anomalies indexes in patients who underwent unilateral orchectomy and preventive radiotherapy. Eur J Obstet Gynecol Reprod Biol. 1998;80:247–50.
13. WHO. WHO laboratory manual for the examination of human semen and sperm-cervical mucus interaction. Cambridge: Cambridge University Press; 1999.
14. Thomson LK, Fleming SD, Aitken RJ, de Iuliis GN, Zieschang JA, Clark AM. Cryopreservation-induced human sperm DNA damage is predominantly mediated by oxidative stress rather than apoptosis. Hum Reprod. 2009;24:2061–70.
15. Thomson LK, Fleming SD, Barone K, Zieschang JA, Clark AM. The effect of repeated freezing and thawing on human sperm DNA fragmentation. Fertil Steril. 2010;93:1147–56.
16. Thomson LK, Fleming SD, Schulke L, Barone K, Zieschang JA, Clark AM. The DNA integrity of cryopreserved spermatozoa separated for use in assisted reproductive technology is unaffected by the type of cryoprotectant used but is related to the DNA integrity of the fresh separated preparation. Fertil Steril. 2009;92:991–1001.
17. Engelmann U, Krassnigg F, Schatz H, Schill WB. Separation of human X and Y spermatozoa by free-flow electrophoresis. Gamete Res. 1988;19:151–60.

Chapter 9
Magnetic-Activated Cell Sorting of Human Spermatozoa

Enver Kerem Dirican

Magnetic Nanoparticles in Cell Separation

Magnetic Nanoparticles Are Highly Biocompatible

The history of cell separation is long, dating back to the 1950s and 1960s [1, 2]. Since then, the success in the synthesis of magnetic particles has empowered a plethora of exciting biotechnological applications [2].

Magnetic cell sorting allows large numbers of viable cells to be isolated with high purity and yield [3]. The superparamagnetic microbeads used in magnetic cell separation are amorphous or semicrystalline structures [2] and are small enough (20–100 nm) to be colloidal, i.e., they remain dispersed due to the random bombardment of Brownian motion. The magnetically susceptible core is small enough that the particles do not retain any residual magnetism when removed from the field. These properties facilitate both the preparation of antigen-specific reagents and separation of specific cell types [3].

In the context of the emerging concern about the potential toxicity of nanoparticles, it is noteworthy that magnetic iron oxide particles are highly biocompatible, as the iron cell homeostasis is well controlled by uptake, excretion, and storage, and the iron excess is efficiently cleared from the body [2]. Although there are few reports on the negative effects of magnetic fields in male reproduction and semen quality [4], several studies have been carried out, and none of them identified any decreased fertility for either males or females [5]. And it is accepted that the process does not cause physical damage to the cell and the magnetic particles do not affect the rate of growth of cell cultures [6]. Therefore, even introduction of these particles inside a living cell is considered as a viable process [3, 6].

E.K. Dirican, PhD (✉)
Department of Embryology, Memorial Hospital of Antalya, Antalya 07020, Turkey
e-mail: kerem@dirican.tr.tc

Magnetic Nanoparticles Are Widely Used in Research and Clinical Protocols of Various Biomedical Disciplines

Magnetic separation has been successfully applied to many aspects of biomedical and biological research. It has proven to be a highly sensitive technique for the selection of rare tumor cells from blood and is especially well suited to the separation of low numbers of target cells [7]. This has, for example, led to the enhanced detection of malarial parasites in blood samples either by utilizing the magnetic properties of the parasite [8] or through labeling the red blood cells with an immunospecific magnetic fluid [9]. It has been used as a preprocessing technology for polymerase chain reactions, through which the DNA of a sample is amplified and identified [10]. Cell counting techniques have also been developed using magnetic technologies [11, 12].

Today, magnetic nanoparticles are widely used in separation of macromolecules or cells from various cell suspensions or homogenates [2] and also in protein purification [13] and nucleic acid applications [14].

Magnetic cell sorting is widely used in many clinical areas in cellular therapies [15] including human autoimmunity diseases like rheumatoid arthritis [16], diabetes [17], multiple sclerosis [18], and systemic lupus erythematosus [19], in nucleic acid transfer as a transfection method [20] and to optimize conditions for viral-mediated gene delivery (therapy) by magnetofection [21].

In the last decade, several studies have been carried out on the use of magnetic cell sorting in human reproduction, for decontamination of testicular cell suspensions in cancer patients [22] and for elimination of apoptotic spermatozoa from human semen samples [23–25].

Apoptosis and Reactive Oxygen Species in the Human Spermatozoa

Defining the "Good" Sperm

In the era of human assisted reproduction where the main choice of treatment for the severe male infertility is intracytoplasmic sperm injection (ICSI), quality of gametes is one of the factors that help to determine the success.

With the innovation of strict Tygerberg criteria, a consensus regarding the importance of sperm morphology assessment in human assisted reproduction seems to be reached. After the breakthrough in human assisted reproduction by ICSI, the raised question about the future need of extended sperm analysis as well as sperm function tests evoked [26, 27].

Infertile men with poor sperm motility and morphology were found to have increased sperm DNA fragmentation compared with individuals with normal semen parameters [28]. Men with normal semen analysis may also have a high degree of

Table 9.1 Common characteristics of a *good* sperm for ICSI

Feature	Desired	Undesired
Morphology	Classified as "normal" in Tygerberg criteria	Vacuoles, elongation, acrosomeless forms, megalo, or duplicated
Motility	Progressive	Immotile, agglutinated
Maturity	Fully matured, not aged	Cytoplasmic droplets, short tails
Functionality	Hypo-osmotic tail swelling (HOS) present	HOS absent
Biochemistry	Low ROS (reactive oxygen species)—high AC (antioxidant capacity)	High ROS—low AC
Nucleus	DNA not fragmented, euploidy	DNA fragmented, aneuploidy
Cellular viability	Nonapoptotic, viable	Apoptotic, necrotic

sperm DNA fragmentation, which can be a major cause of unexplained infertility, and sperm DNA fragmentation may result from aberrant chromatin packaging during spermatogenesis [29], defective apoptosis before ejaculation [30], or excessive production of reactive oxygen species (ROS) in the ejaculate [31]. Exposures to environmental or industrial toxins [32], genetics [33], or lifestyle [34] are also known factors that may cause sperm DNA fragmentation and infertility.

Although the factors present in the paternal genome that may have an impact on poor reproductive outcome are still not well defined, there is accumulating evidence linking sperm nuclear DNA abnormalities to poor reproductive outcome, and one of the most suspected organelle is the sperm nucleus. Studies reveal that severe teratozoospermia results in high preimplantation embryo aneuploidy [35, 36] and the interchromosomal effect is related to impaired semen parameters [37]. Studies have also shown that immature sperms have increased rates of lipid peroxidation and bear poor morphometric and morphological attributes, zona pellucida-binding properties, and fertility [38]. The ROS-induced lipid peroxidation is involved in the mechanisms by which spermatozoa are damaged in many cases of male infertility. Studies show a significant correlation between sperm morphology attributes and the expressed apoptotic markers like caspases-3 activation and mitochondrial membrane potential integrity [39].

The sperm nucleus, as the carrier of paternal DNA to the oocyte, remains as the greatest contributor to the potential success of reproductive outcome, where sperm nuclear DNA strand breaks, DNA repair mechanisms, apoptosis, and DNA remodeling processes are the main factors to be considered [40]. Table 9.1 shows common characteristics of a *good* sperm.

Why Do Reproductive Technologists Need to Select Sperm Prior to Assisted Reproduction?

The spermatozoa of all placental mammals, including humans, are in a protective state at ejaculation and are incapable of fertilization. Spermatozoa must undergo a subsequent period of final maturation termed capacitation, and spermatozoa in the ejaculate are prevented from undergoing capacitation by some factors that are present in the seminal plasma [41]. This final maturation of the mammalian spermatozoa can be evaluated in three steps: capacitation, hyperactivated motility, and acrosome reaction.

As a common sense, sperm preparation prior to assisted reproduction has three basic advantages:

1. Sperm preparation and wash procedures remove the seminal plasma and help the sperm cells to prepare for capacitation.
2. Sperm preparation methods help to eliminate immotile, dead, and morphologically abnormal spermatozoa and nonreproductive cells, which are the main causes of ROS in the ejaculate.
3. Sperm washing and selection techniques can be used to purify the sperm cells from pathogenic microorganisms.

Since the oocyte selects the best sperm to win the race in natural conception and conventional insemination protocols like intrauterine insemination (IUI) and in vitro fertilization (IVF), the contribution of the healthy paternal genome to embryo development, implantation, and conception is the main problem to be solved in sperm preparation for ICSI.

Current Sperm Preparation Techniques and Limitations in Assisted Reproduction

First, sperm preparation technique was washing the spermatozoa with culture medium followed by centrifugation and resuspension of the pellet. Today, there are a number of different sperm preparation methods available, and they are concentrated on selecting sperms with normal morphology, normal and intact acrosomes, and progressive motility.

Density Gradient Centrifugation

According to the principles of density gradient centrifugation (DGC), when a suspension of particles is centrifuged, the sedimentation rate of the particles is proportional to the force applied. At a fixed centrifugal force and liquid viscosity, the sedimentation rate is proportional to the size of the particle and the difference between its density and the density of the surrounding medium. DGC method uses these principles to select motile sperm with good morphology and a healthy chromatin structure [42]. Although some studies point out that the gradient solutions may damage sperm [43], generally the technique is considered to recover sperm with good morphology and high motility [44].

Swim-Up

Swim-up is the choice of semen processing for IUI and IVF, in cases where no male factor is present to mild male factor infertility. The swim-up from a washed pellet method is the most common version of the technique, and it is characterized by extremely high proportions of motile spermatozoa, a preferential selection for morphologically normal spermatozoa, and an absence of the other cell types and debris commonly seen in human ejaculates [45].

As the indications for IVF treatment were expanded beyond simple tubal factor cases to couples with idiopathic infertility and, ultimately, to male factor cases, the problem of fertilization failures [46] and insufficient motile sperm yields appeared by swim-up techniques.

Other Techniques

A variety of techniques were used in human assisted reproduction for the improvement of selecting the best sperm. Most of these techniques are not in routine clinical use anymore, like Percoll gradients, Nycodenz gradients, affinity chromatography, glass beads, sephadex columns, transmembrane migration, etc.

A number of novel sperm preparation and selection techniques have now been proposed that may assist in limiting the chance of selecting an abnormal spermatozoon prior to ICSI [40]. These include the use of high-magnification microscopes to identify minor morphological defects of the living spermatozoa [46], selection of mature spermatozoa referring to the binding ability of human spermatozoa to hyaluronic acid [47], and eliminating apoptotic spermatozoa prior to ICSI by magnetic-activated cell sorting (MACS) [48].

Principles of Magnetic Selection in Human Spermatozoa

Programmed cell death in animals usually occurs by apoptosis. Cells dying by apoptosis undergo characteristic morphological changes. They shrink and condense, the cytoskeleton collapses, the nuclear envelope disassembles, and the nuclear chromatin condenses and breaks up into fragments. Most importantly, the surface of the cell becomes chemically altered, so that a neighboring cell or a macrophage rapidly engulfs them before they can spill their contents [49].

An especially important change occurs in the plasma membrane of apoptotic cells. The negatively charged phospholipid phosphatidylserine (PS) is normally exclusively located in the inner leaflet of the lipid bilayer of the plasma membrane, but it flips to the outer leaflet in apoptotic cells, where it can serve as a marker of these cells. This process blocks the inflammation associated with phagocytosis. The PS on the surface of apoptotic cells can be visualized with a labeled form of Annexin V protein, which specifically binds to this phospholipid [49].

The Annexin V-coated microbeads are used for the isolation of cells with exposed PS, including sickle cells and apoptotic cells, and removal of dead and apoptotic

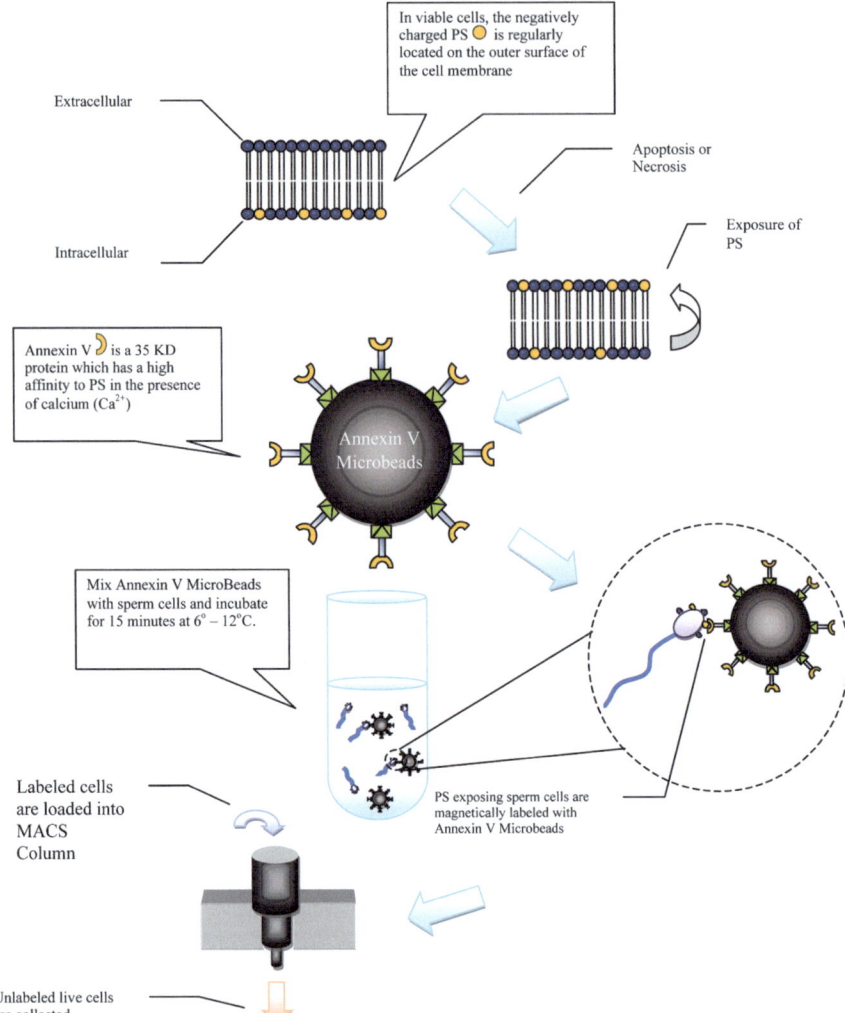

Fig. 9.1 The Annexin V-coated microbeads are used for the isolation of cells with exposed PS, including sickle cells and apoptotic cells, and removal of dead and apoptotic spermatozoa from seminal samples. Briefly, the PS-exposing spermatozoa are magnetically labeled by the protein Annexin V, then the magnetically labeled apoptotic and dead spermatozoa are retained on a MACS column where the unlabeled nonapoptotic spermatozoa are in the flow-through. At the end, magnetically labeled, PS-exposing spermatozoa can be eluted from the column for various cellular tests (Miltenyi Biotec GmbH, Germany)

spermatozoa from seminal samples. Briefly, the PS-exposing spermatozoa are magnetically labeled by the protein Annexin V, then the magnetically labeled apoptotic and dead spermatozoa are retained on a MACS column where the unlabeled nonapoptotic spermatozoa are in the flow-through (Fig. 9.1). At the end, magnetically labeled, PS-exposing spermatozoa can be eluted from the column for various cellular tests (Miltenyi Biotec GmbH, Germany).

Preliminary Studies on Magnetic-Activated Cell Sorting of Human Spermatozoa

Several studies using MACS technique with human spermatozoa have been published over the past 10 years. Interests in these studies were mainly the molecular efficiency of the technique and improving the postpreparation sperm quality.

Efficiency of Magnetic Selection in Conventional Seminal Parameters Was Shown in Some Studies

One of the first studies on the yield of magnetic selection in human spermatozoa came in the mid-2000s. Researchers have evaluated the percentage of sperm recovery following the use of MACS as a sperm preparation technique, and they concluded that the integration of MACS with DGC is an effective sperm preparation technique that does not lead to significant cell loss and separating a distinctive population of nonapoptotic spermatozoa with intact membranes might optimize the outcome of assisted reproduction [50]. Later on, the separation effect of MACS on capacitation and acrosome reaction was investigated in the nonapoptotic sperm fractions. Nonapoptotic human spermatozoa with intact plasma membranes were found to be characterized by superior ability to capacitate and, consequently, by maximum potential to perform acrosome reaction after stimulation [51].

Studies have also shown that nonapoptotic sperm fractions selected by MACS technique have morphologically superior quality [52], higher percentage of motility, viability, and apoptosis indices [53] and routine sperm parameters [54].

Basic Studies Show Improvements in the Markers of Apoptosis and DNA Integrity

At the end of the 1990s, separation of leucocytes from human seminal plasma was successfully performed by magnetic selection [55]. Later on in the early 2000s, scientists focused on studying molecular analyses on human spermatozoa before and after MACS selection. It was shown that spermatozoa with deteriorated membrane and exposed PS are characterized by an increased lysophosphatidylcholine content that is likely generated by phospholipases [56] and also are characterized by an increase in activated caspases, which were found in infertile patients [57].

Reduction of apoptotic spermatozoa within the ejaculate by means of the MACS system results in a distinct reduction of spermatozoa with DNA fragmentation [58], enrichment of spermatozoa free of apoptosis [59], and improvement of sperm viability, motility, and mitochondrial membrane integrity [60].

Cryobiology of Human Spermatozoa with Magnetic Selection Seems to Be Beneficial

The first report on the initiator and effector caspases of the main pathways of apoptosis in ejaculated human spermatozoa came in the early 2000s, and in that study, activated caspases were found especially in spermatozoa with disturbed membranes, where cryopreservation was used as a tool for increasing the number of spermatozoa showing an activation of caspases [61]. Further studies were performed on human sperm cryopreservation and the benefit of MACS on eliminating apoptotic sperm fractions from frozen–thawed semen samples. Studies revealed that MACS separation before cryopreservation results in depletion of spermatozoa which are positive for activated caspases [62], depletes low-quality spermatozoa from cryopreserved semen samples [63], and selects a population of nonapoptotic spermatozoa which optimizes cryopreservation and thawing outcome [64].

MACS from Research Bench to Clinical Application

The integrity of the paternal genome is of a paramount importance in the initiation and maintenance of a viable pregnancy in both natural and assisted reproduction. The need to eliminate nonviable and apoptotic spermatozoa before IVF is therefore one of the factors to improve the outcome of treatment for the infertile couple. Studies have investigated the sperm fertilizing potential using hamster oocyte penetration assay [65], and results suggested that nonapoptotic spermatozoa prepared by MACS display higher fertilization potential following ICSI and this technique should be evaluated in a clinical setting for its impact on ICSI outcomes [66]. Studies also showed a reduced level of apoptotic markers, improved acrosome reaction scores [67], and superior morphological quality [68] after MACS preparation which may contribute to increased implantation and pregnancy rates.

First, assisted reproduction data and clinical pregnancies in the world with the use of MACS as a sperm preparation method in human assisted reproduction were presented in 2006 in a local meeting [69] as a preliminary study of a Turkish group.

A brief step-by-step protocol is as follows:

- Perform all steps under a laminar airflow hood using aseptic techniques. Use only cell culture-tested disposable materials.
- Allow ejaculate to liquefy and evaluate the seminal parameters.
- Prepare 1× binding buffer from 20× stock solution (Miltenyi Biotec GmbH, Germany).
- Centrifuge sperm cells for 10 min at 300 × g. Remove supernatant and resuspend sperm pellet in 80 μL of 1× binding buffer per 10^7 total sperm count.
- Add 20 μL of MACS Annexin V MicroBeads (Miltenyi Biotec GmbH, Germany) per 10^7 total sperm count, mix gently, and incubate for 15 min at 6–12°C, preferably in a temperature-controlled laboratory refrigerator.

- Wash sperm cells by adding 2 mL of 1× binding buffer, centrifuge at 300 × g for 10 min, remove supernatant completely, and resuspend sperm pellet in 500 µL of 1× binding buffer.
- For magnetic sperm separation, use an MS Column (Miltenyi Biotec GmbH, Germany). Place the column in the MACS separator (Miltenyi Biotec GmbH, Germany).
- Prepare column by washing with 500 µL volume of 1× binding buffer.
- Apply sperm suspension in 500 µL amount of 1× binding buffer onto the column. Let the cell suspension pass through drop by drop, then rinse the column with 500 µL of 1× binding buffer 4 times. Collect the sperm suspension and 2 mL binding buffer in the same test tube.
- Evaluate the postseparation sperm values.
- Perform either a DCG or a swim-up preparation on the sperm suspension according to sperm concentration and motility.
- Use the prepared motile sperm cells for ICSI.

Human In Vitro Embryos Cleave Better After MACS

In the 2006 study, MACS preparation did not yield any statistically significant improvement in terms of fertilization and embryo cleavage rates and embryo quality. This was related to the limited number of cases by the authors [69].

In 2007, a prospective study was designed in our program to assess the impact of MACS technique for selection of nonapoptotic spermatozoa on the outcome of ICSI [48]. We compared the cleavage, fertilization, implantation, and pregnancy rates associated with two sperm preparation methods, MACS and DGC, for the ICSI of superovulated women. Especially male factor cases were included in the study to define the effects of MACS preparation, and both MACS and DGC groups had comparable demographic characteristics. The magnetic enrichment of nonapoptotic spermatozoa significantly improved the percentage of sperm with normal morphology.

Although there were no significant differences between two groups in terms of fertilization rates and embryo quality, there was a statistically significant improvement in the cleavage rate of the MACS group embryos. This difference, although fertilization rates are not different from the control group, results in a significantly higher number of embryos on the embryo transfer day, by reducing the number of arrested embryos during in vitro culture [48].

Which embryos arrest in culture? Few studies address the issue in literature. Early embryo arrest is associated with the injection of round spermatids [70], pronuclear morphology, and chromosomal abnormalities [71, 72], which are possible deleterious factors that can be introduced into the human oocyte by spermatozoa [73, 74] and impair the implantation of that embryo. Therefore, it is acceptable to conclude that observed improvement in embryo cleavage rate in our study should be related to better elimination of apoptotic and abnormal spermatozoa by MACS technique.

Does Better Elimination of Apoptotic Spermatozoa Yield Higher Pregnancy Rates in Assisted Reproduction?

Our study demonstrates slightly higher clinical pregnancy and implantation rates after using MACS for preparation of human spermatozoa. Another study from Argentina reported three ongoing clinical pregnancies out of 10 cases by using MACS as a sperm preparation technique [75]. They also represented their first healthy baby born after MACS technique [76].

As apoptotic fractions represent highly abnormal spermatozoa, it should be expected that elimination of these cells would result in better pregnancy and implantation rates in human assisted reproduction.

Since the number of cases in both studies still remains low, further studies should be conducted to better characterize the process of eliminating abnormal spermatozoa and pregnancy rates.

The Future of MACS in Sperm Selection for Assisted Reproduction

A number of studies, including our own, have shown that using spermatozoa prepared with MACS technique significantly improves the quality of spermatozoa in the preparation. These studies indicate that MACS can enrich the sperm population by separating out apoptotic, necrotic, chromosomally abnormal, and DNA-fragmented spermatozoa [48,55-60].

Although our results showed improved sperm morphology and embryo cleavage rates after MACS, the efficiency of this new technique is still not fully evaluated, and the interpretation of ICSI results still remains incomplete. More research is needed to improve our current knowledge in relation to human sperm apoptosis and MACS technique. Additionally, more standardized, large-scale clinical trials are needed to assess the power of MACS technique in assisted reproduction.

On the other hand, development of clinical grade products, manufactured according to good manufacturing practices (GMP), which is absent in the market today, will be useful to carry the MACS technique from research to clinical use in assisted reproduction and will also help to develop the product quality in terms of both clinical results and regulatory status of certain countries.

References

1. Esser C. Historical and useful methods of preselection and preparative scale sorting. In: Recktenwald D, Radbruch A, editors. Cell separation methods and applications. New York: Marcel Dekker; 1998. p. 1.
2. Corchero J, Villaverde A. Biomedical applications of distally controlled magnetic nanoparticles. Trends Biotechnol. 2009;27(8):468–76.

3. Kantor AB, Gibbons I, Miltenyi S, et al. Magnetic cell sorting with colloidal superparamagnetic particles. In: Recktenwald D, Radbruch A, editors. Cell separation methods and applications. New York: Marcel Dekker; 1998. p. 153–61.
4. Li DK, Yan B, Zheng L, et al. Exposure to magnetic fields and the risk of poor sperm quality. Reprod Toxicol. 2010;29(1):86–92.
5. Bernhardt JH, Brix G. Safety aspects of magnetic fields. In: Andrä W, Nowak H, editors. Magnetism in medicine: A handbook. 2nd ed. Weinheim: Wiley-Vch; 2007. p. 80–1.
6. Desai JP, Pillarisetti A, Brooks AD. Engineering approaches to biomanipulation. Annu Rev Biomed Eng. 2007;9:35–53.
7. Liberti PA, Rao CG, Terstappen LWMM. Optimization of ferrofluids and protocols for the enrichment of breast tumor cells in blood. J Magn Magn Mater. 2001;225(1):301–7.
8. Paul F, Melville D, Roath S, et al. A bench top magnetic separator for malarial parasite concentration. IEEE Trans Magn. 1981;17:2822–4.
9. Seesod N, Nopparat P, Hedrum A, et al. An integrated system using immunomagnetic separation, polymerase chain reaction and colorimetric detection for diagnosis of *Plasmodium Falciparum*. Am J Trop Med Hyg. 1997;56:322–8.
10. Hofmann WK, de Vos S, Komor M, et al. Characterization of gene expression of CD34+ cells from normal and myelodysplastic bone marrow. Blood. 2002;100:3553–60.
11. Delgratta C, Dellapenna S, Battista P, et al. Detection and counting of specific cell populations by means of magnetic markers linked to monoclonal antibodies. Phys Med Biol. 1995;40: 671–81.
12. Edelstein RL, Tamanaha CR, Sheehan PE, et al. The BARC biosensor applied to the detection of biological warfare agents. Biosens Bioelectron. 2000;14:805–13.
13. Safarik I, Safarikova M. Magnetic techniques for the isolation and purification of proteins and peptides. Biomagn Res Technol. 2004;2:7.
14. Sarkar TR, Irudayaraj J. Carboxyl-coated magnetic nanoparticles for mRNA isolation and extraction of supercoiled plasmid DNA. Anal Biochem. 2008;379:130–2.
15. Apel M, Heinlein UAO, Miltenyi S, et al. Magnetic cell separation for research and clinical applications. In: Andrä W, Nowak H, editors. Magnetism in medicine: a handbook. 2nd ed. Weinheim: Wiley-Vch; 2007. p. 571.
16. Lande R, Giacomini E, Serafini B, et al. Characterization and recruitment of plasmacytoid dendritic cells in synovial fluid and tissue of patients with chronic inflammatory arthritis. J Immunol. 2004;173:2815–24.
17. Cipolletta C, Ryan KE, Hanna EV, et al. Activation of peripheral blood CD14+ monocytes occurs in diabetes. Diabetes. 2005;54(9):2779–86.
18. Bielekova B, Catalfamo M, Reichert-Scrivner S, et al. Regulatory CD56(bright) natural killer cells mediate immunomodulatory effects of IL-2Ralpha-targeted therapy (daclizumab) in multiple sclerosis. Proc Natl Acad Sci USA. 2006;103(15):5941–6.
19. Köller M, Zwölfer B, Steiner G, et al. Phenotypic and functional deficiencies of monocyte-derived dendritic cells in systemic lupus erythematosus (SLE) patients. Int Immunol. 2004;16(11):1595–604.
20. Plank C, Schillinger U, Scherer F, et al. The magnetofection method: using magnetic force to enhance gene delivery. Biol Chem. 2003;384:737–47.
21. Xenariou S, Griesenbach U, Ferrari S, et al. Using magnetic forces to enhance non-viral gene transfer to airway epithelium in vivo: magnetofection in the mouse nose. Gene Ther. 2006; 13:1545–52.
22. Geens M, Van de Velde H, De Block G, et al. The efficiency of magnetic-activated cell sorting and fluorescence-activated cell sorting in the decontamination of testicular cell suspensions in cancer patients. Hum Reprod. 2007;22(3):733–42.
23. Paasch U, Grunewald S, Fitzl G, et al. Deterioration of plasma membrane is associated with activated caspases in human spermatozoa. J Androl. 2003;24(2):246–52.
24. Paasch U, Grunewald S, Agarwal A, et al. Activation pattern ofcaspases in human spermatozoa. Fertil Steril. 2004;81 Suppl 1:802–9.

25. Said TM, Agarwal A, Grunewald S, et al. Evaluation of sperm recovery following annexin V magnetic-activated cell sorting separation. Reprod Biomed Online. 2006;13(3):336–9.
26. van Dop PA. WHO guidelines for the interpretation of common semen parameters. In: Ombelet W, Bosmans E, Vandeput H, et al., editors. Modern ART in the 2000s: andrology in the nineties. New York: Parthenon; 1998. p. 37–8.
27. Makler A. Human seminology: semen examination and in vitro evaluation of human seminal cells. In: Revelli A, Tur-Kaspa I, Holte J, et al., editors. Biotechnology in human reproduction. New York: Parthenon; 2003. p. 115–30.
28. Chohan KR, Griffin JT, Lafromboise M, et al. Comparison of chromatin assays for DNA fragmentation evaluation in human sperm. J Androl. 2006;27(1):53–9.
29. Manicardi GC, Bianchi PG, Pantano S, et al. Presence of endogenous nicks in DNA of ejaculated human spermatozoa and its relationship to chromomycin A3 accessibility. Biol Reprod. 1995; 52:864–7.
30. Sakkas D, Moffatt O, Manicardi GC, et al. Nature of DNA damage in ejaculated human spermatozoa and the possible involvement of apoptosis. Biol Reprod. 2002;66:1061–7.
31. Cocuzza M, Sikka SC, Athayde KS, et al. Clinical relevance of oxidative stress and sperm chromatin damage in male infertility: an evidence based analysis. Int Braz J Urol. 2007;33(5): 603–21.
32. Uzunhisarcikli M, Kalender Y, Dirican K, et al. Acute, subacute and subchronic administration of methyl parathion-induced testicular damage in male rats and protective role of vitamins C and E. Pestic Biochem Phys. 2007;87:115–22.
33. Saleh RA, Agarwal A, Nada EA, et al. Negative effects of increased sperm DNA damage in relation to seminal oxidative stress in men with idiopathic and male factor infertility. Fertil Steril. 2003;79:1597–605.
34. Agarwal A, Desai N, Makker K, et al. Effects of radiofrequency electromagnetic waves (FR-EMV) from cellular phones on human ejaculated semen: an in vitro pilot study. Fertil Steril. 2009;92(4):1318–25.
35. Cinar C, Yazici C, Ergünsu S, et al. Genetic diagnosis in infertile men with numerical and constitutional sperm abnormalities. Genet Test. 2008;12(2):195–202.
36. Dubey A, Dayal MB, Frankfurter D, et al. The influence of sperm morphology on preimplantation genetic diagnosis cycles outcome. Fertil Steril. 2008;89(6):1665–9.
37. Kirkpatrick G, Ferguson KA, Gao H, et al. A comparison of sperm aneuploidy rates between infertile men with normal and abnormal karyotypes. Hum Reprod. 2008;23(7):1679–83.
38. Huzsar G, Vigue L. Correlation between the rate of lipid peroxidation and cellular maturity as measured by creatine kinase activity in human spermatozoa. J Androl. 1994;15:71–7.
39. Aziz N, Said T, Paasch U, et al. The relationship between human sperm apoptosis, morphology and the sperm deformity index. Hum Reprod. 2007;22(5):1413–9.
40. Sakkas D, Seli E. Sperm DNA and embryo development. In: Elder K, Cohen J, editors. Human preimplantation embryo selection. London: Informa Healthcare; 2007. p. 325–35.
41. Mortimer D. Sperm preparation methods. J Androl. 2000;21(3):357–66.
42. Ng FLH, Liu DY, Baker G. Comparison of Percoll, mini-Percoll and swim up methods for sperm preparation from abnormal semen samples. Hum Reprod. 1992;7(2):261–6.
43. Grab D, Thierauf S, Rosenbusch B, et al. Scanning electron microscopy of human sperms after preparation of semen for in-vitro fertilization. Arch Gynecol Obstet. 1993;252(3):137–41.
44. Yao YQ, Ng V, Yeung WSB, et al. Profiles of sperm morphology and motility after discontinuous multiple-step Percoll density gradient centrifugation. Andrologia. 2009;28(2):127–31.
45. Franken DR, Claassens OE, Henkel RR. Sperm preparation techniques and X/Y chromosome separation. In: Acosta AA, Kruger TF, editors. Human spermatozoa in assisted reproduction. 2nd ed. New York: Parthenon; 1996. p. 277–94.
46. Bartoov B, Berkovitz A, Eltes F. Selection of spermatozoa with normal nuclei to improve the pregnancy rate with intracytoplasmic sperm injection. N Engl J Med. 2001;345(14):1067–8.
47. Huzsar G, Ozenci CC, Cayli S, et al. Hyaluronic acid binding by human sperm indicates cellular maturity, viability, and unreacted acrosomal status. Fertil Steril. 2003;79 Suppl 3: 1616–24.

48. Dirican EK, Ozgun OD, Akarsu S, et al. Clinical outcome of magnetic activated cell sorting of non-apoptotic spermatozoa before density gradient centrifugation for assisted reproduction. J Assist Reprod Genet. 2008;25(8):375–81.
49. Alberts B, Johnson A, Lewis J, et al. Apoptosis. In: Molecular biology of the cell. 5th ed. New York: Garland Science, 2008, p. 1115–30.
50. Said TM, Agarwal A, Grunewald S, et al. Evaluation of sperm recovery following annexin V magnetic activated cell sorting separation. Reprod Biomed Online. 2006;13(3):336–9.
51. Grunewald S, Baumann T, Paasch U, et al. Capacitation and acrosome reaction in nonapoptotic human spermatozoa. Ann NY Acad Sci. 2006;1090:138–46.
52. Aziz N, Said T, Paasch U, et al. The relationship between human sperm apoptosis, morphology and the sperm deformity index. Hum Reprod. 2007;22(5):1413–9.
53. Paasch U, Grunewald S, Glander HJ. Sperm selection in assisted reproductive techniques. Soc Reprod Fertil. 2007;65:515–25.
54. Said TM, Agarwal A, Zborowski M, et al. Utility of magnetic separation as a molecular sperm preparation technique. J Androl. 2008;29(2):134–42.
55. Hipler UC, Schreiber G, Wollina U. Reactive oxygen species in human semen: investigations and measurements. Arch Androl. 1998;40(1):67–78.
56. Glander HJ, Schiller J, Süß R, et al. Deterioration of spermatozoa plasma membrane is associated with an increase of sperm lyso-phosphatidylcholines. Andrologia. 2002;34(6):360–6.
57. Paasch U, Grunewald S, Fitzl G, et al. Deterioration of plasma membrane is associated with activated caspases in human spermatozoa. J Androl. 2003;24(2):246–52.
58. Winkle T, Gagsteiger F, Ditzel N. Reduction of apoptotic spermatozoa within the ejaculate by means of the MACS system. J Fertil Reprod. 2007;17(1):19–21.
59. Grunewald S, Miska W, Miska G, et al. Molecular glass wool filtration as a new tool for sperm preparation. Hum Reprod. 2007;22(5):1405–12.
60. De Vantéry Arrighi C, Lucas H, Chardonnens D, et al. Removal of spermatozoa with externalized phosphatidylserine from sperm preparation in human assisted medical procreation: effects on viability, motility and mitochondrial membrane potential. Reprod Biol Endocrinol. 2009;7:1.
61. Paasch U, Grunewald S, Glander HJ. Transduction of apoptotic signals in ejaculated spermatozoa after cryopreservation via activation of caspases. J Fertil Reprod. 2003;13(2):22–31.
62. Paasch U, Grunewald S, Agarwal A, et al. Activation pattern of caspases in human spermatozoa. Fertil Steril. 2004;81(1):802–9.
63. Paasch U, Grunewald S, Wuendrich K, et al. Immunomagnetic removal of cryo-damaged human spermatozoa. Asian J Androl. 2005;7(1):61–9.
64. Grunewald S, Paasch U, Said TM, et al. Magnetic-activated cell sorting before cryopreservation preserves mitochondrial integrity in human spermatozoa. Cell Tissue Bank. 2006;7(2):99–104.
65. Said T, Agarwal A, Grunewald S, et al. Selection of nonapoptotic spermatozoa as a new tool for enhancing assisted reproduction: an in vitro model. Biol Reprod. 2006;74(3):530–7.
66. Grunewald S, Reinhardt M, Blumenauer V, et al. Increased sperm chromatin decondensation in selected nonapoptotic spermatozoa of patients with male infertility. Fertil Steril. 2009;92(2):572–7.
67. Lee TH, Liu CH, Shih YT, et al. Magnetic-activated cell sorting for human sperm preparation reduces spermatozoa with apoptotic markers and improves the acrosome reaction in couples with unexplained infertility. Hum Reprod. 2010;25(4):839–46.
68. Hoogendijk CF, Kruger TF, Bouic PJ, et al. A novel approach for the selection of human sperm using annexin V-binding and flow cytometry. Fertil Steril. 2009;91(4):1285–92.
69. Dirican EK, Vicdan K, Işık AZ, et al. [Results of the microinjection treatments after eliminating apoptotic spermatozoa] (Article in Turkish: Apoptotik spermlerin elimine edilmesi ile uygulanan mikroenjeksiyon tedavilerinin sonuçları). Second National congress of reproductive endocrinology and infertility. 2006;SS-18:222–3.
70. Kahraman S, Polat G, Samli M, et al. Multiple pregnancies obtained by testicular spermatid injection in combination with intracytoplasmic sperm injection. Hum Reprod. 1998;13(1):104–10.

71. Balaban B, Yakin K, Urman B, et al. Pronuclear morphology predicts embryo development and chromosome constitution. Reprod Biomed Online. 2004;8(6):695–700.
72. Farfalli VI, Magli MC, Ferraretti AP, et al. Role of aneuploidy on embryo implantation. Gynecol Obstet Invest. 2007;64(3):161–5.
73. Sakkas D, Seli E, Bizzaro D, et al. Abnormal spermatozoa in the ejaculate: abortive apoptosis and faulty nuclear remodeling during spermatogenesis. Reprod Biomed Online. 2003;7(4): 428–32.
74. Aitken RJ, De Iuliis GN. On the possible origins of DNA damage in human spermatozoa. Mol Hum Reprod. 2010;16(1):3–13.
75. Rawe VY, Alvarez CR, Uriondo HW, et al. ICSI outcome using annexin V columns to select non-apoptotic spermatozoa. ASRM. 2009;O-250:S73–4.
76. Rawe VY, Boudri HU, Sedó CA, et al. Healthy baby born after reduction of sperm DNA fragmentation using cell sorting before ICSI. Reprod Biomed Online. 2010;20:320–3.

Chapter 10
Polscope-Based Sperm Selection

Luca Gianaroli, Cristina Magli, Andor Crippa, Giorgio Cavallini,
Eleonora Borghi, and Anna P. Ferraretti

The Sperm Cell

The viability of an embryo is strictly related to the competence of the corresponding gametes, and for this reason, an increasing interest in the criteria guiding gamete selection has arisen. The final aim consists in identifying the most viable embryos to increase the chances of implantation with the concomitant reduction in the number of embryos to be either transferred or cryopreserved. Although the oocyte has a preponderant role in determining embryo viability, the identification of the fertilizing sperm for ICSI is of comparable importance, especially in those conditions in which sperm motility and morphology are severely compromised.

The techniques available for the analysis of sperm cells have evidenced that a link exists between the quality of sperm and male infertility with an inverse correlation between sperm indices and the occurrence of numerical and structural chromosome abnormalities that are more frequent in infertile men when compared to the normal population [1, 2].

The highest incidence of abnormalities is detected in patients with severe oligo-asthenoteratospermia (OAT) and azoospermia, and in patients with high levels of

---

L. Gianaroli, MD (✉)
International Institutes of Advanced Reproduction and Genetics,
SISMER, Via Mazzini 12, Bolgona 40138, Italy
e-mail: luca.gianaroli@sismer.it

C. Magli, MSc
Research and Development, SISMER, Bolgona, Italy

A. Crippa, PhD
Andrology Laboratory and Genetics, SISMER, Bolgona, Italy

G. Cavallini, MD • A.P. Ferraretti, MD
Reproductive Medicine Unit, SISMER, Bolgona, Italy

E. Borghi, BSc
Andrology Laboratory, SISMER, Bolgona, Italy

FSH. In these cases, the high proportion of chromosomally abnormal spermatozoa could result in an increased reproductive risk due to the production of embryos with aneuploidy of male origin [3–5].

It is well known that the risk of aneuploid conceptions is mainly associated with maternal age, the contribution of the male gamete being related to a limited number of cases [6]. Nevertheless, ICSI has given the possibility of reproduction to patients that otherwise were destined by nature to remain childless, and it cannot be excluded that the recognized maternal prevalence to the generation of aneuploid fetuses in natural conceptions could be reversed in cases of severe male factor infertility, including azoospermia.

Moreover, as the sperm centrosome is responsible for the organization of the mitotic plates at the first oocyte divisions, the presence of centriolar defects can cause failed cleavage or abnormal cleavage with an abnormal distribution of chromosomes to the resulting blastomeres [7]. Ultra-structural studies have demonstrated that dysfunctional centrioles are present in sperm with altered motility, and the resulting embryos could be highly abnormal [8, 9].

In light of these findings, it is clear that the quality of the sperm sample has an effect not only on the fertilization and implantation rates after ICSI but also on the incidence of abnormalities in the predisposition to chromosomal errors that increase proportionally to the severity of the male factor condition [5, 10–13].

To further improve the sperm selection procedure during ICSI, novel strategies have been proposed that could assist the embryologist in the identification of the most viable spermatozoa without affecting their vitality. One of these techniques is based on the properties of birefringence of sperm cells which permits a meticulous analysis of sperm morphology in vivo, having no adverse effect on sperm motility or on membrane integrity.

Properties of Birefringence in the Sperm Head

Birefringence, or double refraction, is the decomposition of a ray of light into two rays travelling at different velocity (the emerging fast ray and the emerging slow ray) when it passes through an anisotropic material depending on the polarization of the light. The retardance of the slow ray relative to the fast ray generates the birefringence effect.

The sperm cells of many different species, including the human, are naturally birefringent due to the organization of their protoplasmic texture and more specifically the nucleoprotein filaments and the subacrosomal protein filaments which are ordered in rods and longitudinally oriented in the nucleus and in the acrosome, respectively. The same is true for large portions of midpiece and tail (Fig. 10.1).

Comparative studies performed by transmission electron microscopy (TEM) confirm that the presence of birefringence in the sperm head characterizes non-picnotic sperm nuclei and normal acrosomes. Considering that the information provided by the polscope is closer to that derived by TEM than by the conventional

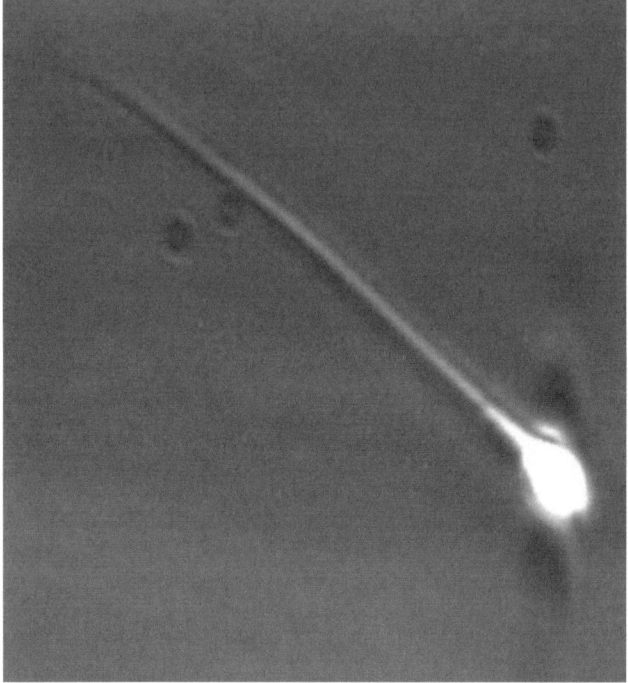

Fig. 10.1 Presence of birefringence in a spermatozoon as observed at the polscope. The birefringence is localized in the acrosomal region, in the nucleus and in the midpiece

phase contrast microscopy, a normal pattern of birefringence is considered to reflect the good health of a sperm cell [14]. Accordingly, it has been found that the fraction of birefringent spermatozoa varies proportionally to the sample concentration, vitality and motility (Fig. 10.2) and that the proportion of birefringent sperm decreases significantly in severe OAT samples and in testicular spermatozoa retrieved by testicular sperm extraction (TESE) compared to normospermic samples (Fig. 10.3). Based on these findings, it has been proposed to perform ICSI in a microscope equipped with a polarizing lens, or polscope, to select sperm cells having an intact organellar organization as reflected by their birefringence appearance.

Polscope-Based Sperm Selection During ICSI

To test the clinical validity of this approach, a prospective randomized study has been designed including 112 sperm samples from patients undergoing ICSI in which sperm were selected for injection on the basis of their birefringent properties (study group). The laboratory and clinical results were compared with those derived

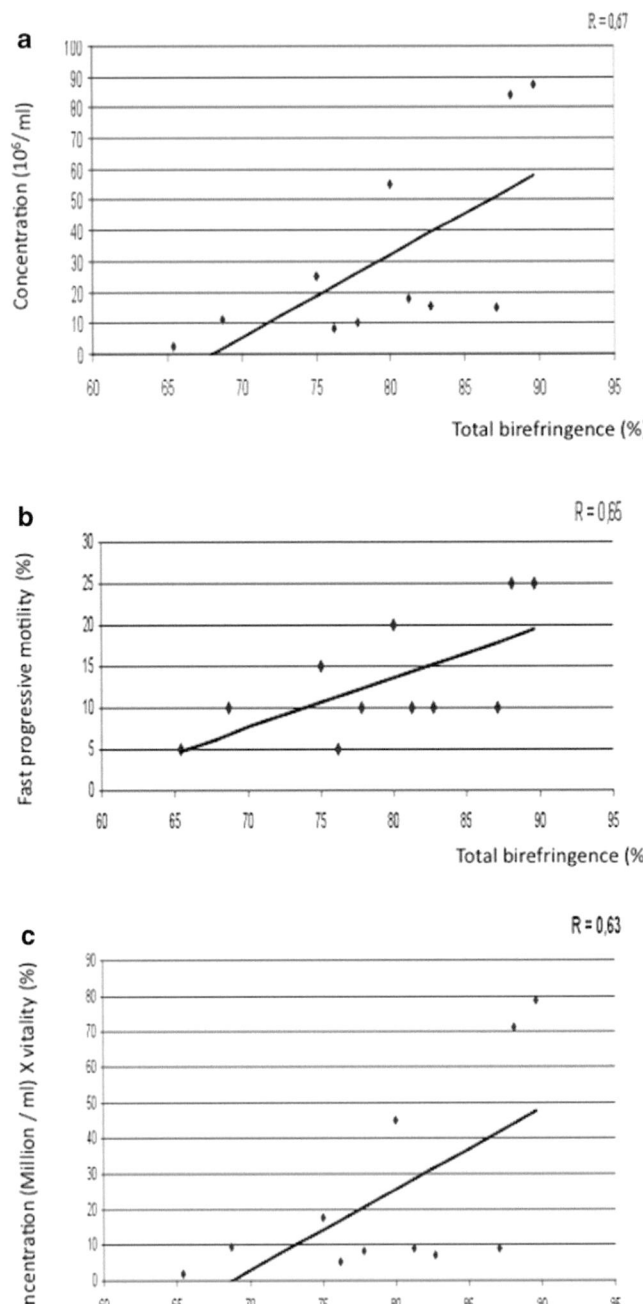

Fig. 10.2 Correlation between the proportion of birefringent spermatozoa and sperm sample parameters. The correlation was positive for sperm concentration (**a**), progressive motility (**b**) and vitality (**c**)

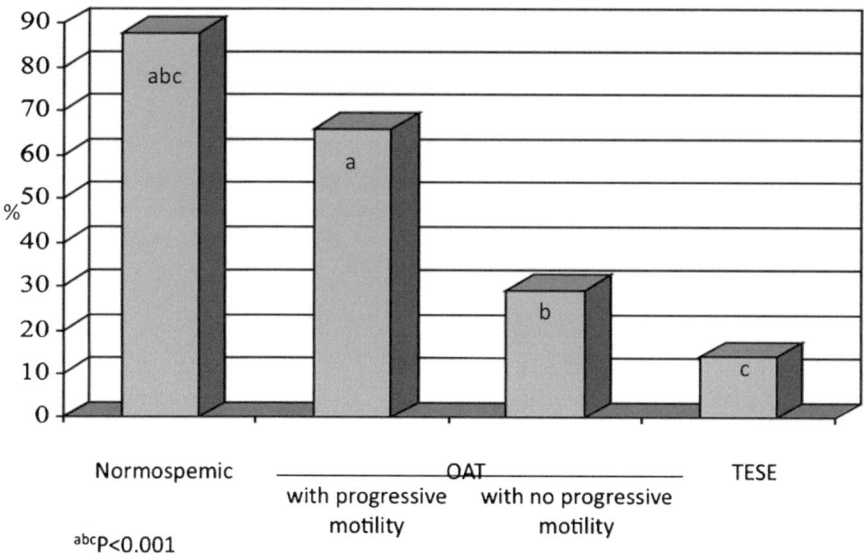

Fig. 10.3 Proportion of spermatozoa with birefringent head in the different sperm types

from 119 patients undergoing conventional ICSI (control group). All included cases presented with various sperm sample characteristics: normospermia, OAT with progressive motility, OAT without progressive motility and TESE, which were equally represented in the study and control group [15]. While fertilization and cleavage rates did not differ between the two groups, the ongoing pregnancy rate was significantly higher in the study group (23%) when compared to the controls (11%; $P < 0.025$) due to a higher incidence of abortions in the controls (41 vs. 16% in the study groups, $P = 0.035$). When analysed according to type of sperm sample, no significant differences appeared in the treatment of normospermic patients and in OAT cases having spermatozoa with progressive motility. Conversely, the ongoing clinical pregnancy rates and implantation rates were significantly increased in the study group compared to the controls in the most severe male factor condition (OAT with no progressive motility and TESE) (Fig. 10.4).

The conclusions of this study support the properties of birefringence as an important criterion for the selection of spermatozoa to be injected. This strategy could represent an accurate and novel method for an improved clinical outcome in patients with extremely severe male factor infertility and azoospermia for which testicular spermatozoa were used.

The use of the polscope has offered also the possibility, confirmed by TEM, to distinguish between spermatozoa that already underwent the acrosome reaction (Fig. 10.5) from those in which the acrosome is still intact (Fig. 10.1). According to a prospective randomization including 71 couples with severe male factor infertility, the polscope was used to select spermatozoa for ICSI based on the pattern of head birefringence. In all, reacted spermatozoa were injected into the oocytes from

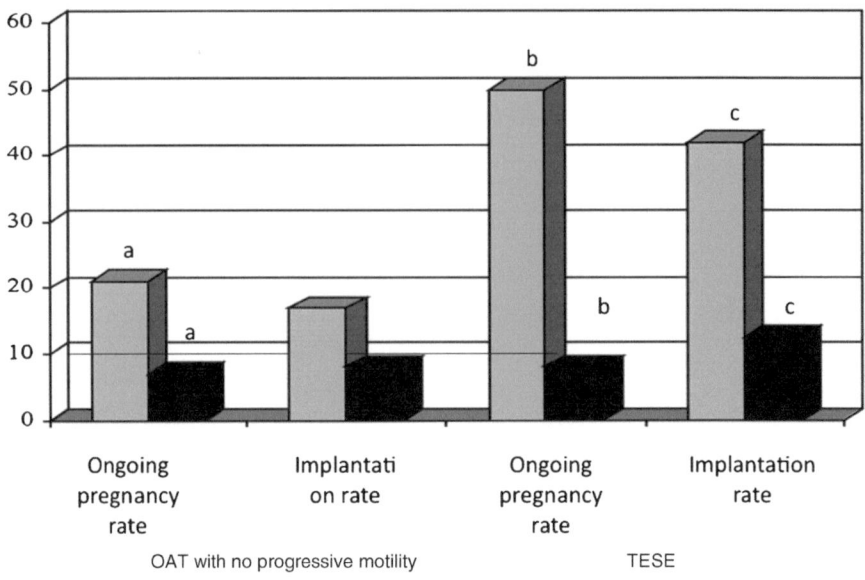

Fig. 10.4 Ongoing pregnancy rate per cycle and implantation rate in OAT patients with no progressive motility and in TESE patients. The study group corresponds to *grey bars* and the control group to *black bars*

[a] P=0.042
[b] P=0.02
[c] P=0.049

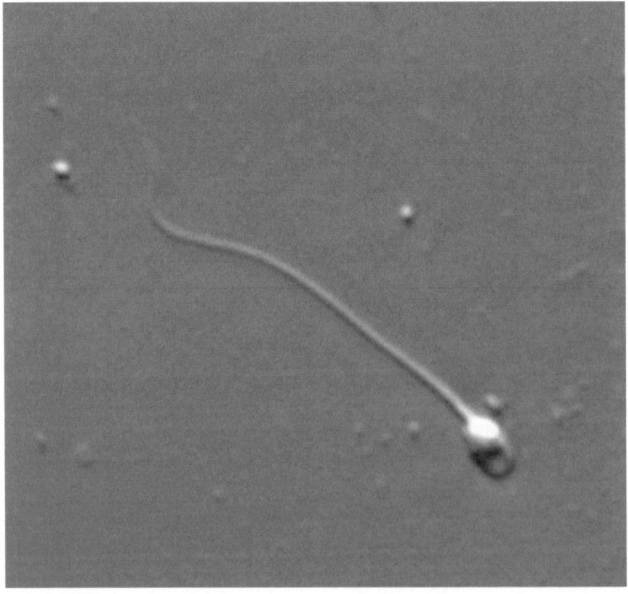

Fig. 10.5 The localization of birefringence in the postacrosomal region indicates that the acrosome is already reacted

23 patients, non-reacted spermatozoa were injected into 26 patients' oocytes, while in 22 patients, both reacted and non-reacted spermatozoa were injected [16]. There was no apparent effect on the fertilization and cleavage rates of either type of sperm, but a higher implantation rate resulted in the group of oocytes injected with reacted spermatozoa (39.0%) vs. those injected with non-reacted spermatozoa (8.6%, $P = 0.002$). In the group of patients in which the type of injected spermatozoa was mixed, the implantation rate (24.4%) was still superior to that detected in the group of non-reacted spermatozoa (8.6%, $P = 0.048$). Most importantly, the delivery rate per oocyte pick-up followed the same trend suggesting that the injection of reacted spermatozoa seems to have higher chances of generating viable embryos. Similar results have been confirmed by others [17].

Birefringence Analysis at High Magnification

In order to evaluate in more detail the morphology of sperm cells during ICSI, the polscope (Leica DMIRB, Leica Microsystem, Wetzlar, Germany) has been equipped with a PL Fluotar L63X objective, and the images are enhanced by digital imaging (Leica Microsystem). The use of the zoom connected to the camera provides a total magnification on the monitor screen between 2,500 and 5,500 × permitting to analyse the characteristics of birefringence in single spermatozoa by observing the corresponding images in real time on the computer screen. In addition, a dedicated software allows to measure sperm dimensions and particularly vacuolar area, providing an accurate classification of sperm morphology in fresh samples assisted by enhanced magnification (Fig. 10.6). In this way, sperm cells can be selected at the same time on the basis of their morphology and birefringence patterns. A recent study has revealed that 7% of motile spermatozoa with normal morphology possess abnormalities in their protoplasmic structure as revealed by the absence of head birefringence. This proportion increases significantly in morphologically abnormal spermatozoa and even more in immotile spermatozoa, where it is close to 40% [18].

Birefringence, Aneuploidy and DNA Integrity

Combining the study of sperm birefringence properties with the assessment of aneuploidy in the same sample, an inverse correlation was observed between the frequency of aneuploidy and the proportion of birefringent spermatozoa [19]. As a result, the selection of birefringent spermatozoa increases the chances of identifying a sperm cell having a normal chromosomal complement. Furthermore, it was found that the proportion of sperm head birefringent spermatozoa is inversely correlated to the incidence of fragmented DNA, suggesting that the selection of birefringent spermatozoa also increases the chances of identifying a vital sperm cell having an

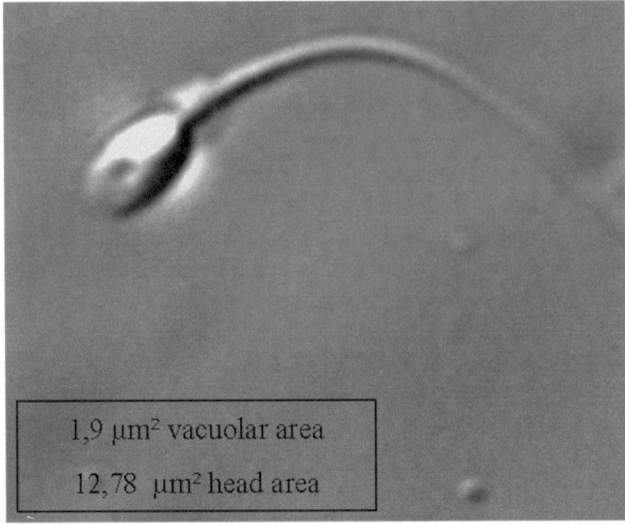

Fig. 10.6 The software allows to measure sperm dimensions and vacuolar area. Therefore, birefringence characteristics and morphology at high magnification are evaluated at the same time

intact DNA strand [20]. Therefore, performing ICSI under a polarizing lens minimizes the risk of selecting spermatozoa having DNA fragmentation as well as an aneuploid condition. These observations could be another reason for the favourable clinical outcome associated to the use of the polscope for sperm selection in severe cases of male infertility.

Conclusions

In a time in which the severe male factor affects at least 50% of infertile couples and ICSI is becoming more and more necessary, refining the selection criteria that help identifying the fertilizing spermatozoon might substantially contribute to the establishment of a healthy pregnancy. The properties of birefringence in the sperm head seem to represent a novel approach aimed at maximizing the viability of the resulting embryos. The clinical data reported are promising and support further application of this strategy.

References

1. Van Assche EV, Bounduelle M, Tournaye H, Joris H, Verheyen A, Devroey P, Van Steirteghem A, Libaers I. Cytogenetics of infertile men. Hum Reprod. 1996;11:1–26.
2. Yoshida A, Miura K, Shirai M. Chromosome abnormalities and male infertility. Assist Reprod Rev. 1996;67:93–9.

3. Egozcue S, Blanco J, Vendrell JM, Gracia F, Veiga A, Aran B, Barri PN, Vidal F, Egozcue J. Human male infertility: chromosome anomalies, meiotic disorder, abnormal spermatozoa and recurrent abortion. Hum Reprod Update. 2000;6:93–105.
4. Bernardini LM, Costa M, Bottazzi C, Gianaroli L, Magli MC, Venturini PL, Francioso R, Conte N, Ragni N. Sperm aneuploidy and recurrent pregnancy loss. Reprod Biomed Online. 2004;9:312–20.
5. Bernardini LM, Calogero AE, Bottazzi C, Lanteri S, Venturini PL, Burello N, De Palma A, Conte N, Ragni N. Low total normal motile count values are associated with increased sperm disomy and diploidy retes in infertile patients. Int J Androl. 2005;28:328–36.
6. Koehler KE, Hawley RS, Sherman S, Hassold T. Recombination and non-disjunction in humans and flies. Hum Mol Genet. 1996;5:1495–504.
7. Sathananthan AH, Kola I, Osborne J, Trounson A, Ng SC, Bongso A, Ratnam SS. Centrioles in the beginning of human development. Proc Natl Acad Sci U S A. 1991;88:4806–910.
8. Palermo G, Munné S, Cohen J. The human zygote inherits its mitotic potential from the male gamete. Hum Reprod. 1994;9:1220–5.
9. Silber S, Escudero T, Lenahan K, Abdelhadi I, Kilani Z, Munné S. Chromosomal abnormalities in embryos derived from testicular sperm extraction. Fertil Steril. 2003;79:30–8.
10. Bartoov B, Berkovitz A, Eltes F, Kogosowski A, Menezo Y, Barak Y. Real-time fine morphology of motile human sperm cells is associated with IVF-ICSI outcome. J Androl. 2002;23:1–8.
11. Calogero AE, Burrello N, De Palma A, Barone N, D'Agata R, Vicari E. Sperm aneuploidy in infertile men. Reprod Biomed Online. 2003;6:310–7.
12. Gianaroli L, Magli MC, Cavallini G, Crippa A, Nadalini M, Bernardini L, Menchini-Fabris GF, Voliani S, Ferraretti AP. Frequency of aneuploidy in spermatozoa from patients with extremely severe male factor infertility. Hum Reprod. 2005;20: 2140–52.
13. Gianaroli L, Magli MC, Ferraretti AP. Sperm and blastomere aneuploidy detection in reproductive genetics and medicine. J Histochem Cytochem. 2005;53:261–8.
14. Baccetti B. Microscopical advances in assisted reproduction. J Submicrosc Cytol Pathol. 2004;36:333–9.
15. Gianaroli L, Magli MC, Collodel G, Moretti E, Ferraretti AP, Baccetti B. Sperm head's birefringence: a new criterion for sperm selection. Fertil Steril. 2008;90:104–12.
16. Gianaroli L, Magli MC, Ferraretti AP, Crippa A, Lappi M, Capitani S, Baccetti B. Birefringence characteristics in sperm heads allow for the selection of reacted spermatozoa for intracytoplasmic sperm injection. Fertil Steril. 2010;93:807–13.
17. Chattopadhyay R, Ghosh S, Goswami SK, Goswami M. Selection of birefringent sperm head under polscope and its effect on outcome of ICSI in azoospermia and complete asthenozoospermia. Hum Reprod. 2009;24 Suppl 1:i71.
18. Boudjema E, Magli MC, Crippa A, Baccetti B, Ferraretti AP, Gianaroli L. Correlation between sperm morphology and birefringence properties in human spermatozoa: implications for sperm selection at ICSI. Hum Reprod. 2009;24 Suppl 1:i72.
19. Crippa A, Gianaroli L, Ferraretti AP, Baccetti B, Cetera C, Magli MC. Chromosomal status and characteristics of birefringence in sperm cell heads. Hum Reprod. 2008;23 Suppl 1:i112.
20. Crippa A, Magli MC, Paviglianiti B, Boudjema E, Ferraretti AP, Gianaroli L. DNA fragmentation and characteristics of birefringence in human sperm head. Hum Reprod. 2009;24 Suppl 1:i95.

Part III
Micromanipulators and Micromanipulation

Chapter 11
Hydraulic Manipulators for ICSI

Hubert Joris

Micromanipulation of cells started more than a century ago. Already in 1859, a description of some kind of microdissector has been made. The first studies on combined micromanipulation of oocytes and embryos appeared around 100 years later. Research on early events of fertilization was the main reason for these studies. In this 100 years between the first description of micromanipulation and the use of this technique for the study of fertilization events, the technologic evolution changed our society completely also improving conditions for such research.

Medical treatments did benefit a lot from scientific progress. Helping infertile couples to conceive was also part of this progress. The birth of Louise Brown in 1978 has been a milestone that changed the world of assisted reproductive technology (ART). The use of IVF evolved rapidly from treatment of female infertility to treatment of male infertility. However, it was obvious that the number, motility, and morphology of the spermatozoa present in the ejaculate largely affected the success rates of IVF. The idea to assist fertilization by bringing sperm cells closer to the egg vestments was already studied in animals in the early 60s. These techniques have been evaluated and used in humans to assist the fertilization process. This evolution is the subject of other chapters in this book. However, for these studies, the instruments developed over the years to study and manipulate different types of cells showed to be very valuable to manipulate gametes.

Different types of manipulators have been developed and used. The main purpose of this equipment is to bring movements from a macroscale to a microscale without affecting the viability of the material worked with. To transfer the movement from a macroscale to a microscale can be done in different ways. This can be done mechanically, hydraulically, and electronically. The use of mechanical and electronic manipulators and their use in ART is subject of different chapters.

H. Joris (✉)
Vitrolife Sweden AB, Göteborg, Sweden
e-mail: HJoris@vitrolife.com

At UZ Brussel, research on assisted fertilization started in the late 1980s aiming for the establishment of a clinical-assisted fertilization program. Assisted fertilization by subzonal insemination (SUZI) in the mouse was successful and demonstrated a correlation between the level of acrosome-reacted sperm cells and fertilization after insertion of a single spermatozoon under the zona pellucida [1]. Micromanipulation of gametes was initially performed with mechanical manipulators (Leica, Wetzlar, Germany). After careful evaluation of different possibilities, they were replaced by a combination of electrical and hydraulic manipulators (Narishige, Japan). This micromanipulation system was used at the start of the clinical-assisted fertilization program. The initial clinical experience by SUZI [2] was soon followed by the first report on intracytoplasmic sperm injection (ICSI) pregnancies [3]. The combination of electrical and hydraulic manipulators showed to be a very successful combination. The aim of this chapter is to describe more in detail the function and characteristics of this micromanipulation system for the ICSI procedure.

Mounting Micromanipulation Systems on Microscopes

Manipulation of cells smaller than what can be observed by the human eye requires the use of microscopes magnifying the cells to a level allowing proper observation of its characteristics. Manipulation of these cells requires a system that allows a firm, steady movement that successfully executes the required action without damaging the biological material submitted to the manipulations. To visualize human oocytes to a level where morphological details can be observed, a magnification of 200× to 400× is very common. Sperm cells are much smaller, and details cannot easily be observed at that magnification. Movement of tools small enough to manipulate these cells without vibration requires a very steady and firm system. Independent of the way micromanipulators are driven, they need to be mounted so that vibration is minimal. Depending on the microscope available and the choice of the micromanipulation system, manipulators are built on the microscope, on the microscope table or placed next to the microscope. These mounting systems allow a very steady positioning of the manipulators but do not necessarily avoid vibration. Several possibilities of equipment absorbing vibration are available and can be installed at different levels. This can be under the table, under the table surface, or directly under the microscope. However, such antivibration systems have a limited capacity, and certain vibrations will not be absorbed. Avoiding vibration is an important aspect to consider when establishing a new laboratory or when installing a new micromanipulation system.

Micromanipulation System

Micromanipulators transfer movements from the macrolevel to the microlevel scale. This involves a transition from a movement at the centimeter scale to a movement at the millimeter or micrometer scale. Movements executed with the control units

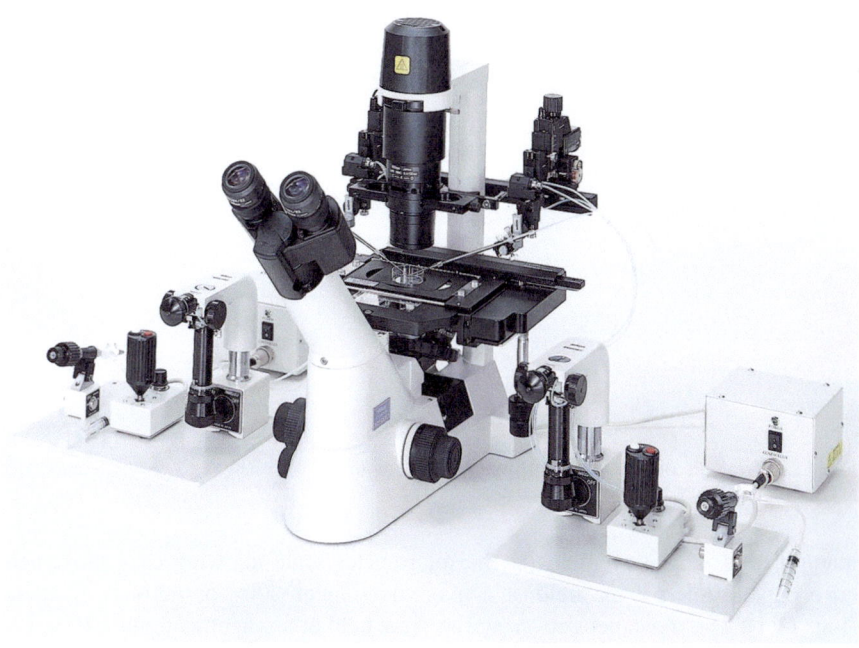

Fig. 11.1 Example of setup for ICSI with electrical coarse manipulators and hydraulic manipulators for fine movements (courtesy of Nikon, Melville, NY, USA)

are transferred to the drive units on which tools or tool holders are mounted. For IVF purposes, cells are manipulated by glass tools mounted in a holder, which is then fixed on the drive unit of the manipulator. These tools are usually made from borosilicate glass capillaries. Using a pipette puller, microforge and if required a grinder allows production of microtools with specific characteristics.

For ICSI purposes, a holding and injection pipette is required. Commercially available products are used mostly nowadays. The micropipettes are fixed in the holder, and the holder is mounted on the universal joint of the drive unit. Before the actual manipulation can start, the tools have to be positioned and aligned allowing easy manipulation procedures. The position of the tools before starting the alignment can be considered the *starting position*. Practically, it is important that tools can easily return to their starting position, e.g., when dishes are replaced. For this purpose, course manipulators are used. These allow easy movements at the centimeter scale that can be driven mechanically or electrically. Details of the alignment procedure using this manipulator system are described later.

Probably, the most commonly used set of micromanipulators for ICSI is from Narishige. These micromanipulators were initially developed for research purposes and are still commonly used in different areas of research [4]. Different types of manipulators have different ranges in their movements and are used for different applications. As such a system had proven to be successful for ICSI [5, 6], it has been introduced in many IVF clinics all over the world. For use in IVF, a combination of coarse manipulators allowing movements in the centimeter range and fine

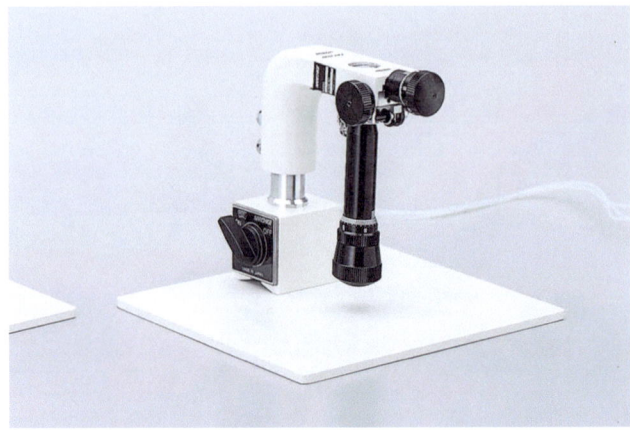

Fig. 11.2 Example of control unit of hydraulic manipulator with hanging joystick (courtesy of Nikon, Melville, NY, USA)

manipulators with movements at the micrometer scale allowing easy movement covering the microscope field at a magnification of 200× or 400× is adequate (Fig. 11.1). The movement covering the view field at a magnification of 400× is a movement of around 500 µm.

The coarse manipulators allow movements at the centimeter scale. These movements can be driven mechanically or electrically. A possible advantage of a mechanical system is presence of less electrical cables in the laboratory, but it requires significant movements with the arms each time these manipulators are used. The major advantage of the electrical coarse control manipulator is the presence of the joystick next to the microscope. This allows performance of all different manipulation steps within reach and without losing visual control over the biological material visible under the microscope.

Hydraulic Micromanipulators

Besides the coarse manipulator, a manipulator for fine movements is required. This manipulator is the most important one. The combination presented here uses a hydraulic micromanipulator for fine movements. Similar to the electrical manipulator, a major advantage of such a manipulator is that the joystick can be placed close to the microscope and next to other joystick(s) or injector(s) avoiding excessive movements during the manipulation procedures. The hydraulic manipulator exists of two main parts, namely the control unit and the drive unit. The control unit (Fig. 11.2) is placed close to the microscope. Its base consists of a magnetic stand, and it is usually fixed on a metal plate by the magnetic switch. In this way, it remains steadily in the same position and allows easy maneuvering of the joystick. The parts of the control unit used during the manipulations are the joystick allowing movements in two dimensions and the three rotating knobs each allowing movement in one

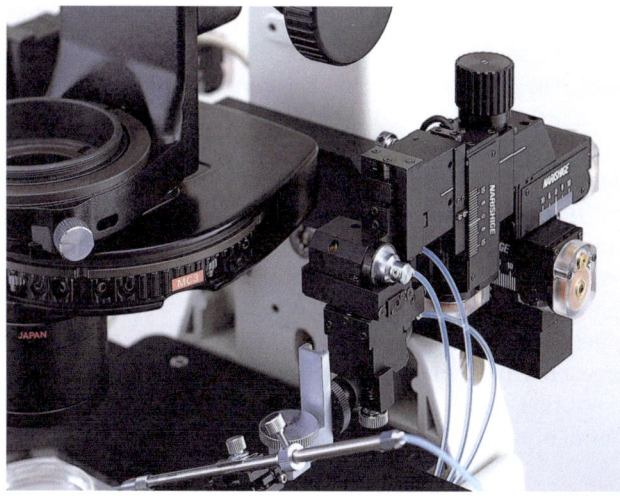

Fig. 11.3 Example of drive unit of hydraulic manipulator (connected to control unit by tubing) mounted on electrical coarse control manipulator and universal joint for mounting of the tool holder (courtesy of Nikon, Melville, NY, USA)

dimension. One of the rotating knobs is positioned at the end of the joystick. The two other rotating knobs are positioned above the joystick. The three rotating knobs can be rotated over a certain range. At the 0 level, there is no hydraulic pressure from the system on the moving parts. Rotation of each of the knobs creates movement in one axis. The length of the movement caused by one complete rotation of the knob depends on the characteristics of the manipulator used. Manipulations can be performed using the rotating knobs individually. However, the major advantage of the manipulator used here is that movements in three dimensions can be controlled simultaneously by using the joystick and the rotating knob at the end of the joystick simultaneously. The amplitude of the joystick movement during the manipulations can be regulated using the *movement ratio adjustment ring*. The sensitivity of the movement can be regulated with the *tension adjustment ring*. This three-dimensional movement is an important feature during the different steps of the manipulation procedures performed on human oocytes, embryos, or sperm cells.

The joystick can be in a hanging or upright position. In the early 1990s, the hanging joystick could be used only in combination with Nikon microscopes. Later on, this has been changed. Hanging joysticks are now available for different brands of microscopes. Compared to the joystick in an upright position, the hanging joystick gives important advantages when it comes to ergonomics. Since the embryologist may spend hours at the microscope, this is an important aspect. A hanging joystick allows maintaining the hands at the same level when switching between the electrical course manipulator, the hydraulic manipulator, and the injector and allows supporting with the wrist on the table while working with the hydraulic manipulator.

The second part of the hydraulic manipulator is the drive unit (Fig. 11.3). This is mounted on the course manipulator and connected with the control unit by three tubings filled with oil. The tool holder can be fixed in the universal joint that is mounted in the drive unit. As such, movement of the drive unit is transferred directly to the microtool. The movement of the knobs or the joystick creates pressure, and this pressure is transferred by the oil to the moving parts of the drive unit. The pressure created results in an immediate response and causes movement of the drive unit that is in proportion to the amplitude and speed executed on the joystick and/or rotating knobs. It is this movement that is the most crucial in the manipulation process. This direct and proportional transfer of movement performed at the control unit and delivered to the drive unit gives a perception of direct control. This is a very important feeling giving confidence to the operator.

Adjusting the amplitude by the ratio adjustment ring to cover the complete view field at the largest magnification ICSI that is performed at starting with the joystick in the neutral position creates a very comfortable working area and allows continuous visual control of the tools during the manipulation steps.

Alignment of Microtools

Proper positioning and alignment of the microtools before starting the injection procedure is crucial for successful ICSI. Although ICSI is considered a routine procedure, it still occurs that micromanipulators are not used optimally and tools are positioned in a way that this can affect results. Like certain knowledge about the use and adjustment of CO_2 incubators is required for control of proper functioning during culture, certain minimal knowledge about the characteristics and possibilities of the manipulators is necessary.

Considering the possibilities this equipment has, there is not just one-way positioning and alignment that is performed correctly. The procedure described hereafter is a procedure used during the many years worked in the IVF lab of UZ Brussel.

Before starting the procedure, it is safe to check that both the coarse and the fine manipulator are more or less in a central position. This avoids a procedure that has to be interrupted during the ICSI procedure because one of the manipulators reached the limit of its movement possibility in one of the different directions. The procedure then starts with mounting ICSI and holding pipette in the tool holder and fixing the tool holder on the universal joint. Holding and injection pipette are placed on the left hand side and right hand side, respectively. The tubings connecting the tool holder with the injector as well as the ones between the control unit and the drive unit of the hydraulic manipulator should be free and without any excessive bending that can possibly interfere with correct transfer of the command to the manipulator or microtool.

The design of the universal joint allows positioning of the tool holder in numerous different positions (Fig. 11.3). The older version of the universal joint had two changeable parts while more recent types have three different parts that can be moved or rotated. As this material was not designed for IVF purposes only, movement in a large spectrum was necessary. However, if ICSI is the only procedure

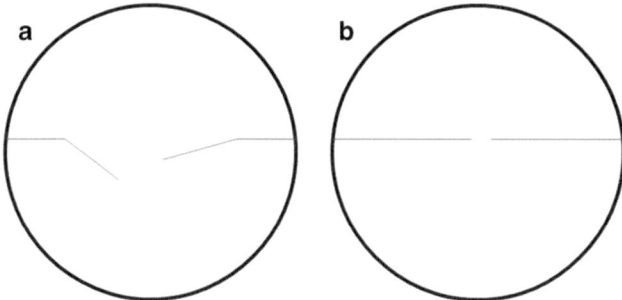

Fig. 11.4 Top view of microtools before initial alignment (**a**) and after initial alignment (**b**). Holding pipette on the left hand side, injection pipette on the right hand side

performed, limited adjustments are required once a more or less optimal position is established. Although produced under strictly controlled conditions, individual microtools may vary slightly for certain characteristics requiring different settings of the universal joint.

Once the holders are fixed in the universal joint, the tip of the microtool can be moved in the light beam of the microscope. The moving and rotating parts of the universal joint may be used for this if required. Depending on the type of microscope used, it may be useful to do this initial positioning (start position) high enough above the microscope stage allowing dishes to be removed and placed under the microtools easily. More recent models of microscopes have a tilting arm on which the manipulators are mounted. By tilting the arm, the complete manipulation system is lifted. This facilitates movements with dishes when microtools are mounted.

For all manipulations related to IVF applications, microtools with similar basic characteristics are used meaning that capillaries with a diameter of around 1 mm are formed into tools with different specifications. In the vast majority of the cases, tools are shaped so that the end part of the glass needle is bent to an angle of between 20 and 40°. This allows easy positioning of the microtools with the final bent part being positioned almost horizontally once fixed on the universal joint.

Once the two needles are brought in the light beam of the microscope, positioning and alignment controlled via the image in the microscope starts. Easiest is to start these steps using the objective with the lowest magnification (often 4×). Without changing the view plane, using the coarse manipulators, the microtools are lowered until they reach the plane where they can be seen clearly (Fig. 11.4a). If required, by rotation of the tool holder, the microtools are rotated until the bent part is positioned in a line going from the 3 o'clock to the 9 o'clock position. Both needles are moved to the center of the image. An ideal alignment brings both microtools in one straight line from the 3 o'clock to the 9 o'clock position (Fig. 11.4b). Further detailed positioning is performed after changing the objective stepwise to 10×, 20× and finally 40×. Whether the bent part is placed horizontal or deviates from the optimal position (Fig. 11.5) is not always that clear in this image for less experienced operators. When placing the microtools in a medium droplet of

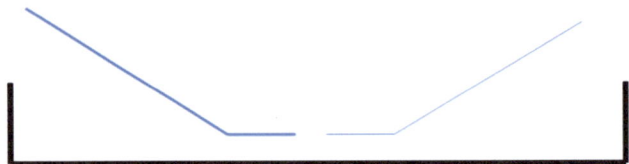

Fig. 11.5 Correct position of microtools at the start of the ICSI procedure. The bent tip is positioned horizontally

a dish, this can be seen more easily. This positioning is performed by using the coarse manipulators for the large movements and the hydraulic manipulators for the fine movements. When using only the rotation knobs of the hydraulic manipulator during these steps, the joystick remains in the neutral position allowing optimal movement ratio once working at larger magnification.

The way the drive unit and universal joint are constructed and mounted allows positioning of the tool holder in almost unlimited different ways. As mentioned before, slight variation in the angle of individual microtools may require adjustment of the angle for an optimal injection procedure. It is at this stage that modification of the position of the tool holder can easily be performed. After having lifted the tool holders to the starting position, one can easily modify the angle of the tool holder and bring the bent part in a more favorable position. Correct adjustment to place the tools in an optimal position will allow an easy procedure and plays a role in the success rates obtained. In the early days of ICSI, these changes were made by using the different possibilities of the universal joint and required some extra manipulation. Nowadays, improvements of the universal joint allow fine changes in certain axes by simply turning a small screw on the universal joint without additional manipulation of the tool holder (Fig. 11.6).

Ideally, the bent part of the microtools should be in an almost completely horizontal position after alignment (Fig. 11.5). Incorrect positioning of the microtools will affect the manipulation process and can result in positions as shown in Fig. 11.7. Touching the bottom of the dish with the tip of the pipette is not possible when the needle is placed as shown in Fig. 11.7, number 2. This results in difficulties fixing the oocyte when it is the case for the holding pipette or does not allow aspiration of a sperm cell from the bottom of the dish nor to immobilize a sperm cell with the tip of the needle in case the injection pipette is positioned in this way. In cases where the tip is placed as shown in Fig. 11.7, number 3, one may not have sufficient support of the holding pipette during the penetration of the ICSI pipette in case it is the holding pipette that is placed like this, or one may not make a straightforward movement when injecting a sperm cell into the oocyte. If a tip is aligned as shown in position 3, only the very end of the tip is in focus while the rest of the pipette cannot be seen sharp in the same view plane. When working at the microscope, we have a two-dimensional image while working in three dimensions. Except for the changes in sharpness of the tools when looking at a certain view plane, deviation from the horizontal position of microtools is not visible. However, minimal trauma to the

11 Hydraulic Manipulators for ICSI

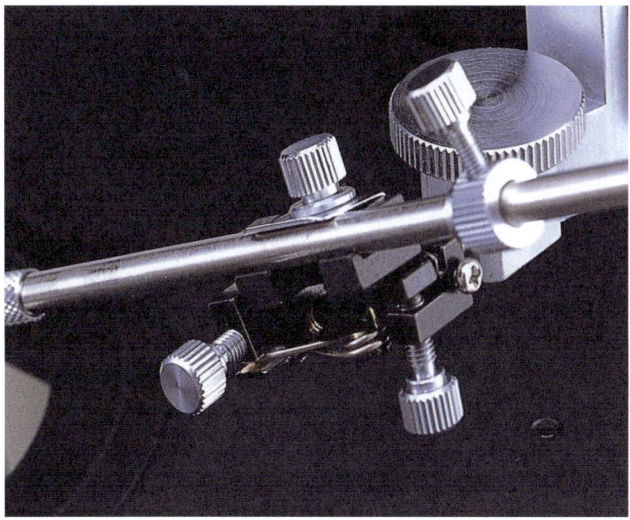

Fig. 11.6 Example of a more recent type of universal joint where changes in position can be made by simple rotation of screws with mounted tool holder (courtesy of Nikon, Melville, NY, USA)

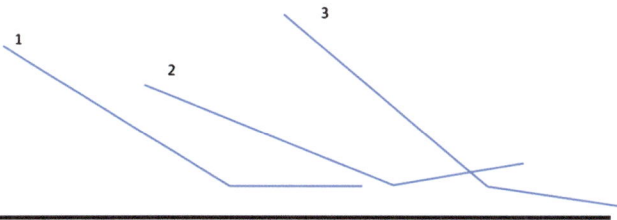

Fig. 11.7 Different positions of microtools. *1*: correct position; *2*: tip of the pipette cannot reach bottom of the dish; *3*: only the very end of the tip touches the bottom of the dish

oocyte is created only if the tip of the injection pipette is horizontally. It may not be easy to quantify the effect of suboptimal positioning on the microtools. However, like for all other aspects of IVF, attention to details makes the difference. This is not different when it comes to ICSI. Once microtools are positioned correctly, the ICSI procedure can start.

As for any type of equipment used in the lab, the manipulation system requires maintenance. Maintenance of the moving parts using certain types of grease (performed by technicians trained by the company) results in continuous normal functioning of the manipulators. As the movement from the joystick to the drive unit is a hydraulic system, this part of the system may need to be changed but only after a very long time of use. It is the authors' experience that it took more than 10 years of intensive daily use until the pressure of the hydraulic system became insufficient, and reparation was required in one of the hydraulic manipulators. One can easily significantly increase the life span of the manipulator by turning the three rotating knobs to the 0 (zero) position at the end of each working day. This releases the pressure in the system.

In summary, hydraulic manipulators are usually only part of a complete micromanipulation system. The combination of mechanical or electrical coarse manipulators and hydraulic manipulators for fine movements is used extensively for IVF applications. The combination of the rotating joystick and the rotation knob that are driven together by hand allows easy three-dimensional movement. The hydraulic pressure results in a movement of the microtool that is in proportion to the amplitude and speed executed on the joystick. This gives a sensation of direct control over the manipulation. Furthermore, the way the manipulators and tool holder are designed offers a large scale of possibilities and allows easy adjustment to the type of tool used and kind of manipulation performed.

Acknowledgment The permission of Nikon to use pictures showing different manipulators is greatly acknowledged.

References

1. Palermo G, Van Steirteghem A. Enhancement of acrosome reaction and subzonal insemination of a single spermatozoon in mouse eggs. Mol Reprod Dev. 1991;30:339–45.
2. Palermo G, Joris H, Devroey P, et al. Induction of acrosome reaction in human spermatozoa used for subzonal insemination. Hum Reprod. 1992;7:248–54.
3. Palermo G, Joris H, Devroey P, et al. Pregnancies after intracytoplasmic injection of single spermatozoon into an oocyte. Lancet. 1992;340:17–8.
4. Company information about use of micromanipulation tools. http://narishige-group.com/profile/en/index.html. Accessed 10 June 2011.
5. Van Steirteghem AC, Liu J, Joris H, et al. Higher success rates by intracytoplasmic sperm injection than by subzonal insemination. Report of a second series of 300 consecutive treatment cycles. Hum Reprod. 1993;8:1055–60.
6. Van Steirteghem AC, Nagy Z, Joris H, et al. High fertilization and implantation rates after intracytoplasmic sperm injection. Hum Reprod. 1993;8:1061–66.

Chapter 12
Research Instruments Micromanipulators

Steven Fleming and Catherine Pretty

History and Overview

Company Foundation and Development

In response to the requirement for integrated circuit testing by microelectronic companies such as GEC, Research Instruments (RI) was established by Mike Lee and Vince Grispo in 1964. Following an approach by Dr Simon Fishel during the 1980s, RI adapted their product output in order to meet the needs of assisted reproduction practitioners attempting to perfect new techniques for male factor infertility, such as partial zona dissection (PZD) and sub-zonal insemination (SUZI).

Instrumentation Principles

The earliest purely mechanical micromanipulators manufactured by RI, such as the TCV500 that was released in 1964, featured individual levers with three axes of movement and movement reduction from 100:1 to 500:1. The TLO500 was introduced in the 1980s, incorporating flexural hinges in order to improve stability and reliability. The subsequent development of the classic TDU500 enabled

---

S. Fleming, BSc (Hons), MSc, PhD (✉)
Assisted Conception Australia, Greenslopes Private Hospital, Brisbane, QLD 4120, Australia
e-mail: Steven.fleming@acaivf.com.au

C. Pretty, PhD
Assisted Conception Services, Nuffield Health Woking Hospital, Woking, Surrey, UK

mounting onto an inverted microscope and extremely ergonomic manipulation. Accessory instrumentation, including the *Sonic Sword*, was also introduced at this time to facilitate penetration of the *zona pellucida* (ZP), primarily for the SUZI technique.

In the early 1990s, following the successful application of intracytoplasmic sperm injection (ICSI) to the human [1], RI modified their micromanipulators to introduce a number of useful features. The first of these allowed rapid raising and lowering of micromanipulators, avoiding accidental damage to the micropipettes and, therefore, was referred to as a *home function*. An innovative feature, a laser-guided setting up device (LASU) launched in 1994, facilitated correct alignment of micropipettes. Another of the features added during the 1990s were tool holder angle adjustment indicators for more accurate alignment of a range of micropipettes with various known degrees of bend between the tip and the shank.

Precisely controlled heated plates were integrated into the mechanical stage in 1999, culminating in a major modification of the TDU500, known as the *Integra*. RI introduced semicircular handrests to further improve ergonomics. The current version of the Integra is known as the IntegraTi as it was originally manufactured using titanium for the microscope stage plate. It incorporates a mechanical stage, TDU5000 micromanipulators, touch-screen four-channel independent control of heated plates, a one-touch *home* function, one-touch micropipette angle adjustment and a unique touch-screen digital help menu (Fig. 12.1).

Consistent with original company policy, the TDU5000 micromanipulators remain purely mechanical and are directly controlled, the joysticks providing proportional movement. This policy is based upon the principles that direct proportional movement provides greater control and that simple mechanical components are ready to use, are more reliable and are less likely to require routine servicing and maintenance.

Installation and Set-Up of the IntegraTi™

Installation of the IntegraTi is extremely simple, quick and straightforward as the system comes largely pre-assembled in a purpose-built dispatch case. However, it is still necessary to exercise some care when removing the Integra from its dispatch case in order to avoid potential damage to the micromanipulator mechanism from any inadvertent severe shock. An installation manual is available from RI in Adobe Acrobat format on the company's website (www.research-instruments.com). The IntegraTi can be adapted to a range of inverted microscopes supplied by the *big four* manufacturers, Leica, Nikon, Olympus and Zeiss using just four screws (Fig. 12.2).

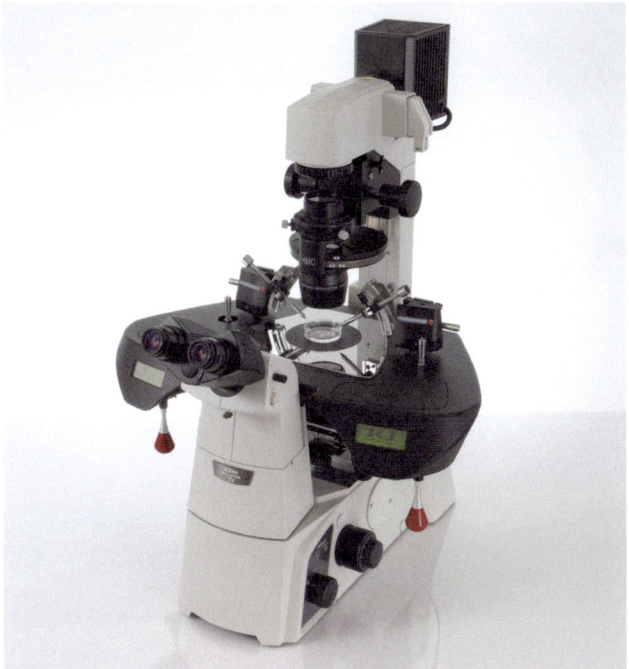

Fig. 12.1 The IntegraTi

Micromanipulators

The micromanipulators on the IntegraTi incorporate both fine and coarse controls in the one compact unit. Both fine and coarse control levers should be set to their vertical positions before making further adjustments. In common with the classic TDU500 micromanipulator, the joysticks of the TDU5000 also extend downwards but now from within the microscope stage of the Integra. Rotation of the fine control knob actuates up to 5 mm of movement within the z-axis, so, in order to avoid running out of travel mid-procedure, it is recommended to set its travel of movement at the midpoint prior to use.

Tool Holders, Micro-Tool Holders and Micropipettes

RI's PL30 tool holders are supplied with the IntegraTi and are calibrated and actuated using a single screw to enable accurate adjustment to a range of micropipette

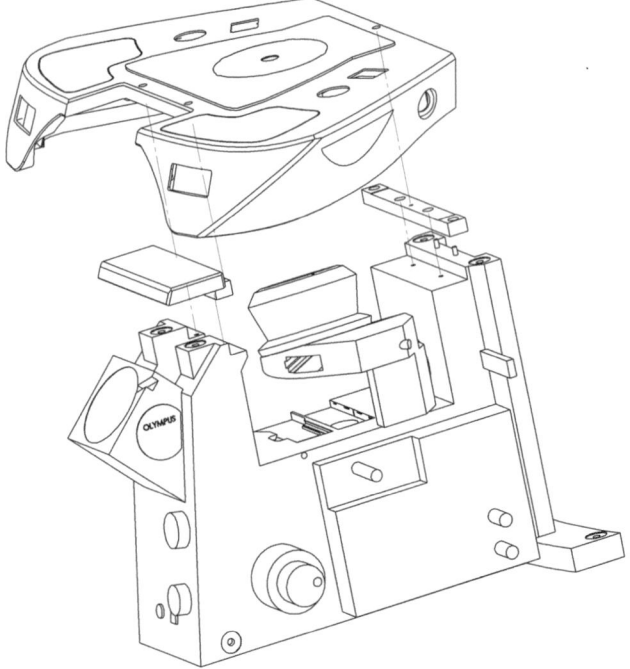

Fig. 12.2 Installation diagram for the IntegraTi to the Olympus IX71

bend angles, from 15 to 40° (Fig. 12.3). This is important to ensure an optimal angle at which a micropipette is employed respective to the procedure being undertaken so as to achieve effective manipulation while minimising shear stress. A unique feature of the PL30 tool holder is that the tip of the micropipette does not move when the angle is changed, allowing alterations of pipette angle to be made mid-procedure. Once the angle of the tool holder has been set to correspond to the bend angle of the micropipette to be used, RI's MPH micro-tool holders can be clipped into place onto the PL30 tool holders (Fig. 12.3). Once fitted to each other, vertical, axial and rotational movement of the micropipette is possible, allowing rapid set-up. When adjusted using an additional objective lens and spacer (supplied by RI), micropipettes can be aligned 14 mm above the microscope stage, minimising the likelihood of damage to them.

A one-off initial set-up of the tool holder is achieved as follows: A scratch is made on the inner surface of a Petri dish using a hypodermic needle, and the dish is placed onto the microscope stage of the IntegraTi. Using the ×4 objective lens, the scratch is brought into focus to establish the set focal length for tool holder set-up and is not adjusted further. A holding micropipette is fitted to the micro-tool holder, and with the vertical movement lever of the tool holder in the fully raised position, the objective lens is changed over to the RI ×4 objective lens with spacer which allows the micropipette to be brought into focus in this raised position. Check that

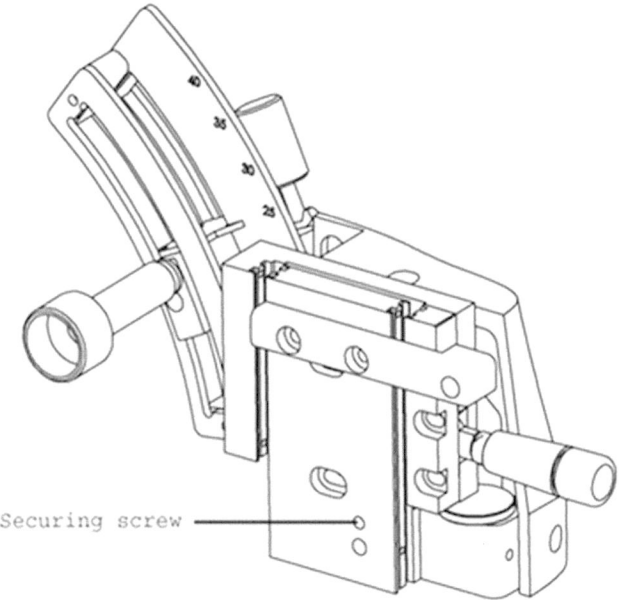

Fig. 12.3 PL30 tool holder

the micromanipulator is set to the middle of its vertical travel and that both fine and coarse control levers are positioned in their vertical axis. Drive the MPH micro-tool holder forward until the tip of the micropipette is directly above the objective lens. Rotate the micro-tool holder until the micropipette vertically bisects the objective light path, as viewed with the naked eye, and then tighten the bottom securing screw of the PL30 tool holder. This adjustment effectively sets the detent position of the micro-tool holder to its central position.

For routine micropipette set-up, next use the axial drive mechanism of the PL30 tool holder to position the micropipette within the centre of the field of view and rotate it axially using the rotating wheel at the distal end of the MPH micro-tool holder to obtain a perfectly vertical orientation of the micropipette—precise alignment is best achieved with the aid of the inverted microscope, viewing the micropipette using the ×4 or ×10 objective lens and using the fine control lever to bring its tip into focus. If necessary, move the ×4 objective lens back into place and fully lower the vertical lever on the PL30 tool holder—the scratch on the Petri dish should still be in focus. Because the micropipette is positioned slightly above the surface of the Petri dish, it will now appear slightly out of focus. If desired, the distance between the tip of the micropipette and the surface of the microinjection dish can be minimised by increasing the distance travelled when lowering the vertical lever on the PL30 tool holder. This adjustment is achieved using the small silver thumbwheel located on the side of the PL30 tool holder. These steps are repeated when setting up the injection, zona drilling or biopsy micropipette on the opposite side of the micromanipulation rig. As an optional extra for those wishing to biopsy

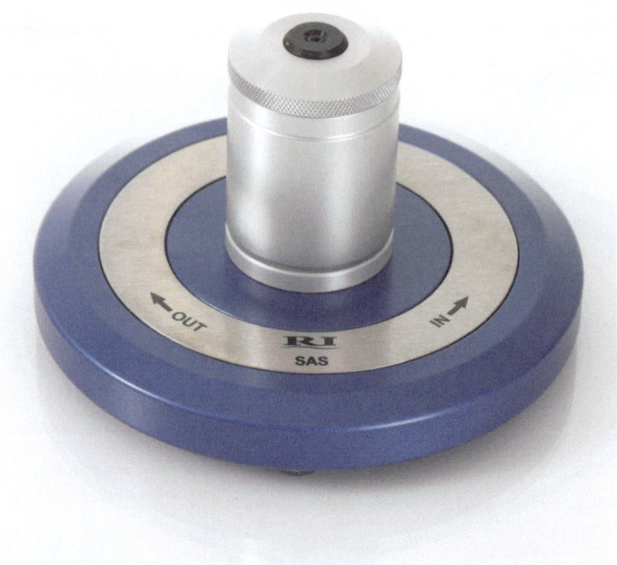

Fig. 12.4 SAS air injector with equilibration button

embryos for the purpose of pre-implantation genetic diagnosis (PGD), RI also supplies a double tool holder that enables independent movement of both micropipettes.

Microinjectors

The RI screw-actuated syringes (SAS) supplied as standard with the IntegraTi are air-assisted microinjectors that are sometimes referred to as *mushrooms* due to their design. By virtue of their heavy circular base, they are very stable, yet they occupy a relatively small footprint. With an extremely low dead space and a capacity of 10 mL, they can generate high aspiration and pressure. The SAS air injector also benefits from incorporating a pressure release button situated on top of the screw control that enables rapid equilibration of internal and external pressure (Fig. 12.4). This is particularly useful for stabilising capillary flow and for rapid cessation of aspiration pressure applied to rupture the oolemma during ICSI. An extra smooth chrome special edition of the SAS microinjector is available from RI as an optional extra. For those that prefer to use an oil microinjector, RI will supply a micrometre-actuated sealed oil syringe (SOS) mounted upon a sturdy, non-slip base.

The SAS microinjectors come supplied with hard polythene tubing for connecting them to the MPH micro-tool holders. It is a simple procedure to attach the tubing at one end to the metal nozzle underneath the SAS microinjector and, at the other end, to the proximal end of the MPH micro-tool holder. Once the tubing has been connected and a micropipette fitted to the MPH micro-tool holder, the micropipettes must be primed with media, and the SAS microinjectors equilibrated prior to use. For the holding micropipette, this procedure simply requires the micropipette to be lowered into a drop of micromanipulation medium and the SAS to be rotated slowly anticlockwise until media rushes in, at which point, the pressure release button can be pressed down in order to equilibrate the pressure inside and outside of the micropipette, thereby halting the influx of medium. Priming and equilibrating an injection micropipette is a slightly longer process. Firstly, the SAS needs to be rotated fully clockwise to its lowest position, and the pressure release button pressed. Secondly, the micropipette can be lowered into a drop of micromanipulation medium or a 7–10% polyvinylpyrrolidone (PVP) solution and the SAS rotated several turns anticlockwise, approximately 50% of its travel upwards. It may then be necessary to wait for up to 5 min in order for the media to be aspirated into the micropipette until it almost reaches the un-pulled shank. At this point, the pressure release button can be pressed down to ensure equilibration of the pressure and so prevent unwanted drift of media up or down the micropipette. For those using older SAS models that do not incorporate a pressure relief button, it is necessary to disconnect and reconnect the tubing at the SAS microinjector in order to achieve equilibration during priming of micropipettes.

Heated Stages

The IntegraTi incorporates an independent four-channel temperature control system that is accurately calibrated to within 0.05°C of the desired set point. One of these channels controls the temperature of the central metal insert in the microscope stage. As an optional upgrade, RI will supply a central glass heated stage. Two of these channels control two other heated stages, either side of the central insert, towards the front of the microscope stage. These have been designed for temperature maintenance of microinjection dishes additional to that being worked on at any given time, e.g. in those circumstances where it is necessary to have a testicular sperm prep in one dish and oocytes ready to be injected in another. The fourth channel can be used to control the temperature of an external heated plate or the heated stage of an adjacent stereo dissecting microscope. The four channels are controlled via a touch-screen panel incorporated into the IntegraTi (Fig. 12.1). Since the heated stages come already installed, no set-up other than adjustment of the temperature set points is necessary.

Mechanical Stages

On the IntegraTi, the standard mechanical stages of the *big four* microscope manufacturers have been replaced by a custom-designed built-in XY mechanical stage. It comes as standard and incorporates a stainless steel stage plate. Each turn of the stage control moves the stainless steel stage plate 28 mm in either the *X* or *Y* plane, with 40 mm full travel. Since the mechanical stage is supplied already fitted to the IntegraTi, no set-up is required.

Standard Applications

Zona Drilling and Assisted Hatching

Zona drilling is the technique of creating a hole in the ZP surrounding the oocyte or pre-implantation embryo, originally described in 1986 [2]. The most widely used application of zona drilling in assisted reproduction, termed *assisted hatching*, is based upon the assumption that the blastocyst will more readily *hatch* from the ZP if previously breached by drilling a hole or cutting a slit in it. A variety of factors, including excessive thickness of the ZP and zona hardening following embryo culture, were originally proposed as one cause of recurrent implantation failure, due to an inability of blastocysts to *hatch* [3]. Various means have been employed to achieve *assisted hatching* including the use of acids, enzymes and lasers to dissolve the ZP, no single method proving universally better than another [4]. It can be achieved by chemical means through controlled and directed application of acidified Tyrode's solution (pH 2.3–2.5) or pronase, using a drilling micropipette attached to a microinjector. For the flow of acidified or enzymatic media to be precisely controlled, a drilling micropipette should be fire-polished to an internal diameter of 5–10 μm, which is much smaller than the internal diameter of a holding micropipette. Contact and non-contact lasers, operating in either the ultraviolet or infrared spectrum, may also be applied to the ZP at a single point or at several adjacent points, depending upon the length of hole desired. Lasers dissolve the ZP by generating heat, so non-contact lasers, especially those operating within the infrared spectrum, are generally considered safer for use with human oocytes and embryos. Zona drilling has also been used for other applications such as fragment removal from early cleavage stage embryos and embryo biopsy for PGD.

Partial Zona Dissection

One of the earliest applications of zona *drilling* in the human, termed zona tearing or PZD, was to create a conduit for access to the oocyte by spermatozoa deemed incapable of binding to and penetrating the ZP [5, 6]. In this approach, micropipettes are employed to physically cut a slit-like hole in the ZP while holding the oocyte firmly onto a holding micropipette.

Sub-zonal Insemination

At around the same time that PZD was developed, the PZD technique was being combined with the use of large microinjection pipettes in order to introduce spermatozoa directly into the sub-zonal perivitelline space [7, 8]. Originally termed *microinjection sperm transfer* (MIST), the technique later became known as SUZI. Once the manufacture of fine, sharp microinjection pipettes had been perfected, PZD became redundant for the purposes of SUZI.

Intracytoplasmic Sperm Injection

The technique known as ICSI represents the ultimate evolution of experimental methods to alleviate male factor infertility, such as PZD and SUZI [1, 9]. The vastly superior efficiency of ICSI in achieving monospermic fertilisation of the oocyte resulted in its rapid replacement of the SUZI technique. Successful application of ICSI depends upon an appreciation that it must mimic the latter stages of fertilisation that occur in vivo [10]. As with gamete fusion, the sperm plasmalemma and oolemma have to be temporarily broken. Hence, the microinjection pipette should be set-up at such an angle that the sperm plasmalemma can be ruptured using the tip of the pipette, illustrated by a permanent kink in the sperm tail. Likewise, the tip of the microinjection pipette must be sharp enough that the oolemma ruptures when aspirated onto it using a microinjector, as evident by sudden free flow of ooplasm into the microinjection pipette. Modifications of ICSI, such as laser-assisted ICSI [11], could feasibly result in improvements to the technique, though their relative benefits and risks need to be considered further.

Oocyte, Embryo and Blastocyst Biopsy

Following zona drilling, cells can be removed from the oocyte, early cleavage embryo and blastocyst as biopsy material for the purpose of PGD, this technique having been pioneered soon after that of *assisted hatching* [12]. Since the majority of aneuploidies occur during oocyte maturation [13], the first polar body (PB) represents a useful source of material for PGD, so methods have been developed to perfect PB biopsy. However, since post-zygotic aneuploidy is also possible, although less common, blastomere biopsy of early cleavage embryos at the 8-cell stage has tended to be the approach preferred by those testing for sex-linked disease and other genetic mutations. More recently, partly because of the possibility of misdiagnosis due to mosaicism in the early cleavage stage embryo, trophectoderm biopsy of the blastocyst has assumed greater importance.

Biopsy micropipettes should have an internal diameter of 40–50 μm. If a laser is not available for zona drilling, it will be necessary to fit drilling and biopsy micropipettes to a double tool holder that allows rapid interchange between the two during a biopsy procedure. For the purposes of blastomere biopsy, the optimal size hole to be drilled in the ZP should be only just large enough to allow a biopsy micropipette to enter the perivitelline space. One or two blastomeres may be removed from a 7-cell or 8-cell embryo, two blastomeres providing greater control for the potential for a misdiagnosis. With trophectoderm biopsy of the blastocyst, a commonly applied method is to allow a small portion of trophectoderm to herniate from the ZP following zona drilling and then to use a laser to separate the extruded trophoblast.

Troubleshooting

Micromanipulators

If it proves impossible to bring the injection micropipette into focus at the surface of the microinjection dish, the most likely reason for this is that the angle of alignment of the micropipette is too obtuse, causing it to be *heel down* and pushing the pipette tip upwards and out of the microscope's focal range at high magnification. NB. Attempting to raise the focal plane will bend the micropipette further until it eventually snaps. The remedy for this problem is to lower the focal plane until the micropipette is clear of the surface of the microinjection dish and then use the angle compensation screw of the PL30 tool holder to adjust the pitch angle to a steeper position.

If the micropipette fails to move smoothly in either the X or Y planes, the most likely reason for this is that its tip is scraping along the surface of the microinjection dish, resulting in a juddering movement. This is simply remedied by raising the micropipette off the surface of the microinjection dish using the fine control lever of the micromanipulator. If there is no movement in the Z plane in response to rotation of the fine control lever of the micromanipulator, the most likely reason for this is that the control lever has reached the limit of its travel. This is simply remedied by resetting the fine control lever to its midpoint by rotating it in the opposite direction in order to free the locked movement. If the fine or coarse control levers are too stiff/loose, the most likely reason for this is that the ball joint is out of adjustment. The remedy for this is to loosen/tighten the screws in the plate that retains the ball joint in place using the appropriately sized hexagonal wrench supplied with the IntegraTi.

Microinjectors

Should it prove impossible to control the sperm's position within the injection micropipette, the most likely cause of this is incorrect priming and equilibration of the micropipette. In this event, it will be necessary to repeat the steps described above in the installation section on microinjectors.

Should there be drifting of the sperm's position following correct priming and equilibration of the injection micropipette, then the most likely cause of this is an air leak. In this case, check the tightness of both the MPH micro-tool holder and microinjector seals. If necessary, cut a 10 mm length off the end of the polythene tubing and reconnect it to create a fresh seal. If this fails to resolve the problem, remove the top of the SAS microinjector, replace the O-ring inside the barrel and lubricate the O-ring using the special lubricant supplied by RI.

Heated Stages

If the touch-screen display shows a '?' message, the most likely reason for this is a malfunction of one of the heated plates. There is no remedy for this, other than repair or replacement by RI.

References

1. Palermo G, Joris H, et al. Pregnancies after intracytoplasmic injection of single spermatozoon into an oocyte. Lancet. 1992;340:17–8.
2. Gordon JW, Talansky BE. Assisted fertilization by zona drilling: a mouse model for correction of oligospermia. J Exp Zool. 1986;239(3):347–54.
3. Cohen J, Elsner C, et al. Impairment of the hatching process following IVF in the human and improvement of implantation by assisting hatching using micromanipulation. Hum Reprod. 1990;5(1):7–13.
4. Balaban B, Urman B, et al. A comparison of four different techniques of assisted hatching. Hum Reprod. 2002;17(5):1239–43.
5. Cohen J, Malter H, et al. Implantation of embryos after partial opening of oocyte zona pellucida to facilitate sperm penetration. Lancet. 1988;2(8603):162.
6. Gordon JW, Grunfeld L, et al. Fertilization of human oocytes by sperm from infertile males after zona pellucida drilling. Fertil Steril. 1988;50(1):68–73.
7. Laws-King A, Trounson A, et al. Fertilization of human oocytes by microinjection of a single spermatozoon under the zona pellucida. Fertil Steril. 1987;48(4):637–42.
8. Ng SC, Bongso A, et al. Pregnancy after transfer of sperm under zona. Lancet. 1988;2(8614):790.
9. Lanzendorf SE, Maloney MK, et al. A preclinical evaluation of pronuclear formation by microinjection of human spermatozoa into human oocytes. Fertil Steril. 1988;49(5):835–42.
10. Fleming SD, King RS. Micromanipulation in assisted conception: a user's manual and troubleshooting guide. Cambridge: Cambridge University Press; 2003.
11. Abdelmassih S, Cardoso J, et al. Laser-assisted ICSI: a novel approach to obtain higher oocyte survival and embryo quality rates. Hum Reprod. 2002;17(10):2694–9.
12. Handyside AH, Kontogianni EH, et al. Pregnancies from biopsied human preimplantation embryos sexed by Y-specific DNA amplification. Nature. 1990;344(6268):768–70.
13. Hassold T, Hunt P. To err (meiotically) is human: the genesis of human aneuploidy. Nat Rev Genet. 2001;2(4):280–91.

Chapter 13
Eppendorf Micromanipulator: Setup and Operation of Electronic Micromanipulators

Ehab Abu-Marar and Safa Al-Hasani

History and Overview

In 1945 after World War II, two German scientists Dr. Hans Hinz and Dr. Heinrich Netheler founded a small company in Hamburg Eppendorf University Hospital. The demolition of the hospital and destruction of medical equipment during the war necessitated the founding of the company so that the physicians could repair broken devices and develop new ones. The workshop was established under the supervision of both scientists in order to return the hospital to a functioning state. The team succeeded in repairing many devices and invented new ones like Thermorapid and Eppendorf photometer. Since then, Eppendorf AG, Hamburg, Germany, has created many devices and tools which are now considered breakthroughs in the field of laboratory applications. The importance of micromanipulators appeared before assisted reproductive technology (ART) proved its effectiveness. In the 1960s, different groups were experimenting with fertility in animal models. Hiramoto found that microinjection of spermatozoa into unfertilized sea urchin oocytes did not induce activation of the oocyte or condensation of the sperm nucleus, whereas others demonstrated the opposite in frog oocytes. Ryuzo Yanagimachi and his group later demonstrated that isolated hamster nuclei could develop into pronuclei after microinjection into homologous eggs, and a similar result was obtained when freeze-dried human spermatozoa were injected into a hamster egg [1]. After the amazing success of ART, scientists began thinking about how to overcome the difficulties faced in fertilizing oocytes. At that time, conventional IVF gave unsatisfactory results.

E. Abu-Marar, MD (✉)
IVF Unit, Department of Obstetrics and Gynecology, University of Schleswig-Holstein,
Campus Lübeck, Schleswig-Holstein 23538 Lübeck, Germany
e-mail: ehababumarar@hotmail.com

S. Al-Hasani, DVM, PhD
IVF Unit, Frauenklinik, Lübeck Schleswig-Holstein, Germany

In those days, conventional IVF produced unsatisfactory results in a number of cases. In some of those cases the number of progressively motile spermatozoa with normal morphology was lower than the desired threshold and more assistance was needed for the spermatozoa to reach the ooplasma and for fertilization to take place.

All the efforts were aimed at embracing these cases of limited number of progressively motile sperm with normal morphology. That goal was attained after bypassing or penetrating the barriers which prevent the fertilization (like zona pellucida) and was achieved by partial zona dissection (PZD) and subzonal insemination (SUZI). After that, fertilization, pregnancy, and birth were reported [2–4]. Following these trials, intracytoplasmic sperm injection (ICSI) was adopted by many and showed its effectiveness in 1992 [5]. A micromanipulator's main usage in ART was for assisted fertilization, but many other procedures could be performed with it, especially operations requiring proportional movement like ICSI which became successful worldwide.

Description

Components

The Eppendorf micromanipulator (Fig. 13.1) is composed of three main components: motor module unit, control board, and main power supply.

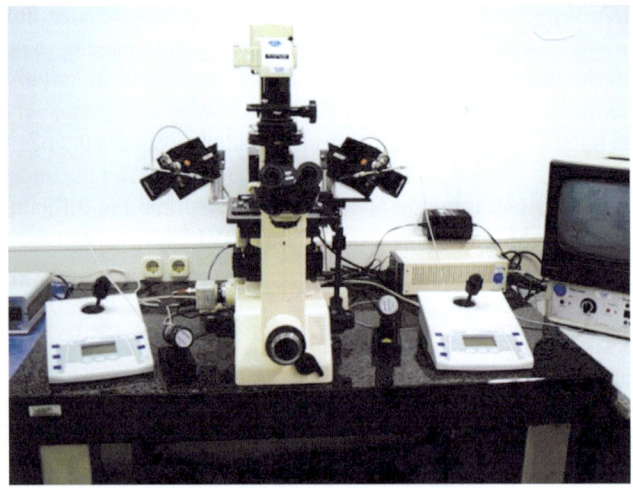

Fig. 13.1 The Eppendorf micromanipulator is composed of three main components: motor module unit, control board, and main power supply

Motor Module Unit

The motor module unit can be fixed on any microscope on any side, but for the best results, especially for ICSI procedures or any cell surgery, the motor modules are mounted via a microscope-specific adapter on both sides of the microscope.

The motor module consists of two main parts attached to each other through a wire and a straight guide fixed with a screw. One part is for Y and Z axis movements (Y/Z module) and the other one serves X axis movements (X module), and this part ends up with X head angle adjuster. Figure 13.2 shows a mounted motor module with attached capillary holder.

Control Board

The upper part of the control board contains:

- The joystick which enables the user to make horizontal and vertical movements in a proportional way and controls position and speed depending on the settings. The joystick can also be disabled by pressing and holding down the joystick top button. The position can be changed to another saved position by pressing the button twice, and clockwise and counterclockwise movements are available. One of the main advantages of the Eppendorf micromanipulator is that it is user friendly even for brand new users. It can save certain positions and limit pipette movements downward and can maintain the same surface level as the Petri dish. This feature is not found in other brands of micromanipulator and greatly reduces pipette breakage by inexperienced and experienced users.
- The display which illustrates the axis coordinates and the options chosen.

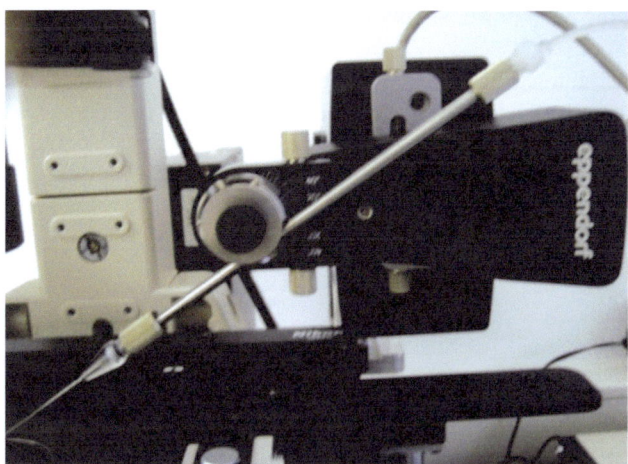

Fig. 13.2 Mounted motor module with attached capillary holder

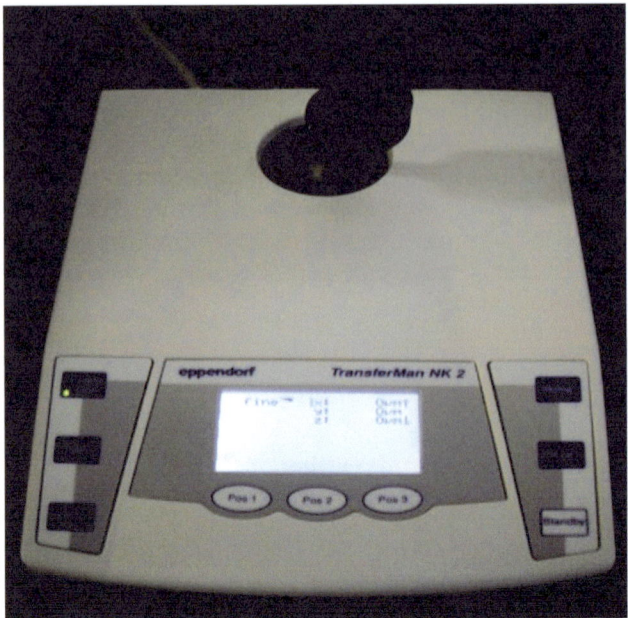

Fig. 13.3 Control board of Eppendorf micromanipulator

- The multifunctional keypad which gives the desired function when the button is pressed or released and allows multiple positions to be saved (Fig. 13.3).

  The control board which has a wheel for radius settings on one side.

  The underside of the control board which has the connector sockets for the module unit and the main power supply as well as the serial port and the connection for an optional foot switch.

  The home button which can save the last position while the user prepares for other functions like changing the Petri dish or preparing more oocytes without losing the last position.

ICSI Procedure

Preparation

Preparation for the ICSI procedure starts by proper selection of patients. Because of the high ICSI success rate, it is widely used even in patients who have not been thoroughly screened.

Here are some cases that we believe might benefit from the ICSI procedure:

- After recurrent failure of conventional IVF treatment, ICSI is advised especially in unexplained fertilization failure.
- In patients who undergo an oncology treatment, as ICSI might enhance the fertilization chances especially for patients having cryopreserved tissue.
- In cases of immunological factors impairing fertility.
- For PGD cases to prevent sperm contamination of the sample.
- For almost all cases of male sub- or infertility like oligozoospermia, cryptozoospermia, asthenozoospermia, teratozoospermia, globozoospermia, azoospermia, and cases of retrograde ejaculation, paraplegic patients after TESE, and CABVD where PESA, TESA, or TESE could be done.

After making sure that the necessary equipment and materials are available, it is important to make sure that the micromanipulator and the work station are ready as well.

Make sure that the work place is comfortable then check that the controls are functioning properly. One of the important advantages of the Eppendorf micromanipulator is that it offers the opportunity of saving in memory certain preferred positions so that they can be recalled at any time. For accurate results, you must make sure that there are no bubbles present. We recommend using a vibration-free work station, to enhance the reliable performance by protecting sensitive instruments and equipment from faulty operation or failure. The heating stage of the microscope should be assessed for suitable temperature before starting the procedure.

After oocyte retrieval, cumulus and corona cells should be dispersed by enzymatic and mechanical methods including incubation for 1 min in Sage medium with about 60 IU hyaluronidase/mL. Then aspiration of the cumulus-corona-oocyte complexes takes place with 250–300 and 200 μm opening pipette respectively. After that, all complexes should be transferred in a 5-mL Falcone tube with 1 mL preequilibrated Sage medium.

Oocyte rinsing comes next in Sage medium after observation under inverted microscope to check for germinal vesicles and polar body presence as well as zona pellucida assessment.

After this, we usually incubate the oocytes in 25 μm microdrops of Sage medium covered by mineral oil at 37°C in an atmosphere of 5% CO_2 in air, and then make the metaphase II oocytes selection for the ICSI procedure.

Semen analysis and selection is performed to make sure that a sufficient number of spermatozoa are available for the ICSI procedure. Ejaculated sperm preparation involves seminal fluid removal by washing using medium and centrifuging twice at $500 \times g$ for 5 min, followed by supernatant removal. We then suspend them for the swim-up or mini swim-up method [6]. Others might use a procedure of passing the specimen through 2–3 layers of discontinuous Percoll gradient, ending by centrifugation [7, 8].

Epididymal sperm is recovered by microsurgery then dealt with as the ejaculated ones are. Freshly recovered from the epididymis proximal caput, some sperm could be frozen to avoid surgery in future cycles [9–11]. Testicular spermatozoa were isolated from a testicular biopsy specimen. The tissue was then transferred into a

Petri dish with Sage medium and torn into pieces during the heated stage of a stereomicroscope, then removed and medium centrifugation at 300 × g for 5 min. The pellet was then resuspended for ICSI [7, 12–15].

Technique Description

The ICSI procedure should be performed with the assistance of two bent needles angled at 30–40 degrees, at 200–400 magnification microscopy at a heated stage. Oocyte fixation is done as it is attached gently but firmly to the holding pipette with the help of negative pressure created by the CellTram Air device and then keeping the polar body at 6 or 12 o'clock, after which the single live spermatozoon is immobilized either by a quick movement of the TransferTip (ICSI) capillary via the tail, or by pressing the tail of the sperm cell against the bottom of the dish, then aspirating it (tail-first) into the injection pipette. Move the spermatozoon along the pipette and bring it to rest at its very tip by rotating the knob of the CellTram vario. The injection pipette containing the spermatozoon is introduced at the 3 o'clock position into the cytoplasm through the zona pellucida. Then the spermatozoon is released to pass into the cytoplasm with the smallest amount of medium [16].

After the procedure is completed, the oocyte washing takes place in 25 µL microdrops of B2 medium in a Petri dish and is then stored at 37°C in an incubator containing 5% CO_2 in air.

Good preparation and technique are important in order to make the ICSI service available to a wide number of laboratories [17]. It is also important to make it more comfortable for patients. For troubleshooting tips and error message remedies, consult the TransferMan NK 2 Operating Manual (Eppendorf).

Future Aspects and Considerations

The following considerations and suggestions are offered to tune and streamline the process with the goal of improving the ICSI procedure:

- Smaller microscope and manipulators could be developed to reduce the space requirement.
- The number of the manipulators per microscope might be increased to facilitate more operations to be performed.
- Development of one complete compatible station which includes the microscope, manipulator, temperature adjusting system, comfortable stool, camera, and monitor will help make the station work more smoothly.
- Forming a team taskforce comprised of representatives of the laboratory, manufacturing company, and physicians to assist in idea exchange and technology advancement.

- Robotic micromanipulation might be invented to make distance work possible and make movements coordinate with each other like human fingers.
- More tactile movements are better and more meticulous for this type of cell surgery.
- Foot pedal functions might help the manual part and decrease the pressure on it.
- A more ergonomically efficient workspace that keeps the operator from having to move when taking new dishes and discarding dishes that are not needed anymore.
- Better flexibility and bigger axis diameter to the device movement.
- Better position for the operator to decrease the stress and effort on the eyes and neck.
- More training sessions on the manipulators to produce more skilled operators.

References

1. Elder K, Dale B. In vitro fertilization. 2nd ed. Oxford: Cambridge University Press; 2000. p. 228.
2. Cohen J, Alikani M, Adler A, Berkely A, Davis O, Farrara TA, Graf M, Grifo J, Liu HC, Malter HE, Reing AM, Suzman M, Talansky BE, Trowbridge J, Rosenwaks Z. Microsurgical fertilization procedures: the absence of stringent criteria for patient selection. J Assist Reprod Genet. 1992;9:197–206.
3. Fishel S, Timson J, Lisi F, Rinaldi L. Evaluation of 225 patients undergoing subzonal insemination for the procurement of fertilization in vitro. Fertil Steril. 1992;57:840–9.
4. Ng SC, Bongso A, Ratnam SS. Microinjection of human oocytes: a technique for severe oligoasthenoteratozoospermia. Fertil Steril. 1991;56:1117–23.
5. Palermo G, Joris H, Devroey P, Van Steirteghem AC. Pregnancies after intracytoplasmic injection of single spermatozoon into an oocyte. Lancet. 1992;340:17–8.
6. Al-Hasani S, Kupker W, Baschat A, Sturm R, Bauer O, Diedrich Ch, Diedrich K. Mini-swim up: a new technique of sperm preparation for intracytoplasmic sperm injection. J Assist Reprod Genet. 1995;12(7):428–33.
7. Liu J, Nagy Z, Joris H, Tournaye H, Devroey P, Van Steirteghem AC. Intracytoplasmic sperm injection does not require special treatment of the spermatozoa. Hum Reprod. 1994;9:1127–30.
8. Van Steirteghem AC, Joris H, Nagy Z, Bocken G, Vankelecom A, Desmet B, et al. Protocol for intracytoplasmic sperm injection. Hum Reprod Update 1995;1(3):CD-ROM.
9. Silber SJ, Nagy ZP, Liu J, Godoy H, Devroey P, Van Steirteghem AC. Conventional in-vitro fertilization versus intracytoplasmic sperm injection for patients requiring microsurgical sperm aspiration. Hum Reprod. 1994;9:1705–9.
10. Tournaye H, Devroey P, Liu J, Nagy Z, Lissens W, Van Steirteghem AC. Microsurgical epididymal sperm aspiration and intracytoplasmic sperm injection: a new effective approach to infertility as a result of congenital bilateral absence of the vas deferens. Fertil Steril. 1994;61:1045–51.
11. Devroey P, Silber SJ, Nagy Z, Liu J, Tournaye H, Joris H, Verheyen G, Van Steirteghem AC. Ongoing pregnancies and birth after intracytoplasmic sperm injection with frozen-thawed epididymal spermatozoa. Hum Reprod. 1995;10:903–6.
12. Rabe T, Diedrich K, Runnebaum B, editors. Manual on assisted reproduction. Heidelberg: Springer; 1997. p. 312–22.
13. Devroey P, Liu J, Nagy Z, Tournaye H, Silber SJ, Van Steirteghem AC. Normal fertilization of human oocytes after testicular sperm extraction and intracytoplasmic sperm injection. Fertil Steril. 1994;62:639–41.

14. Nagy Z, Liu J, Janssenswillen C, Silber S, Devroey P, Van Steirteghem AC. Using ejaculated, fresh and frozen-thawed epididymal and testicular spermatozoa gives rise to comparable results after intracytoplasmic sperm injection. Fertil Steril. 1995;63:808–15.
15. Silber SJ, Van Steirteghem AC, Liu J, Nagy Z, Tournaye H, Devroey P. High fertilization and pregnancy rate after intracytoplasmic sperm injection with spermatozoa obtained from testicle biopsy. Hum Reprod. 1995;10:148–52.
16. Nagy ZP, Liu J, Joris H, Bocken G, Desmet B, Van Ranst H, Vankelecom A, Devroey P, Van Steirteghem AC. The influence of the site of sperm deposition and mode of oolemma breakage at intracytoplasmic sperm injection on fertilization and embryo development rates. Hum Reprod. 1995;10:3171–7.
17. Al-Hasani S, Ludwig M, Karabulut O, Al-Dimassi F, Bauer O, Sturm R, Kahle D, Diedrich K. Results of intracytoplasmic sperm injection using the microprocessor controlled TransferMan Eppendorf manipulator sytem. Middle East Fertil Soc J. 1999;4(1):41–4.

Chapter 14
The Leica Microsystems' IMSI System

Christiane Wittemer, Bruno Laborde, Frederic Ribay, and Stephane Viville

In 2001, Bartoov and collaborators introduced a new concept for observing spermatozoa called *motile-sperm organelle morphology examination* (MSOME) [1]. This technique allowed examination of the fine nuclear morphology of motile spermatozoa in real time at a magnification of up to ×16,000. The same authors consequently established a new intracytoplasmic sperm injection procedure called intracytoplasmic morphologically selected sperm injection (IMSI) and reported on the benefit of selecting spermatozoa using such a technique [2].

Like many other IVF teams, we were immediately interested in this new technique and its possible implications for the treatment of infertility. However, unlike the original system described by Bartoov, we wanted a practical, easy-to-use system, which allowed a single person both to select spermatozoa at a high magnification level and to inject these sperm into the oocytes, without having to change the Petri dish or the microscope. With this goal, we started a productive collaboration with Leica Microsystems, which resulted in a new user-friendly workstation that we have used successfully since 2005 and which is described in this chapter.

C. Wittemer, PhD (✉)
ART Centre, 8 rue des Recollets, 57000 Metz, France
e-mail: christiane.wittemer@neuf.fr

B. Laborde
ART Centre, SIHCUS-CMCO, Schiltigheim, France

F. Ribay
Leica Microsystems DSA/Clinical EU, Leica Microsystems SAS, Nanterre, France

S. Viville, Pharm D, PhD
Department of Biology of Reproduction, Hospital of the University of Strasbourg, Schiltighein, France

Overall Description of the System

This workstation is comprised of the components shown in Fig. 14.1:

- The Leica DMI6000 B microscope (equipment labelled 1 in Fig. 14.1) is fully motorized for its different functions: the field depth and aperture diaphragms; the condenser S 28 with its slits and Wollaston prism; the stage X/Y movement, fine and fast; the nosepiece with its different objectives (×10 and ×20 dry, ×20 and ×100 immersion oil) and the turret of the Wollaston objective prisms. A magnification changer allows an additional optical magnification of ×1.6. The different contrast methods, bright field, integrated modulation contrast (IMC), and differential interference contrast (DIC), can be activated through the Leica Application Suite software © (LAS) installed on a PC (equipment labelled 2 in Fig. 14.1), which displays all the microscope functions, or by pressing simple knobs placed on the microscope stand. The motorized stage is equipped with a heated insert (diameter 30 mm) connected to a temperature controller (equipment labelled 3 in Fig. 14.1). A remote controller, the SmartMove (equipment labelled 4 in

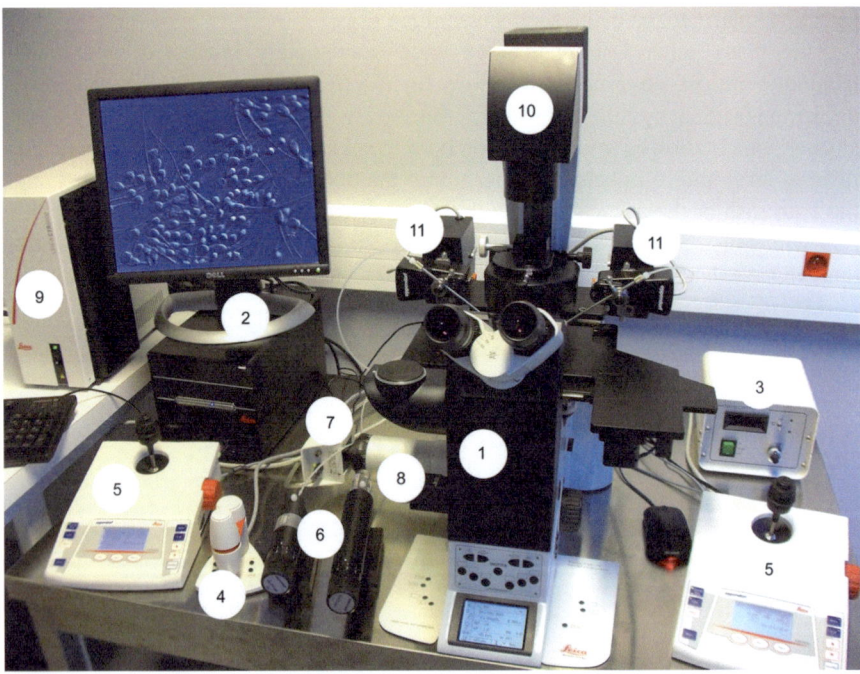

Fig. 14.1 The different components of the LEICA AM6000 working station: (1) Leica DMI6000 B microscope, (2) PC with LAS software, (3) temperature controller, (4) SmartMove, (5) micromanipulators, (6) microinjectors, (7) camera, (8) Vario Zoom, (9) CTR6000 controller, (10) microscope's column, (11) pipettes' motors

Fig. 14.1), allows the operator to focus and control the stage movements without touching the microscope itself.
- A set of two Leica AM6000 electrical micromanipulators (equipment labelled 5 in Fig. 14.1) (developed in partnership with Eppendorf).
- A set of two Eppendorf microinjectors (equipment labelled 6 in Fig. 14.1): Cell®Tram Oil, for the injection pipette, and Cell® Tram Air, for the holding pipette.
- A digital camera (equipment labelled 7 in Fig. 14.1) (DFC 290) connected to a PC fully controlled by the LAS. A continuous zoom is applied to the camera through the Vario Zoom (equipment labelled 8 in Fig. 14.1). This optical component easily provides magnification on the screen varying from 1,000 to 12,500 times.

The Step-by-Step Protocol of an IMSI Procedure

Preparation of the Workstation

Switching on the Components in a Precise Order

- Switch on the microscope with the CTR6000 controller (equipment labelled 9 in Fig. 14.1) and wait for the complete end of the microscope initialization.
- Use the X-Y controls of the SmartMove to set the motorized heating stage in the centre of the circular hole above the ×10 dry objective.
- First, switch on the right micromanipulator and then the left one.
- Switch on the PC and then launch the LAS Software.

Installation of the Pipettes

- Put the column (equipment labelled 10 in Fig. 14.1) of the microscope to its backward position and the two stands of the pipettes' motors (equipment labelled 11 in Fig. 14.1) on the side in order to have convenient access to place the pipettes.
- Mount the holding pipette (30° angle from Conception Technologies, USA) in the Cell® Tram Air grip head and the injection pipette (30° angle, provided by Humagen, USA) in the Cell® Tram Oil grip head.
- Place the stands of the pipettes' motors to their initial position, and using the manipulators, bring the tip of the pipettes in the bright field above the ×10 dry objective.
- First, adjust the position of the holding pipette until it appears in a horizontal, central and clear position on the screen. Then record this upper position by pressing the button POS1 on the control unit of the micromanipulator until you see P1 for recording the position.
- Adjust and register the high position of the injection pipette as previously described.

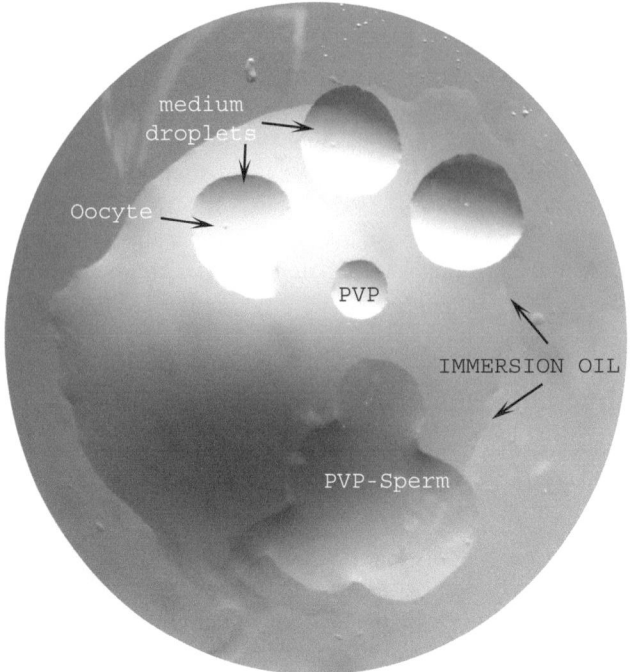

Fig. 14.2 The glass bottom dish with the different drops of medium

Preparation of the Dish (see Fig. 14.2)

- For IMSI, glass bottom dishes are required to obtain a high image quality using immersion objectives. We used WPI—FluoroDish 20090330, 0.17 mm thick, mouse embryo-tested, sterile single use (Gynemed, Germany).
- Turn the dish upside down and cover with immersion oil (Cargille type DF, Formula Code 1261, USA) until reaching a circular working area of 2 cm. Carefully avoid air bubbles.
- Turn the dish again and put it on the overturned lid to avoid contact between the immersion oil and the worktop.
- Several droplets of 3 microliters of FertiCult™Flushing medium with HEPES (FertiPro, Belgium) are placed next to an elongated polyvinylpyrrolidone drop (PVP Clinical Grade, MediCult, Denmark). The sperm suspension obtained after routine preparation through a two-layer density gradient (Sil-Select, FertiPro, Belgium) is deposited at one end of the PVP drop in order to allow the motile sperm to swim up.
- Place one drop of pure PVP between the HEPES medium drops to store the selected spermatozoa (Fig. 14.2).

- The drops are carefully covered with 2 mL of sterile mineral oil (FertiPro, Belgium).
- Before placing the prepared dish on the microscope stage, the immersion objectives ×20 and ×100 are covered with a droplet of immersion oil.
- Place the dish on the microscope stage and mark the 6 o'clock position on the side with a pen for reference.

Practical remark. According to our experience, a sperm concentration between 0.3 and 10 million/mL in the original droplet is recommended to retrieve enough motile sperm in the PVP droplet at a 10,000 magnification level. Due to the glass bottom, the medium droplets are very unsteady and the dish must always be handled very carefully to avoid mixing the drops.

Preliminary Settings

- The PVP-sperm drop is macroscopically placed above the ×20 immersion objective using the SmartMove. The objective comes in contact with the bottom of the dish and is then progressively lowered using the Z fine movement of the SmartMove until the sperm can be clearly seen in the oculars. Focus on the edge of the PVP-sperm drop and register its X and Y positions with the LAS.
- Repeat the same procedure to register the position of the pure PVP drop.
- Keeping the PVP drop focused in the oculars, bring the injection pipette in the observation field by lowering it with the coarse function of the manipulator. When the pipette appears in the field, switch to the fine function to precisely adjust the position. Then record this low position as POS 2 (P2) by using the control unit of the micromanipulator.
- Bring back the pipette to its upper position, and using the LAS, move to the registered position of the PVP-sperm drop.
- Switch to the ×100 immersion objective and DIC contrast and get the focus right. Tune the live streaming on screen by varying the light intensity, contrast and brightness directly on the LAS. Then record this position which can be called back by double-clicking on the icon, which looks like symmetrical triangles reflected over a horizontal line.
- Check the lower position of the injection pipette by pressing the button P2 on the manipulators and adjust the focus. If necessary, record a new lower position by pressing P2 again.
- The LAS allows precise control of the parameters of brightness, contrast, colour, exposure and all camera features.

Practical remark. Even if these preliminary settings are time-consuming, they are extremely important and have to be made carefully for they allow an easier and more efficient sperm selection and IMSI procedure.

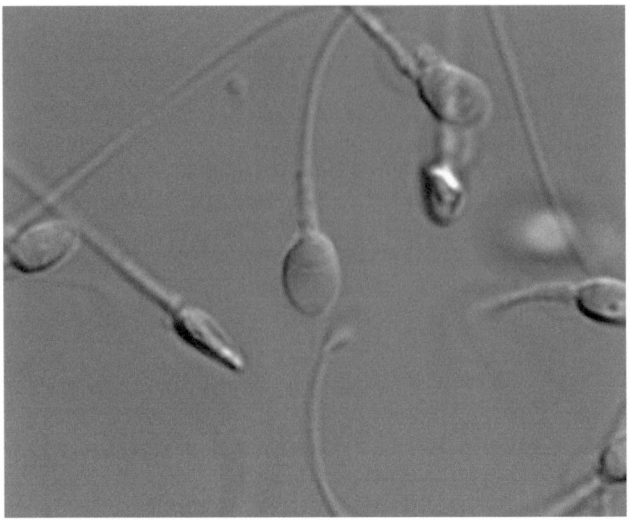

Fig. 14.3 Spermatozoa grade 0: no vacuole

Selection of Motile Sperm for IMSI

- A first evaluation of the overall semen quality is performed using the immersion objective ×100. This observation takes about 15 min and evaluates the PVP-sperm drop in order to estimate the best quality of spermatozoa to expect in the sample and to define a minimal threshold of abnormalities which must be expected throughout the selection procedure.
- If possible, spermatozoa that are selected display a normal oval head shape as well as absence of tail defect. Since the influence of the size and number of vacuoles has been well described [3, 4], we classify the spermatozoa into four categories (Figs. 14.3–14.6): grade 0, no vacuole at all; grade 1, one or two small vacuoles; grade 2, more than two small vacuoles or at least one large; and grade 3, several large vacuoles more or less associated with other morphological abnormalities. Small or large vacuoles are defined according to the analysis made by Bartoov and colleagues [2].
- The characterization of the vacuoles is made easier by using the Wollaston prism which gives a three-dimensional aspect.
- A first selection of motile sperm fitting to the minimal threshold defined during the preliminary evaluation is performed at an optical magnification of ×1,600 (objective ×100, magnification changer ×1.6 and ocular ×10).
- The selected sperm is aspirated into the injection needle and stabilized inside it. Still keeping the sperm in view, move the pipette to the drop of pure PVP using the joystick of the micromanipulator.

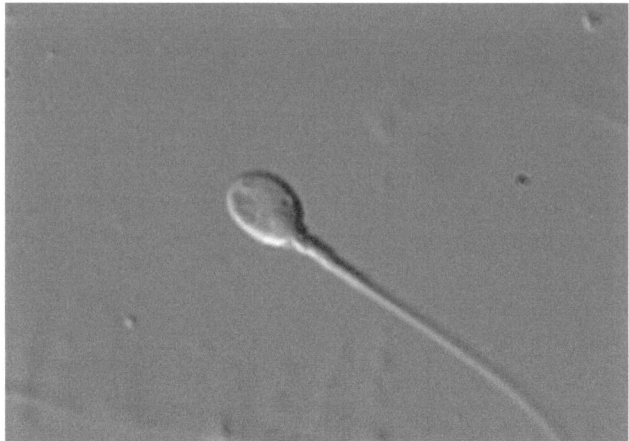

Fig. 14.4 Spermatozoa grade 1: one or two small vacuoles

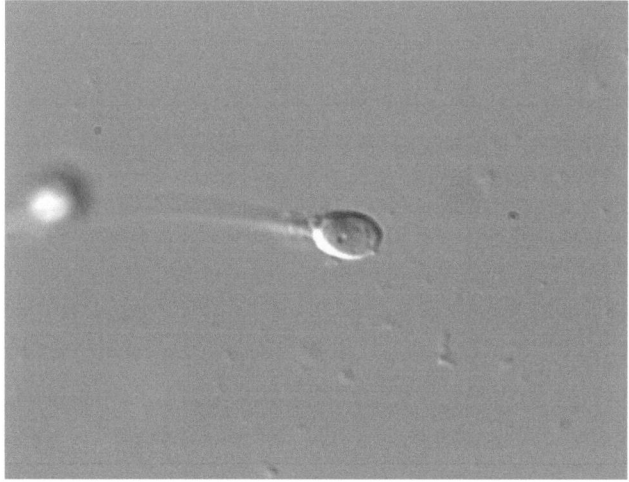

Fig. 14.5 Spermatozoa grade 2: more than two small or one large vacuole

- The selected sperm is deposited into the PVP drop (position called back on the LAS) and gently moved to the glass bottom by a smooth pressure on the tail, without immobilizing the sperm.
- Collect as many sperm as necessary, usually 1.5 times more than the number of oocytes to be injected.
- A more precise observation of the preselected sperm is then performed by using the Vario Zoom which allows magnification up to ×12,500. By using the

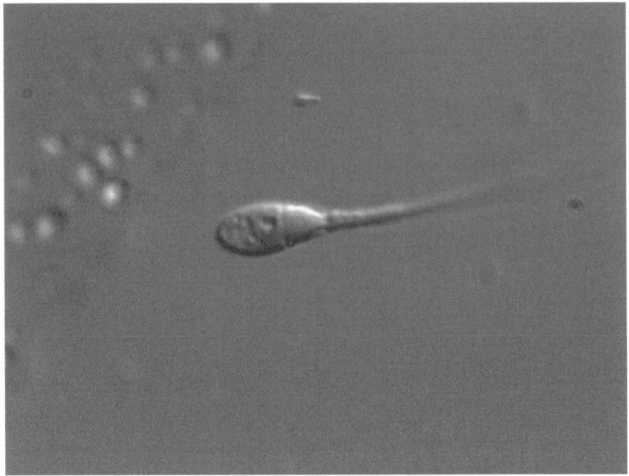

Fig. 14.6 Spermatozoa grade 3: more than one large vacuole

Wollaston prism again, some minimal defects can be detected and cytoplasm heterogeneity can be distinguished from vacuoles.
- Each sperm is carefully examined and selected for ICSI or otherwise discarded.

Practical remark. All the described selection procedures are performed at room temperature in order to avoid the negative impact of temperature on sperm fine morphology [5].

It is very important that the selected sperm remains motile until the injection procedure itself. The aspiration into the pipette and the release into the PVP drop must be very gently carried out in order to avoid a premature spermatozoa immobilization which could compromise the fertilization process.

Good management of the drops' position with the LAS and the pipette's position with the micromanipulator allows precise and efficient control of the steps in the sperm selection process without losing any of the precious motile spermatozoa.

The Intracytoplasmic Sperm Injection

Preliminary Settings

- Put the column of the microscope to its backward position and the two stands of the pipettes' motors on the side in order to carefully remove the dish containing the selected spermatozoa. Put the dish on its lid and place it into an incubator at

37°C, long enough to be sure that the medium drops reach the required temperature (about 15 min).
- Switch on the controller of the heating stage in order to perform the ICSI procedure at 37°C (see practical remarks below).
- Switch to the ×20 immersion DIC contrast objective and cover it again with a new droplet of immersion oil.
- After incubation at 37°C, the dish is removed from the incubator, and a maximum of five oocytes are placed into the prepared drops of HEPES medium using a stereomicroscope (see Fig. 14.2).
- The dish is then deposited on the heated stage of the microscope by placing the reference mark at the 6 o'clock position in front of the oculars.
- The column of the microscope and the two stands of the pipettes' motors are moved to their working position.

Practical remark. The temperature displays on the heating controller must be adjusted in advance in order to be sure that the drop itself reaches 37°C. In our case, only when the controller is settled on 45°C is the temperature inside the drops under oil measured at 37°C.

The Injection Procedure

- First, the PVP drop containing the selected sperm must be reached again. Thanks to the reference mark on the side of the dish, the initial recorded position is usually very close to the new position. If necessary, record this new position again on the LAS.
- The position of each drop containing one oocyte is recorded and named on the LAS. The injection procedure can now start.
- In the PVP drop, one sperm is gently removed from the bottom of the dish, immobilized as usual during ICSI, and aspirated tail first into the injection pipette.
- Move to the first oocyte by calling back its registered position on the LAS.
- Bring the holding pipette to its lower position and record it by pressing POS 2 (P2) on the control unit of the micromanipulator. Adjust this position with the fine control.
- Bring the injection pipette to its lower position and check that the selected sperm is still at its tip.
- Aspirate the oocyte with the holding pipette and inject the sperm by the standard procedure.
- Remove the two pipettes to their upper position (P1).
- Repeat these steps for all the oocytes.
- At the end of the injection procedure, put the column of the microscope to its backward position and the two stands of the pipettes' motors on the side and carefully remove the dish containing the injected oocytes.

- Using a stereomicroscope, each injected oocyte is deposited into one 30 µL drop of culture Medium (Global®, LifeGlobal) covered with sterile mineral oil (FertiPro, Belgium) and incubated in 37°C, 5%O_2, 6% CO_2.

Practical remark. The injection procedure is performed using only the ×20 immersion objective. As the insert hole of the heated stage is small, a maximum of five drops can be positioned around the PVP drop. If more than five oocytes have to be injected, repeat the procedure of injection, using the previous injection drops.

Switch Off the Workstation

- Clean the microscope optics. After each use, an effective cleaning of the immersion objectives is mandatory. Medical wound cotton sticks are required to clean the lens. An alcohol-soaked tissue (avoid lint residues) is used to clean the lens surface and the objectives' body.
- Put the two stands of the pipettes' motors on the side.
- First, switch off the right micromanipulator and then the left one.
- Switch off the LAS Software and then the PC.
- Switch off the Leica DMI6000 B microscope.

Discussion

The development of new tools like the IMSI system Leica AM6000 leads to the discovery of the fine morphology of the living spermatozoa and the presence of the so-called *vacuoles*. The nature of these nuclear vacuoles is unclear, and their number, size and location are extremely different from one sperm to another. Spermatozoa with large vacuoles have a clearly demonstrated detrimental effect on ICSI outcomes [3] probably related to DNA damage [6, 7]. It has been recently suggested that the small vacuoles mostly located in the anterior part of the sperm head could be of acrosomal origin [8].

The selection of spermatozoa without vacuoles appears to be positively associated with pregnancy rates in couples with previous implantation failures ([2, 3, 9], and our own unpublished data) in patients with an elevated degree of DNA fragmented spermatozoa [10] and in patients with severe oligoasthenoteratozoospermia [6]. To evaluate the possible benefit of IMSI compared to ICSI for infertile couples with a moderate oligoasthenoteratozoospermia during their first attempt, a prospective randomized study is still in progress in France.

Apart from IMSI, the MSOME evaluation of sperm represents a much stricter evaluation criteria for sperm morphology than routine methods (WHO or Tygerberg classification) [11, 12] and could be included in the routine laboratory semen analysis and conventional IVF and ICSI procedure.

Conclusion

The Leica IMSI system is a very efficient tool for examining the fine morphology of spermatozoa at a very high magnification level (up to ×12,500) with excellent image quality on the PC screen. Due to good ergonomic design of the components, this workstation allows a single operator to complete the entire IMSI procedure and to easily conduct traditional ICSI without immersion objectives, thanks to the replaceable objectives which can be attached to the nosepiece.

References

1. Bartoov B, Berkovitz A, Eltes F. Selection of spermatozoa with normal nuclei to improve the pregnancy rate with intracytoplasmic sperm injection. N Eng J Med. 2001;345:1066–7.
2. Bartoov B, Berkovitz A, Eltes F, Kogosovsky A, Yagoda A, Lederman H, Artzi S, Gross M, Barak Y. Pregnancy rates are higher with intracytoplasmic morphologically selected sperm injection than with conventional intracytoplasmic injection. Fertil Steril. 2003;80:1413–9.
3. Berkovitz A, Eltes F, Ellenbogen A, Peer S, Feldberg D, Bartoov B. Dos the presence of nuclear vacuoles in human sperm selected for ICSI affect pregnancy outcome? Hum Reprod. 2006;21:1787–90.
4. Vanderzwalmen P, Hiemer A, Rubner P, Bach M, Neyer A, Stecher A, Uher P, Zintz M, Lejeune B, Vanderzwalmen S, Cassuto G, Zech N. Blastocyst development after sperm selection at high magnification is associated with size and number of nuclear vacuoles. Reprod Biomed Online. 2008;17:617–27.
5. Peer S, Eltes F, Berkovitz A, Yehuda R, Itsykson P, Bartoov B. Is fine morphology of the human sperm nuclei affected by in vitro incubation at 37°C. Fertil Steril. 2007;88:1589–94.
6. Franco J, Baruffi R, Mauri A, Petersen C, Oliveira J, Vagnini L. Significance of large nuclear vacuoles in human spermatozoa: implications for ICSI. Reprod Biomed Online. 2008;17: 42–5.
7. Boughali H, Wittemer C, Viville S. Intérêt de l'analyse de la morphologie fine et de la qualité nucléaire des spermatozoïdes dans le cadre des techniques d'AMP. Andrologie. 2006;16: 38–45.
8. Kacem O, Sifer C, Barraud-Lange V, Ducot B, De Ziegler D, Poirot C, Wolf JP. Sperm nuclear vacuoles, as assessed by motile sperm organellar morphological examination, are mostly of acrosomal origin. Reprod Biomed Online. 2010;20(1):132–7.
9. Antinori M, Licata E, Dani G, Cerusico F, Versaci C, d'Angelo D, Antinori S. Intracytoplasmic morphologically selected sperm injection: a prospective randomized trial. Reprod Biomed Online. 2008;16:835–41.
10. Hazout A, Dumont-Hassan M, Junca AM, Cohen Bacrie P, Tesarik J. High-magnification ICSI overcomes paternal effect resistant to conventional ICSI. Reprod Biomed Online. 2006;12:19–25.
11. Bartoov B, Berkovitz A, Eltes F, Kogosowski A, Menezo Y, Barak Y. Real-time fine morphology of motile human sperm cell is associated with IVF-ICSI outcome. J Androl. 2002; 23:1–8.
12. Oliveira J, Massaro F, Mauri A, Petersen C, Nicoletti A, Baruffi R, Franco J. Motile sperm organelle morphology examination is stricter than Tygerberg criteria. Reprod Biomed Online. 2009;18:320–6.

Chapter 15
Automated Robotic Intracytoplasmic Sperm Injection

Zhe Lu, Xinyu Liu, Xuping Zhang, Clement Leung,
Navid Esfandiari, Robert F. Casper, and Yu Sun

Overview of Robotic Microinjection

Conventionally, oocyte injection has been conducted manually; however, long training, low throughput, and low success rates from poor reproducibility and inconsistency among technicians in manual operations call for the reduction of human involvement and automated injection systems. The past decade has witnessed significant efforts to automate oocyte injection using automation and robotics approaches. Several systems have been reported for robotically assisted oocyte injection [1–5].

These systems all borrowed the architecture directly from manual operation and automated a few procedures. Commonalities include (1) a holding micropipette for immobilizing an oocyte, (2) an injection micropipette for penetrating the oocyte and

Z. Lu, PhD • X. Zhang, PhD • Y. Sun, PhD (✉)
Department of Mechanical and Industrial Engineering, University of Toronto,
Toronto, ON, Canada
e-mail: zhe.lu@utoronto.ca

X. Liu, PhD
Department of Mechanical Engineering, McGill University, Montreal, QC, Canada
e-mail: xinyu.liu@mcgill.ca

C. Leung, BASc
Department of Electrical and Computer Engineering, University of Toronto,
Toronto, ON, Canada

N. Esfandiari, DVM, PhD
Andrology and Immunoassay Laboratories, Division of Reproductive
Endocrinology and Infertility, Department of Obstetrics and Gynecology,
University of Toronto, Toronto, ON, Canada

R.F. Casper, MD
Department of Obstetrics and Gynecology, University of Toronto, Toronto, ON, Canada

depositing materials, and (3) microrobots for positioning the holding and injection micropipettes. Research emphases were placed upon precise microrobotic motion control, development of computer vision algorithms for localization and visual tracking of oocyte and micropipettes, visual servo control of the micropipette, or integration of visual and haptic interfaces.

However, there exist several difficulties that prevent these systems or automation techniques from practical use for microinjection. In the state-of-the-art oocyte immobilization process, a robot mimics a human operator to control a holding micropipette to search, hold, and release individual oocyte ($\sim$100 μm for mouse and $\sim$150 μm for human). The procedures pose tremendous difficulties to a robotic system to achieve a high speed and reliability. Consequently, switching from one oocyte to another has been conducted manually, making robotically assisted oocyte injection cumbersome and time-consuming.

Furthermore, microinjection usually requires that the polar body be positioned away from the penetration site to avoid polar body damage and increase the chance of further cellular development [6]. In existing systems, oocyte orientation is achieved by repeated releasing and holding or rotating using micropipette until the polar body is located on the 6 or 12 o'clock position. Therefore, orienting oocyte can be a slow and trial-error process. Thus, oocyte orientation is also manually conducted in robotically assisted systems, further decreasing the value of the limited number of automated procedures.

Picking up materials into a micropipette is also a bottleneck in the automation of robotic microinjection due to its complexity. Intracytoplasmic sperm injection (ICSI) is a procedure in which an individual sperm cell is selected, immobilized, and loaded into an ICSI pipette, then injected into an oocyte. There are several challenges in automating sperm manipulation. For example, in sperm tracking, the computer vision algorithm should be robust to variations in sperm motion (e.g., sperm moving in and out of focus; and overlapping of multiple sperm trajectories). In sperm immobilization, the positions of the ICSI pipette and sperm need to be coordinately controlled to properly tap/break sperm tails. Aspiration and depositing single sperm cell also requires the manipulation of sub-picoliter fluids and fast dynamic response of a system.

To overcome the above difficulties in robotically assisted oocyte injection system, we recently developed an automated ICSI system prototype featuring fast oocyte immobilization, automatic oocyte orientation control, automated sperm tracking and immobilization, and oocyte injection. A minimal amount of human involvement remains in the system to ensure system reliability and permits a user to make certain decisions, such as sperm selection. The system is independent of operator skills and immune from human fatigue and/or errors. It has demonstrated a high success rate and a high degree of consistency in mouse zygote injection and is undergoing human ICSI trials. As the first-of-its-kind system, it aims to standardize clinical automated ICSI.

Automated Intracytoplasmic Sperm Injection

System Architecture

The automated ICSI system (Fig. 15.1) consists of a standard inverted microscope (Bright field imaging, 20× objective, Nikon Ti-S), a CMOS camera (601f, Basler), an in-house developed vacuum-based cell holding device for immobilizing multiple oocytes, an in-house developed precision vacuum pump, an in-house developed motorized rotational stage placed on a motorized X–Y translational stage (ProScan™, Prior Scientific Inc.) for oocyte positioning and orientation control, a straight ICSI micropipette (MIC-50-0, Humagen™) connected to a 25-µL glass syringe (Hamilton), filled with mineral oil, and mounted on a linear stage (eTrack, Newmark System Inc.) for computer-controlled sperm aspiration and deposition, a three degrees-of-freedom motorized micromanipulator (MP285, Sutter Inc.) for positioning the ICSI micropipette (45° tilting angle) to diagonally penetrate oocyte, a heating stage (THN-60-10, LINKAM) to maintain oocytes and sperm at 37°, a host computer for controlling multiple motion control devices and processing images in real time, a vibration isolation table (9100 series, KSI), and a dissect microscope (SZX 12, Olympus) for loading oocytes and sperm onto the cell holding device.

Overall Operation Sequence

System operation starts with depositing sperm and oocytes onto the cell holding device under the dissect microscope. The application of a low vacuum immobilizes each oocyte on top of a through-hole on the cell holding device. The culture medium consisting of gamete is then covered with mineral oil.

The cell holding device is then transferred onto the rotational stage on the inverted microscope. Through moving the X–Y translational stage, the first oocyte is positioned at the image center. A straight ICSI micropipette is lowered until the tip of the micropipette roughly appears in the image. The system integrates a vision-based contact detection algorithm to automatically determine the vertical position of the micropipette tip and device surface in the oocyte area. The micropipette is then moved automatically to the sperm area to perform contact detection to determine the vertical position of the micropipette tip and device surface in the sperm area. The position of the sperm area is also recorded by the system.

To inject a sperm cell into an oocyte, the user first selects a sperm cell by mouse-clicking the sperm cell head on the monitor of the host computer. The system tracks the motion of the sperm cell and taps its tail for immobilization automatically.

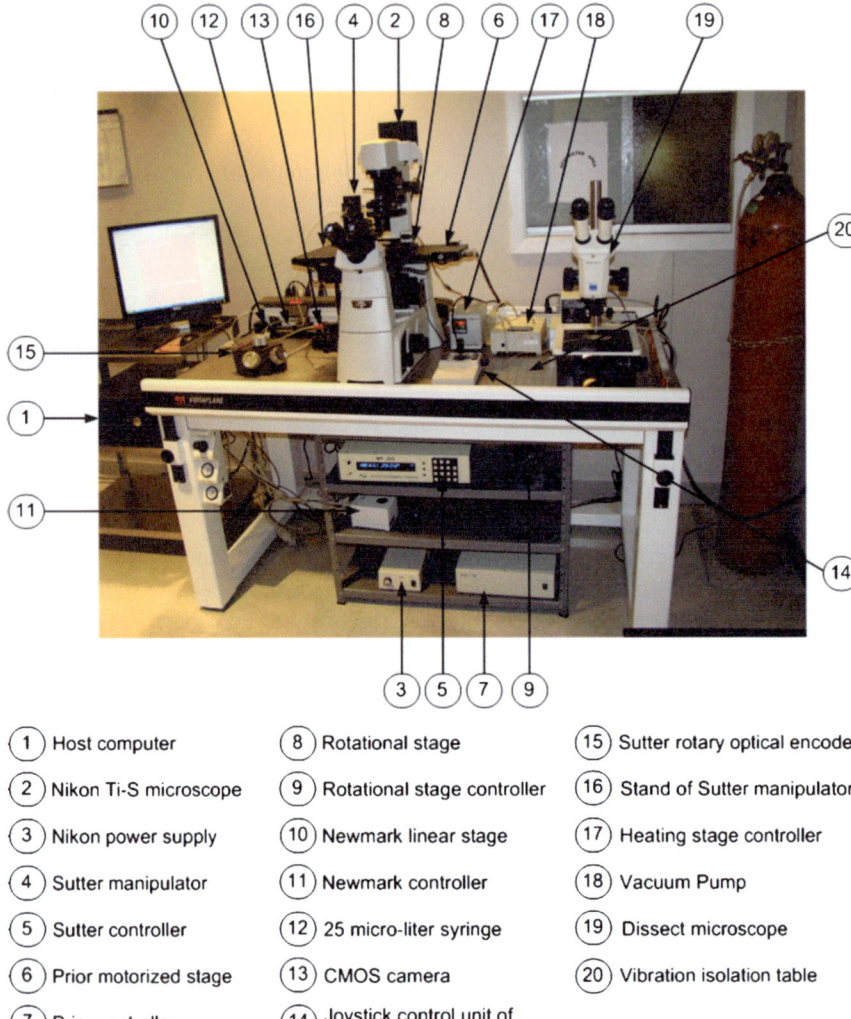

Fig. 15.1 Automated ICSI system

1. Host computer
2. Nikon Ti-S microscope
3. Nikon power supply
4. Sutter manipulator
5. Sutter controller
6. Prior motorized stage
7. Prior controller
8. Rotational stage
9. Rotational stage controller
10. Newmark linear stage
11. Newmark controller
12. 25 micro-liter syringe
13. CMOS camera
14. Joystick control unit of Prior motorized stage
15. Sutter rotary optical encoder
16. Stand of Sutter manipulator
17. Heating stage controller
18. Vacuum Pump
19. Dissect microscope
20. Vibration isolation table

Then the user aspirates the sperm cell into the micropipette through the control program interface. When the sperm cell is positioned in the proximity of micropipette opening, an oocyte is automatically brought into the field of view. The user identifies the position of the polar body on the monitor, and if needed, the system automatically rotates the polar body away from the penetration site. The system performs penetration, sperm cell deposition, and micropipette retraction all through computer control. For the next injection, the system moves the sperm area into the field of view for the user to select the next sperm cell for injection. This process is repeated until all the held oocytes are injected.

At the end of ICSI, the cell holding device is taken off the rotational stage and put under the dissect microscope. A low positive pressure is applied to release the held oocytes for collection. The oocytes are then transferred to proper culture medium for further culture.

Devices for Oocyte and Sperm Manipulation

Devices were developed for simultaneously immobilizing multiple oocytes (vs. a conventional holding pipette that immobilizes a single oocyte at a time), orienting an oocyte, and aspirating and depositing a single sperm cell. Related components include a vacuum-based cell holding device with an array of through-holes via which fine vacuum is applied for immobilizing oocytes, a precision vacuum pump, a computer-controlled motorized syringe for sperm aspiration and deposition, and a motorized rotational stage for polar body orientation (Fig. 15.2).

Vacuum-Based Cell Holding Device

Immobilizing multiple oocyte into a regular pattern permits the system to automatically switch from one oocyte to the next, eliminating the need for random oocyte searching. Figure 15.2a shows a vacuum-based cell holding device developed for the automated ICSI system. Evenly spaced through-holes (diameter 70 μm, pitch 500 μm for human oocytes and a diameter of 35 μm for mouse zygotes) are formed on the top layer of the device. The numbers of through-holes are designed to adapt the requirements of mouse, hamster, and human. A vacuum chamber is formed between the top and bottom layer of the device. Upon placing oocytes onto the device, a sucking pressure enables each through-hole to trap a single oocyte. The device proves to be highly effective for rapid, parallel immobilization of many oocytes. A separate area is integrated on the device to contain sperm. The distance between the sperm area and the oocyte area is ~10 mm.

Precision Vacuum Pump

A portable and stand-alone precision vacuum pump was developed to provide pressure ranging between −2.5 and 2.5 kPa for holding and releasing oocytes (Fig. 15.2b). The pressure system has a resolution of 10 Pa. It consists of two air rotary micropumps. One pump supplies positive pressure, while the other supplies negative pressure. A miniature pressure sensor is integrated to monitor pressure output.

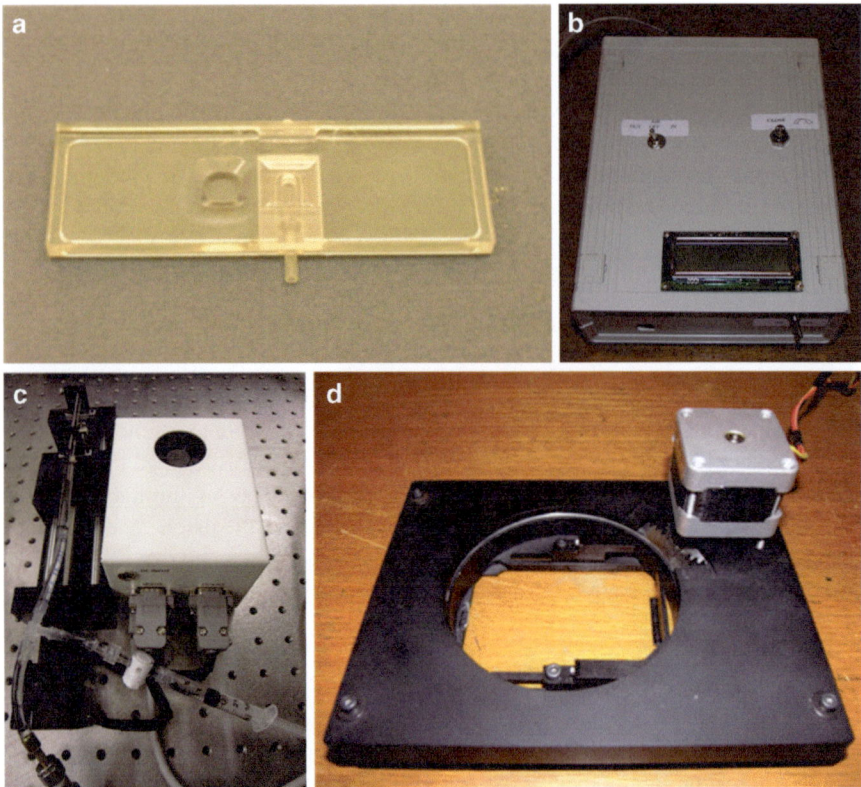

Fig. 15.2 Devices developed for robotic ICSI System: (**a**) cell holding device, (**b**) precision vacuum pump, (**c**) computer-controlled motorized syringe, and (**d**) motorized rotational stage

Motorized Syringe

Aspirating and dispensing a single sperm cell requires precision volume control of liquid at varying flow velocities. A computer-controlled linear stage is used to control the motion of the plunger inside a microliter syringe for precisely aspirating a sperm and dispensing an extremely small volume of culture medium when depositing the sperm cell into an oocyte (Fig. 15.2c).

Motorized Rotational Stage

A motorized rotational stage was specifically developed for inverted microscopy use to orient the polar body of an oocyte away from the injection site (Fig. 15.2d). The rotational stage is capable of orienting oocyte with a positioning resolution of 0.08 degree and a rotational speed of 30 degree/s. A clamping mechanism is designed on the rotational stage to fit the cell holding device and make it close enough to the microscope objective. During oocyte orientation, the polar body of oocyte is tracked by a computer vision algorithm. An image-based visual servo controller is used to keep the first target oocyte in the field of view during orientation, when on-line calibration of coordinate transformation between the cell holding device frame and the motorized X–Y stage frame is realized. High-speed oocyte orientation is then achieved on the rest of oocytes in the same batch via coordinate transformation and closed-loop position control.

Methods for Automated ICSI

Vision-Based Contact Detection

A computer vision-based method was developed for the system to detect relative vertical positions of the micropipette tip and cell holding device surface. The fundamental rationale is based on the experimental observation that when contact is established, further vertical motion of the micropipette produces horizontal motion in the image plane. Without requiring the micropipette tip to be in focus, detection starts with the determination of a region of interest and then further detects the contact point using a sub-pixel accuracy method. Experiments demonstrated that the contact detection method is capable of achieving contact detection between a micropipette tip and the cell holding device surface with a sub-micrometer accuracy.

Sperm Cell Tail Tracking and Immobilization

Locating and tracking the sperm cell tail is an important part of sperm immobilization. Thus, the integration of computer vision algorithms for identifying and tracking the sperm cell tail is essential in robotic ICSI. The maximum intensity region (MIR) algorithm for tracking the sperm cell tail has been developed. The algorithm is capable of reliably tracking the sperm cell tail despite the sperm cell tail's fast motion and low contrast under bright-field microscopy.

The sperm cell tail tracking algorithm comprises of three steps. Step 1 exploits the distinctiveness of the sperm cell head to track the position of the sperm cell of interest. To mitigate sperm cell position tracking errors caused by other sperm entering the vicinity of the sperm cell of interest, the sperm cell's movement direction vector is used as a unique identifier that is able to differentiate the sperm cell of interest being tracked from other sperm that are nearby. Step 2 uses the sperm cell head position found in step 1, and the sperm cell's movement direction vector to extrapolate the region in which the sperm cell tail is located. This region, called the sperm tail region of interest (STROI), is approximately from the middle of the sperm cell to the sperm cell tail's tip. Once the STROI is found, the MIR algorithm can be used to locate a position on the sperm cell tail within the STROI.

The MIR algorithm first constructs a flicker image of the STROI by taking the absolute difference between every six consecutive STROI image frames, and summing the resulting differences. The motivation behind this step stems from the fact that an individual frame may not illuminate the structure of the sperm cell tail due to the tail's low contrast and fast motion. However, by utilizing the additive information provided by every six consecutive frames in which the sperm cell is present, the sperm cell tail can be more easily located. After extracting the flicker image, the algorithm locates the region of the flicker image with the highest intensity value. The center point of this region is considered a position on the sperm cell tail.

After the sperm cell tail is located using the MIR algorithm, the sperm cell tail is tracked until its orientation is perpendicular to the micropipette direction. The system then lowers the micropipette and quickly slides over the sperm cell tail and breaks it.

Preliminary Results

The robotic ICSI system was first tested to inject one-cell mouse embryos with phosphate buffered saline (PBS). The injected embryos were cultured inside potassium simplex optimized medium (KSOM) in a 37°C incubator with 5% CO_2 for 72 h to allow the embryos to develop to the blastocyst stage.

During this phase, two measures were defined [7]: *Survival rate*, which was defined as the ratio of the number of injected embryos without lysis to the total number of injected embryos, essentially representing the frequency of the injection-induced embryo lysis. Based on visual inspection of the 240 embryos shortly after injection, the robotic injection system produced a success rate of 98.9%. *Success rate*, which was defined as the ratio of the number of injected embryos developing into the blastocyst stage to the total number of injected embryos, quantitating the negative impact of microrobotic injection on embryo development. System performance on mouse zygote injection was highly satisfactory, as summarized in Table 15.1.

After the preliminary study on mouse embryos, we performed trials on 1,000 sperm from a healthy sperm donor to evaluate the immobilization success rate of the automated system. The sperm motility was lowered in a viscous culture medium (SpermCatch). The system achieved a sperm cell tail visual tracking success rate of 96%, a sperm cell immobilization success rate of 88.2%, and an average time of 2–3 s per immobilization.

Patient trials are planned. The system is presently injecting human sperm into hamster oocytes as a testing model [8] before moving on to clinical ICSI evaluation. Figure 15.3 shows an array of immobilized hamster oocytes (Fig. 15.3a), a human sperm cell being tracked and immobilized (Fig. 15.3b, c), and the sperm cell being inserted into a hamster oocyte (Fig. 15.3d) by the robotic system. We expect the automated system to produce a high success rate and consistency in human ICSI, which together with other features such as skill independence and short learning curve will make the system a useful tool for clinical ICSI.

Table 15.1 Statistics of non-lysis and blastocyst formation rates of mouse embryos with PBS injection using the robotic system. Injected embryos were cultured in KSOM medium

Experiments	1	2	3	4	5	6	7	Overall
Number of injected embryos	18	18	27	27	50	50	50	240
Number of surviving embryos	18	18	26	27	50	49	49	237
Number of blastocysts	16	15	24	23	46	45	44	213
Non-lysis rate (%)	100	100	96.3	100	100	98	98	98.9 ± 0.6 (mean ± s.e.m.)
Blastocyst formation (%)	88.9	83.3	92.3	85.2	92	91.8	89.8	89 ± 1.3 (mean ± s.e.m.)

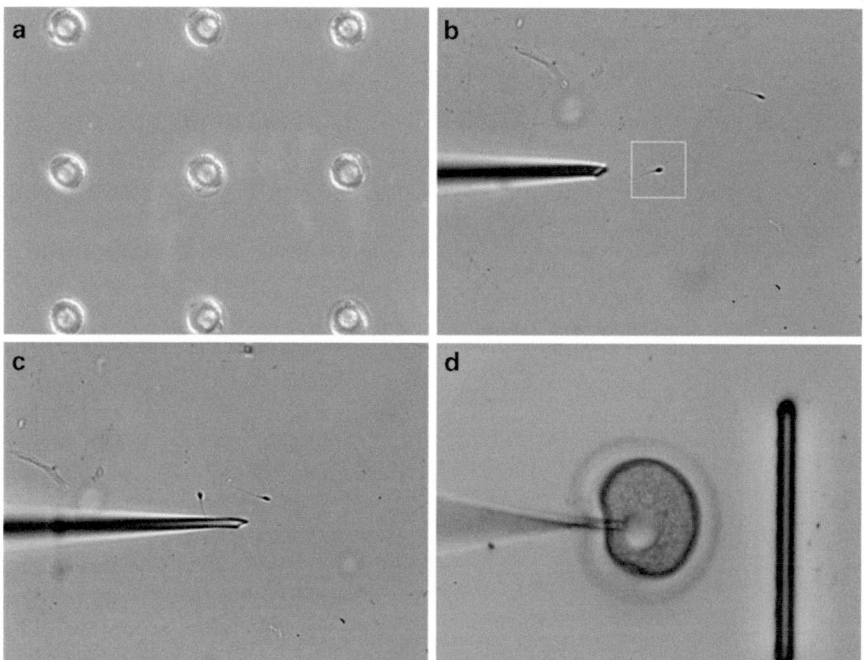

Fig. 15.3 Hamster ICSI: (**a**) an array of immobilized hamster oocytes, (**b, c**) a human sperm cell is being tracked and immobilized, and (**d**) a sperm cell is being inserted into a hamster oocyte

References

1. Kobayashi K, Kato K, Saga M, Yamane M, Rothman C, Ogawa S. Subzonal insemination of a single mouse spermatozoon with a personal computer-controlled micromanipulation system. Mol Reprod Dev. 1982;33:81–8.
2. Sun Y, Nelson BJ. Biological cell injection using an autonomous microrobotic system. Int J Rob Res. 2002;21:861–8.

3. Kumar R, Kapoor A, Taylor RH. Preliminary experiments in robot/human cooperative microinjection. In: Proceedings of IEEE international conference on intelligent robots and systems, Las Vegas; 2003. p. 3186–91.
4. Ammi M, Ferreira A. Realistic visual and haptic rendering for biological-cell injection. In: Proceedings of IEEE international conference on robotics and automation, Barcelona, Spain; 2005. p. 918–23.
5. Mattos L, Grant E, Thresher R, Kluckman K. New developments towards automated blastocyst microinjections. In: Proceedings of IEEE international conference on robotics and automation, Rome, Italy; 2007. p. 1924–9.
6. Nagy A, Gertsenstein M, Vintersten K, Behringer R. Manipulating the mouse embryo—a laboratory manual. 3rd ed. Cold Spring Harbor: Cold Spring Harbor Laboratory Press; 2003.
7. Liu XY, Sun Y. Automated mouse embryo injection moves toward practical use. In: Proceedings of IEEE international conference on robotics and automation, Kobe; 2009. p. 526–31.
8. Gvakharia MO, Lipshultz LI, Lamb DJ. Human sperm microinjection into hamster oocytes: a new tool for training and evaluation of the technical proficiency of intracytoplasmic sperm injection. Fertil Steril. 2000;73:395–401.

Chapter 16
Oocyte Treatment and Preparation for Microinjection

Thomas Ebner

It must be emphasized in advance that two major problems must be solved in preparation for intracytoplasmic sperm injection (ICSI). First of all, it has to be ensured that temperature is constantly kept at physiological ranges (approximately 35–37.5°C) throughout the whole process of oocyte collection, denudation, and injection. For this purpose, the temperature of all laboratory devices involved (e.g., heating plate, transportable container, microscope stage, incubator) has to be set higher than the requested temperature in the prevailing incubation medium. The required difference has to be tested individually for each laboratory setup and will be closely related to the volumes of culture medium and/or mineral oil used.

The second prerequisite for an optimal ICSI performance is a well-calculated time schedule. The period between oocyte collection and subsequent ICSI should never exceed 6 h [1, 2] in order to avoid in vitro aging of the oocytes. In this respect, it seems irrelevant whether the cumulus-oocyte complexes (COC) are denuded immediately after collection, leaving denuded eggs in culture for later ICSI, or if the manipulation is performed directly prior to ICSI after a resting period of several hours [1]. However, since oocytes may develop osmotic problems, e.g., an unwanted influx of culture medium, after a prolonged period without cumulus cells attached (unpublished data) and cumulus cells play an important role in maturation of the oocyte, it is recommended to perform processing of the COCs close to the time of injection.

T. Ebner, PhD (✉)
IVF Unit, Landes Frauen and Kinderklinik Linz, Krankenhausstr. 26-30, Linz 4020, Austria
e-mail: Thomas.ebner@gespag.at

Processing of the Cumulus-Oocyte Complex

Harvested COCs are traditionally evaluated by their appearance and by the expansion of the corona radiata and the cumulus complex. Based on these criteria, oocytes within cumulus matrix are roughly categorized as either mature (metaphase II) or immature (pro- and metaphase I). In detail, an expanded and luteinized cumulus complex and a radiant corona radiata suggest completion of nuclear maturation, while the absence of expanded cumulus or corona cells is associated with immaturity [3]. This is in contrast to more recent data which show that nuclear maturation and oocyte quality cannot be predicted adequately by scoring the COCs [4, 5].

Frequently, blood clots or other amorphous clumps [5, 6] are present in the cumulus matrix. Embryologists tend to cut off these areas with the help of two needles. Apart from the fact that this is mechanical stress to the oocyte, particularly if the dysmorphic cells are close to the corona radiata, it is of no use. On the one hand, amorphous clumps, considered to be a sign of postmaturity, did not have any effect on preimplantation outcome, and on the other, COCs showing blood clots have already been harmed during folliculogenesis, and thus, their developmental capacity may not be retained by cutting off the blood clots mechanically [5].

Denudation of the Oocyte

For successful ICSI, it is critical that cumulus cells are adequately removed from the oocyte. Apart from the fact that oocyte maturity and/or quality needs to be checked prior to injection, some technical problems could occur. Theoretically, it could happen that the oocyte cannot be manipulated adequately with the holding pipette if these nutritive cells block the 9 o'clock position. In addition, there is a certain risk to accidentally bring in foreign somatic DNA into the egg if cumulus cells are still attached at the site of injection [7].

It has been established that any denudation process consists of two steps, an initial enzymatic digestion followed by mechanical precision work. Since it has been shown that a dislocation between the first polar body and the meiotic spindle could occur if the mechanical part is performed inadequately, e.g., using pipettes of an inappropriate inner diameter (<140 µm), it is recommended to prolong the enzymatic incubation period. This would definitely help to minimize the mechanical denudation part.

Usually, commercially available hyaluronidase is used to start the denudation process. Hyaluronidase is an enzyme degrading hyaluronic acid which is a major component of the extracellular matrix of the oocyte. Most of the commercially available hyaluronidases have a concentration of 80 IU/L which is only a tenth of the critical threshold above which parthenogenetic activation might occur [8]. For reducing the theoretical risk of harming the oocyte, even further incubation time could be shortened (30 s) or the dilution could be changed to 40 IU/L (1:1 mixture with culture medium). Ultimately, it seems to be sufficient to put few drops of hyaluronidase in the well containing the COCs, but in such a case, the exposure time will naturally need to be prolonged to approximately 10–15 min (P. Vanderzwalmen, personal communication). Alternatively, plant (Coronase™, Bio-Media, Boussens, France) or recombinant human products (ICSI Cumulase™, Origio, Måløv, Denmark) could be applied [9]. It has been argued that due to the reduced toxicity of these enzymes, exposure time is not critical anymore.

The question remains if it is at all necessary to completely denude the female gametes. Our study group could demonstrate that coculture using homologous cumulus cells in situ (partial denudation) is associated with an enhanced rate of in vitro maturation, embryo quality, and blastocyst formation [10]. Obviously, leaving numerous cumulus cells attached to the zona pellucida mimics the in vivo situation and utilizes the stimulatory effect of the somatic cells during the first days of preimplantation development. However, due to their varying stage of maturity, oocytes do not present a standardized pattern of cumulus cell attachment. Younger oocytes (from the time ovulation induction) show a more homogeneous pattern with cumulus cells involving the whole surface of the gamete which makes ICSI somewhat difficult since there is almost no cumulus cell-free access to the zona.

Catching the Spermatozoa

In parallel to the processing of the COCs, the ejaculate produced under sterile conditions has to be processed for further usage. This can either be done using a centrifuge combined with a swim-up procedure (e.g., Percoll, density gradient, Sephadex columns, glass wool column) or sperm isolation without centrifugal stress (Zech-Selector, microfluidics).

Since in most of the patients a certain proportion of sperm is motile, embryologists are faced with the problem of catching these gametes prior to immobilization and injection. This procedure can be performed in three different milieus: culture medium, polyvinylpyrrolidone (PVP), or a more physiological viscous solution.

Naturally, catching sperm in the same balanced culture medium in which the oocytes are cultured (different drop) would be the most natural approach. Loading a processed sperm sample into medium drops on an ICSI dish has the benefit that motile sperms will automatically separate from immotile gametes, somatic cells, and other debris by their motility. This makes the purity of the whole drop much higher and minimizes theoretical contamination. However, this mode of catching sperms has the drawback that without a viscous solution covering the inner surface of the injection pipette, sperm manipulation during injection is not a smooth process but much rather a jerky one. This problem cannot be overcome, but it can be reduced by either washing the ICSI tool with PVP or by slightly changing the injection technique [11]. It is recommended that a minimum volume of medium is placed in the ICSI pipette (border between medium and oil/air should be below the knee of the

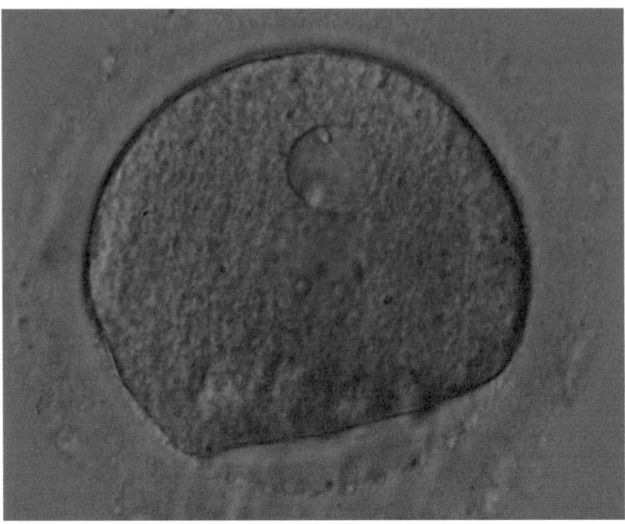

Fig. 16.1 Artificially created vacuole (V) after ICSI (day 1) resulting in a monopronuclear (Pn) zygote. Please note that sperm is located within the vacuole

pipette) and that the sperm is placed in the foremost third of the visible part of the glass tool. These precautions will facilitate stabilization of the sperm and help further manipulation. Embryologists using this setup often tend to aspirate the sperm with its headfirst since this is much easier and less time-consuming than trying to aspirate a hypermotile sperm from its tail end. Although ICSI in reverse has been found to be of similar outcome [12], there is a much higher risk of artificially creating vacuoles at zygote stage [13] since the larger volume (as compared to sperm headfirst ICSI) of medium entering the oocyte frequently becomes encapsulated (Fig. 16.1).

For these reasons, most embryologists regularly use a viscous water-soluble polymer (PVP) of the monomer *N*-vinylpyrrolidone to facilitate manipulation of sperms (and to coat the injection pipette). In contrast to the usage of culture medium, PVP that enters the oocyte cannot be actively removed through membrane channels due to its rather high molecular weight (between 40,000 and 360,000). Thus, larger volumes of PVP could alter intracytoplasmic pressure and/or osmotic behavior of the oocyte. It has to be mentioned that PVP per se is not toxic at all, e.g., it is used in personal care products, such as toothpaste, contact lens solutions, and shampoo. However, there is no denying the fact that it is an unphysiological liquid.

This circumstance led several companies to introduce more physiological solutions for sperm manipulations. Currently, two such products are on market, SpermSlow™ (Origio, Måløv, Denmark) and SpermCatch™ (Nidacon, Mölndal, Sweden). Both are based on the finding that a naturally occurring major component of the cumulus cell matrix called hyaluronate (polymeric chain of glycosaminoglycans) slows down the movement of spermatozoa and could act as a natural alternative to PVP [14]. Hyaluronate has a relatively high negative charge and a high hydration capacity which allow for the preparation of solutions with adequate viscosity for ICSI. It has been reported that its effect on sperm motility is reversible, and its use does not affect the outcome of the treatment cycles in terms of fertilization, pregnancy, and live birth rates [15]. However, it has to be noted that hyaluronate-based products do not have the same effect on the ease of sperm modulation as PVP probably due to its rather low content of hyaluronate (approximately 1%).

Immobilization of the Spermatozoon

Once the spermatozoon is caught, it appears necessary to immobilize it prior to injection [16]. Regardless of the fact that under normal in vivo conditions no sperm tail enters the oocyte, immobilization of the sperm has two beneficial effects: on the one hand, any possible damage to the cytoskeleton caused by motile sperms is theoretically negligible, and on the other, permeabilization of the sperm membrane will ensure that a soluble oocyte-activating factor (phospholipase C zeta) immediately enters the ooplasm [17].

Sperm immobilization is usually performed toward the end of the tail (back half); however, permeabilizing alternative sites is also possible. Yong et al. [18] successfully damaged the head membrane of porcine spermatozoa. This is also possible in the human since sperm chromatin is tightly complexed to protamines (approximately 85%) and histones (approximately 15%) and further stabilized by the formation of intramolecular-intermolecular disulphide cross-links between the cysteine residues of the protamine molecules [19]. Thus, any suggested mechanical harm to sperm DNA is only of theoretical nature.

However, sperm immobilization can be performed using four different methods. The most common approach would be a mechanical one, e.g., pressing the tail of the spermatozoon to the bottom of the ICSI dish by use of the injection pipette [16]. This is in line with the work of Palermo et al. [20] who found a more aggressive mechanical immobilization process in epididymal sperms helpful in order to increase fertilization rate from 48 to 82%.

Sometimes, the angle of the ICSI pipette is suboptimal, permitting no adequate manipulation of the spermatozoon. In such cases, repeated aspiration in and out the injection pipette has found to be helpful to immobilize sperms. However, only 16% of the corresponding oocytes showed 2Pn as compared to conventional mechanical breakage (90%) of the sperm membrane [16].

Montag et al. [21] introduced laser-assisted permeabilization of the sperm membrane into the field of assisted reproduction. Our study group [22, 23] successfully used this mode of immobilization as a routine procedure. In detail, spermatozoa were immobilized with a noncontact diode laser (1.48 μm wavelength) applying a double shot strategy. Two successive laser irradiations were applied per spermatozoon, the first aimed near the middle of the tail (1.5 mJ) and the second directly at the end of the tail (1.0 mJ). This strategy minimized the total energy dose male gametes were exposed to. In addition, laser shots were placed far from the head which made laser application for immobilization a presumably safe process.

A fourth alternative is piezoelectric manipulation of the motile sperm [24]. The same authors [25] published that the piezo method shows the most rapid onset of Ca^{2+} oscillations of all techniques (except laser immobilization) and, thus, may have caused the most damage to the sperm membrane. The method of sperm immobilization may be important for the rapid release of sperm factors that initiate oocyte activation.

Selection of Spermatozoa

Whatever method appears convenient, special care should be taken to select spermatozoa with best prognosis in terms of fertilization and further preimplantation development. Optimal selection of male gametes is a prerequisite for a successful ICSI program and should at least be performed at a magnification of ×400 if not at much higher magnification [26]. Not only should embryologists accurately evaluate normal sperm morphology [27, 28] in order to use gametes of optimal prognosis, but it is also of utmost importance that these cells reveal a high grade of maturity and genetic stability.

Huszar et al. [29] reported that a hyaluronate receptor is expressed in mature spermatozoa only after plasma membrane remodeling during spermiogenesis and that hyaluronate is an ideal medium for sperm selection for ICSI. Thus, hyaluronic acid (HA) has recently been used as *physiologic selector* for spermatozoa prior to ICSI as a convergence to a more physiological fertilization [15, 30, 31]. Spermatozoa bound to HA show a significant reduction in DNA fragmentation and a significant improvement in nucleus normalcy compared with spermatozoa immersed in PVP. Furthermore, injection of HA-bound spermatozoa significantly improved embryo quality and development [15], whereas zygote score was unaffected [30].

It should be noted that HA-ICSI requires special preparation of the ICSI dish. In detail, a small (e.g., 2 μL) droplet with suspension of spermatozoa has to be connected with a pipette tip to a slightly larger (e.g., 5 μL) droplet of HA-containing medium and allowed to incubate for 15 min at 37°C under oil. Thereafter, spermatozoa bound to HA in the junction zone of the two droplets can be detected, easily detached by the injection pipette, and subsequently used for injection.

A similar mode of selection aiming toward more mature spermatozoa utilizes spermatozoa previously bound to the zona pellucida of an immature egg [32]. This specific binding induces the acrosome reaction and, theoretically, should provide for better ICSI outcome. Indeed, embryo quality was found to be increased, although fertilization rate was unaffected [32].

In practice, it has been suggested [32] that a processed sperm sample (ca. 1×10^6 motile spermatozoa per ml) should be incubated with one MI-oocyte in buffered culture medium. After a 2-h incubation period, the eggs should be carefully washed to dislodge sperms loosely adhering to the surface of the zona pellucida. Spermatozoa bound to the MI-oocyte zona pellucida are presumed to be mature and can be removed with a microinjection needle for subsequent ICSI. However, since MI-gametes did not finish either nuclear or cytoplasmic maturation, it is questionable whether immature eggs express a zona pellucida selecting for the same male gametes as a MII-oocyte. Another technical limitation is the rather strong binding between sperm head and zona. Anyone having tried to detach bound sperm from the outer shell of an ovum will have realized that this requires rather strong suction forces by the ICSI pipette. Moreover, the sperm tail is still intensely motile since this step has to be performed in culture medium and not in viscous solutions.

Although both methods, using zona- or HA-bound spermatozoa for ICSI, will increase the percentage of genetically intact spermatozoa, there is currently no way to completely remove a DNA strand break-free from a given processed sperm sample. Recently, our study group (unpublished data, submitted) evaluated the efficiency of a particular sperm selection chamber (Zech-Selector™, AssTIC Medizintechnik GmbH, Leutasch, Austria) with respect to its selection properties in terms of DNA damage. Interestingly, it turned out that these glass or polyethylene chambers exclusively accumulate strand break-free spermatozoa which for the first time ensures elective usage of DNA-intact sperms for ICSI. Since the Zech-SelectorTM strictly separates spermatozoa according to their motility/velocity without exposure to centrifugation stress [33], these parameters should be of utmost importance during sperm selection. Obviously, once DNA damage has occurred, both nuclear and mitochondrial DNA will be affected. Any impact on the latter could reduce ATP production and as a consequence sperm motility.

Immotile Sperm

This selection criterion can of course not be applied if all spermatozoa of an ejaculate are immotile (e.g., Kartagener syndrome, cryopreserved sperm, testicular sperm extraction [TSE] material). In this particular case, embryologists have to be aware that it is of serious consequence if they cannot distinguish between immotile and nonviable sperms, although immotility does not preclude viability. Theoretically, one has four options to solve this tricky problem.

Commonly, the most reasonable approach would be to use the ICSI pipette in order to test the elasticity of the sperm tail [34]. A spermatozoon showing an elastic tail (once being manipulated with a glass tool) is presumed to be more viable than those with more rigid ones. Typically, these nonviable sperms show incapacity to resume the initial tail position once touched by the pipette from the side, and they show a characteristic *rolling* motion when touched from above. However, in the final analysis, there is no guarantee that more elastic sperms are viable, e.g., being an osmotically intact cell.

For confirming osmotic capacity, sperms can be incubated in a hypoosmotic swelling solution, e.g., a 150 mOsm NaCl solution [35, 36]. Gametes with a functional membrane will undergo swelling of the cytoplasmic space, and the sperm tail fibers will curl, whereas those gametes with damaged or osmotically inactive membranes do not show these phenomena. It is important to consider that swollen and curled sperms have to be moved to an isoosmotic culture medium prior to injection in order to facilitate original state and osmotic status.

Recently, a third alternative was introduced [37], suggesting usage of a diode laser in order to assess viability in cases of complete asthenozoospermia. Applying a single laser pulse (1.2 ms) at the very end of the sperm tail (direct method) caused a characteristic curling of the tail end. Since nonviable sperm did not show this phenomenon, this new technique helped to identify spermatozoa with functional integrity of its membrane.

The fourth strategy is the only one allowing for partial restoration of original motility [38]. Pentoxifylline and other caffeine derivates such as theophylline (Spermmobil™, Gynemed, Lensahn, Germany) are inhibitors of phosphodiesterase activity, which enhance motility in spermatozoa. They show maximum activity after 10 min and an activity phase of less than 2 h [39]. Because of this immediate and short-term effect, direct addition into the droplet containing the immotile sperms is recommended.

Intracytoplasmic Sperm Injection

Regardless of whether a motile or immotile sperm is available, ICSI should be performed according to a standardized procedure. To perform ICSI, the oocyte is held in place with a holding pipette at 9 o'clock. The first polar body usually is located on the 6 or 12 o'clock position. As soon as the equatorial plane of the oocyte is focused, the ICSI pipette has to be pressed against the zona pellucida, creating a characteristic funnel at 3 o'clock. After penetrating both the zona and the oolemma, a small volume of cytoplasm should be aspirated into the glass tool to activate the egg and to ensure entering of the ooplasm [40]. The single immotile spermatozoa should then be gently placed near the horizontal axis. Withdrawal has to be done carefully to prevent the oocyte from leakage.

Placing the first polar body farthest from the path of the injection needle was thought to protect the meiotic spindle, which is considered to be located in the periphery of the egg subjacent to the first polar body, against mechanical damage [41]. Meanwhile, it has been published that due to the manipulation during denudation, the first polar body is a rather inaccurate marker of the spindle position [42] and that it is almost impossible to harm the dense microtubule structure of the spindle apparatus.

This finding is further supported by data of Blake et al. [43] who analyzed fertilization and embryo development resulting from varying distances between the injected sperm and the polar body associated with the presumed area of the spindle. Among the orientations examined in this chapter, depositions of the sperm in the vicinity of a polar body at 9 o'clock resulted in significantly fewer normally fertilized oocytes and significantly more unfertilized and digynic oocytes.

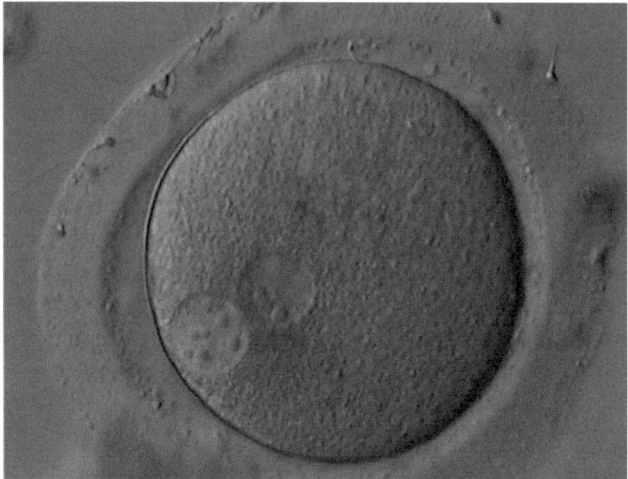

Fig. 16.2 Suboptimal pronuclear formation close to the periphery of the oocyte

All other locations gave similar rates of fertilization and embryo qualities. It appears to be crucial that the immobilized spermatozoon is placed in the very center of the female gamete. Since decondensation of the sperm head and formation of the male pronucleus take place at the site of sperm deposition [44], any deviation from this optimal place, e.g., close to the periphery of the egg, would result in suboptimal pronuclear formation (Fig. 16.2). This scenario is most likely associated with cleavage anomalies or developmental arrest [45].

Intracytoplasmic Sperm Injection Failure

Since ICSI is more invasive than other micromanipulation techniques, there is a higher risk of irreversibly damaging the injected oocyte (lysis, shrinkage, and/or tanning of the egg). The rate of degenerated oocytes after ICSI should be around 1% and not exceed 3%. Though most embryologists have made the experience that a suboptimal injection technique may influence ICSI outcome as they progressed on their learning curve with micromanipulation, only few studies deal with degeneration of oocytes [46]. The main problems found were as follows: (1) spermatozoon remained attached to the ICSI pipette while being released, (2) insufficient immobilization of the spermatozoon (as assessed by subsequent movement of the tail after injection), (3) rejection of spermatozoon into perivitelline space after ICSI (as assessed by the sperm's tail protruding out of the oolemma/zona pellucida), and (4) difficult breakage of oolemma. None of the above mentioned deviations from a presumed optimal injection procedure is significantly correlated with oocyte survival except the latter one.

During ICSI, different responses of the zona pellucida and the membrane to the injection pipette can be observed. In contrast to the very frequent normal response, showing a distinct injection funnel prior to rupture, two rather rare breakage patterns are considered as abnormal [20], namely, sudden breakage without any invagination during injection and difficult breakage characterized by delayed rupture of the oolemma.

It has been shown that additional manipulation in MII-oocytes showing difficult oolemma breakage may cause an increase in degeneration rate [47]. In order to avoid this scenario, a modified injection technique has been suggested [41] combining a pressing and a sucking phase, thus keeping oocyte survival rate at an adequate level.

Laser-Assisted ICSI

To overcome this high risk for degeneration in such oocytes, an alternative laser-assisted ICSI has recently been suggested [48] and successfully applied in patients with diminished oocyte survival in previous cycles [48, 49]. This method involves injection of the oocyte through a small laser-created hole (5–10 µm) in the zona which facilitates penetration of all anatomical structures. As a consequence, oocyte survival is increased significantly, as demonstrated in a larger number of cases [50].

However, none of the above mentioned studies took into account a major problem of laser-assisted ICSI, namely, the impossibility to localize the laser-generated hole at later developmental stages [50]. This phenomenon is particularly evident at the blastocyst stage, when the embryo expands and the zona pellucida gets thinner prior to hatching. Thus, if assisted hatching is applied in such embryos, as recommended in embryos derived from oocytes with difficult penetration of the oolemma [51], an additional opening is unintentionally created which might impair the hatching process per se and/or result in monozygotic twinning [52].

In order to avoid this possible dilemma, Moser et al. [53] decided not to perform ICSI through a relatively small opening but through a zona pellucida area on which laser zona thinning [54] was applied. This approach allows for accurate location of the manipulated zona area at later developmental stages and, theoretically, should combine two advantages, namely, minimal mechanical stress to the oocyte during ICSI (e.g., increased oocyte survival) and assisted hatching. Laser-assisted ICSI suggests that difficult penetration during ICSI is always caused by the zona pellucida and never by the structure of the oolemma. As in zona-free ICSI, no injection funnel forms in laser-assisted approaches and immediate penetration is observed.

Modified ICSI

Considering the complexity of the fertilization process may help to understand its susceptibility to disturbances potentially causing complete fertilization failure (in spite of the presence of a presumably normal spermatozoon). The frequency of total fertilization failure cycles is up to 3% with most of them being the result of impaired semen characteristics or a very low number of eggs collected. In such cases, repeated ICSI treatment proved useful [55]; however, some patients will have to face repeated fertilization failure in spite of normal sperm parameters and good ovarian response.

In order to rescue such cycles, Tesarik et al. [56] reported a modified ICSI technique mainly based on a repeated dislocation of central ooplasm to the periphery, thus increasing the intracellular concentration of free calcium by either creating an influx of calcium ions or a considerable release of calcium stored in cell organelles.

Taking into account a possible negative effect of this rather vigorous injection technique on further preimplantation development, another modified ICSI version was developed [57] which is based on the hypothetical accumulation of high-polarized mitochondria, e.g., showing a high inner mitochondrial membrane potential [58], from pericortical regions (9 o'clock) to the center of the oocyte, thus supplying more energy (ATP) directly to the place where the spermatozoon is normally injected. In this respect, it proved helpful that aggregation patterns of mitochondria correspond well to the light-microscopical appearance of the oocyte [59]. In 17 cases of complete fertilization failure after ICSI, we [57] could achieve a 54% fertilization rate and a 33% clinical pregnancy rate, respectively. However, it must be emphasized that the positive effect of our modified ICSI that could be shown in cases of previous fertilization failure after standard ICSI could not be demonstrated in cases without this problem since fertilization rate and further development were comparable. This implies that a minimum baseline of functionally active mitochondria must have been present in oocytes without impaired fertilizability [60].

More recently, an additional modified ICSI technique has been suggested [61], namely, increasing the effectiveness of ICSI by piezoelectric activation. In 50 patients with more than one previous total fertilization failure after ICSI, as many as 48% eggs could be fertilized resulting in a 44% clinical pregnancy rate.

Since all these techniques to overcome fertilization failure after ICSI are either rather invasive or require certain technical skills or equipment, usage of a calcium ionophore, e.g., Calcimycin (CULT-aktiv™, Gynemed, Lensahn, Germany) can be recommended in such patients [62]. This ready-to-use solution (Ca^{2+}-ionophore in DMSO and culture medium) opens membrane channels and facilitates entrance of extracellular Ca^{2+} from the culture medium which is a prerequisite for oocyte activation and fertilization. In practice, immediately after ICSI (since the ionophore might alter the constitution of the zona), injected oocytes are incubated in a bath of ionophore (approximately 15 min), whereafter the ionophore has to be removed by carefully washing the ova several times.

Conclusion

ICSI is undoubtedly one of the most severe manipulation techniques in IVF laboratories. Not only that it requires a certain learning curve, but it is also particularly dependent on oocyte quality which is governed by individual patient response and other stimulation details. It is a fact that suboptimal ICSI results in an impaired oocyte survival and reduced preimplantation development [46, 63]. It is a prerequisite to use ICSI pipettes of standardized quality which show a relative sharp spike (Gynemed, Lensahn, Germany; Humagen, Charlottesville, VA, USA). These tools combined with the individual skills of the embryologist will maximize fertilization rate and outcome, particularly if only a limited number of female gametes are available. In difficult ICSIs, spontaneous change of the injection technique can rescue the cycle or optimize the results. Additional help may come from the usage of theophylline, Ca^{2+}-ionophore, and (in the case of TESE) collagenase (Gynemed, Lensahn, Germany). To conclude, there is a general tendency toward the application of a more physiological ICSI using PVP substitutes (Origio, Måløv, Denmark; Nidacon, Mölndal, Sweden) and more mature and strand break-free spermatozoa.

References

1. Van de Velde H, De Vos A, Joris H, et al. Effect of timing of oocyte denudation and microinjection on survival, fertilization and embryo quality after intracytoplasmic sperm injection. Hum Reprod. 1998;13:31603164.
2. Dozortsev D, Nagy P, Abdelmassih S, et al. The optimal time for intracytoplasmic sperm injection in the human is from 37 to 41 hours after administration of human chorionic gonadotropin. Fertil Steril. 2004;82:1492–6.
3. Veeck LL. The human oocyte. In: Veck LL, editor. An atlas of human gametes and conceptuses. 1st ed. New York: Parthenon Publishing; 1999. p. 19–24.
4. Ebner T, Moser M, Shebl O, et al. Blood clots in the cumulus-oocyte complex predict poor oocyte quality and post-fertilization development. Reprod Biomed Online. 2008;16:801–7.
5. Rattanachaiyanont M, Leader A, Léveillé MC. Lack of correlation between oocyte-coronacumulus complex morphology and nuclear maturity of oocytes collected in stimulated cycles for intracytoplasmic sperm injection. Fertil Steril. 1999;71:937–40.
6. Daya S, Kohut J, Gunby J, et al. Influence of blood clots in the cumulus complex on oocyte fertilization and cleavage. Hum Reprod. 1990;5:744–6.
7. Stanger JD, Stevenson K, Lakmaker A, et al. Pregnancy following fertilization of zona-free, coronal cell intact human ova. Hum Reprod. 2001;16:164–7.
8. Van de Velde H, Nagy ZP, Joris H, et al. Effects of different hyaluronidase concentrations and mechanical procedures for cumulus cell removal on the outcome of intracytoplasmic sperm injection. Hum Reprod. 1997;12:2246–50.
9. Parinaud J, Vieitez G, Milhet P, et al. Use of a plant enzyme preparation (Coronase) instead of hyaluronidase for cumulus cell removal before intracytoplasmic sperm injection. Hum Reprod. 1998;13:1933–5.
10. Ebner T, Moser M, Sommergruber M, et al. Incomplete denudation of oocytes prior to ICSI enhances embryo quality and blastocyst development. Hum Reprod. 2006;21:2972–7.
11. Hlinka D, Herman M, Veselá J, et al. A modified method of intracytoplasmic sperm injection without the use of polyvinylpyrrolidone. Hum Reprod. 1998;13:1922–7.
12. Woodward BJ, Campbell KH, Ramsewak SS. A comparison of headfirst and tailfirst microinjection of sperm at intracytoplasmic sperm injection. Fertil Steril. 2007;89:711–4.
13. Ebner T, Moser M, Sommergruber M, et al. Occurrence and developmental consequences of vacuoles throughout preimplantation development. Fertil Stertil. 2005;83:1635–40.
14. Barak Y, Menezo Y, Veiga A, et al. A physiological replacement for polyvinylpyrrolidone (PVP) in assisted reproductive technology. Hum Fertil. 1999;4:99–103.

15. Parmegiani L, Cognigni GE, Bernardi S, et al. "Physiologic ICSI": hyaluronic acid (HA) favors selection of spermatozoa without DNA fragmentation and with normal nucleus, resulting in improvement of embryo quality. Fertil Steril. 2010;93:598–604.
16. Van den Bergh M, Bertrand E, Biramane J, et al. Importance of breaking a spermatozoon's tail before intracytoplasmic injection: a prospective randomized trial. Hum Reprod. 1995;10:2819–20.
17. Dozortsev D, Qian C, Ermilov A, et al. Sperm-associated oocyte-activating factor is released from the spermatozoon within 30 minutes after injection as a result of the sperm-oocyte interaction. Hum Reprod. 1997;12:2792–6.
18. Yong HY, Pyo BS, Hong JY, et al. A modified method for ICSI in the pig: injection of head membrane-damaged sperm using a 3–4 μm diameter injection pipette. Hum Reprod. 2003;18:2390–6.
19. Balhorn R. Mammalian protamine: structures and molecular interactions. In: Adolph KW, editor. Molecular biology of chromosome function. New York: Springer; 1989. p. 366–95.
20. Palermo GD, Schlegel P, Colombero LT, et al. Aggressive sperm immobilization prior to intracytoplasmic sperm injection with immature spermatozoa improves fertilization and pregnancy rates. Hum Reprod. 1996;11:1023–9.
21. Montag M, Rink K, Delacrétaz G, et al. Laser-induced immobilization and plasma membrane permeabilization in human spermatozoa. Hum Reprod. 2000;15:546–852.
22. Ebner T, Yaman C, Moser M, et al. Laser assisted immobilization of spermatozoa prior to intracytoplasmic sperm injection in humans. Hum Reprod. 2001;16:2628–31.
23. Ebner T, Moser M, Yaman C, et al. Successful birth after laser assisted immobilization of spermatozoa before intracytoplasmic injection. Fertil Steril. 2002;78:417–8.
24. Yanagida K, Katayose H, Yazawa H, et al. The usefulness of a piezo-micromanipulator in intracytoplasmic sperm injection in humans. Hum Reprod. 1999;14:448–53.
25. Yanagida K, Katayose H, Hirata S, et al. Influence of sperm immobilization on onset of Ca^{2+} oscillations after ICSI. Hum Reprod. 2001;16:148–52.
26. Bartoov B, Berkovitz A, Eltes F, et al. Pregnancy rates are higher with intracytoplasmic morphologically selected sperm injection than with conventional intracytoplasmic injection. Fertil Steril. 2003;80:1413–9.
27. World Health organization. WHO laboratory manual for the examination of human semen and semen-cervical mucus interaction. 4th ed. Cambridge: Cambridge University Press;1999.
28. Kruger TF, Menkveld R, Stander FSH, et al. Sperm morphologic features as a prognostic factor for in in vitro fertilization. Fertil Steril. 1986;46:1118–23.
29. Huszar G, Jak A, Sakkas D, et al. Fertility testing and ICSI sperm selection by hyaluronic acid binding: clinical and genetics aspects. Reprod Biomed Online. 2007;14:650–63.
30. Van Den Bergh MJ, Fahy-Deshe M, Hohl MK. Pronuclear zygote score following intracytoplasmic injection of hyaluronan-bound spermatozoa: a prospective randomized study. Reprod Biomed Online. 2009;19:796–801.
31. Parmegiani L, Cognigni GE, Ciampaglia W, et al. Efficiency of hyaluronic acid (HA) sperm selection. J Assist Reprod Genet. 2010;27(1):13–6.
32. Paes Almeida Ferreira de Braga D, Iaconelli Jr A, Cassia Savio de Figueira R, et al. Outcome of ICSI using zona pellucida-bound spermatozoa and conventionally selected spermatozoa. Reprod Biomed Online. 2009;19:802–7.
33. Ebner T, Moser M, Sommergruber M, et al. Presence, but not type or degree of extension, of a cytoplasmic halo has a significant influence on preimplantation development and implantation behaviour. Hum Reprod. 2003;18:2406–12.
34. De Oliveira NM, Sanchez R, Fiesta S, et al. Pregnancy with frozen–thawed and fresh testicular biopsy after motile and immotile sperm microinjection, using the mechanical touch technique to assess viability. Hum Reprod. 2004;19:262–5.
35. Casper RF, Meriano JS, Jarvi KA, et al. The hypo-osmotic swelling test for selection of viable sperm for intracytoplasmic sperm injection in men with complete asthenozoospermia. Fertil Steril. 1996;65:972–6.

36. Liu J, Tsai YL, Katz E, et al. High fertilization rate obtained after intracytoplasmic sperm injection with 100% nonmotile spermatozoa selected by using a simple modified hypo-osmotic swelling test. Fertil Steril. 1997;68:373–5.
37. Aktan TM, Montag M, Duman S, et al. Use of a laser to detect viable but immotile spermatozoa. Andrologia. 2004;36:366–9.
38. de Mendoza MV, Gonzales-Utor AL, Cruz N, et al. In situ use of pentoxifylline to assess sperm vitality in intracytoplasmic sperm injection for treatment of patients with total lack of sperm movement. Fertil Steril. 2000;74:176–7.
39. Tesarik J, Thebault A, Testart J. Effect of pentoxifylline on sperm movement characteristics in normozoospermic and asthenozoospermic specimens. Hum Reprod. 1992;7:1257–63.
40. Vanderzwalmen P, Bertin G, Lejeune B, Nijs M, Vandamme B, Schoysman R. Two essential steps for a successful intracytoplasmic injection: injection of immobilized spermatozoa after rupture of the oolemma. Hum Reprod. 1996;11:540–7.
41. Nagy ZP, Liu J, Joris H, et al. The influence of the site of sperm deposition and mode of oolemma breakage at intracytoplasmic sperm injection on fertilization and embryo development rates. Hum Reprod. 1995;10:3171–7.
42. Hardarson T, Lundin K, Hamberger L. The position of the metaphase II spindle cannot be predicted by the location of the first polar body in the human oocyte. Hum Reprod. 2000;15:1372–6.
43. Blake M, Garrisi J, Tomkin G, et al. Sperm deposition site during ICSI affects fertilization and development. Fertil Steril. 2000;73:131–7.
44. Payne D, Flaherty SP, Barry MF, et al. Preliminary observations on polar body extrusion and pronuclear formation in human oocytes using time-lapse video cinematography. Hum Reprod. 1997;12:532–41.
45. Van Blerkom J, Davis P, Merriam J, et al. Nuclear und cytoplasmic dynamics of sperm penetration, pronuclear formation und microtubule organisation during fertilization und early preimplantation development in the human. Hum Reprod Update. 1995;1:429–61.
46. Ebner T, Yaman C, Moser M, et al. A prospective study on oocyte survival rate after ICSI: influence of injection technique and morphological features. J Assist Reprod Genet. 2001;18:623–8.
47. Ebner T, Moser M, Yaman C, et al. Prospective hatching of embryos developed from oocytes exhibiting difficult oolemma breakage during ICSI. Hum Reprod. 2002;17:1317–20.
48. Rienzi L, Greco E, Ubaldi F, Iacobelli M, Martinez F, Tesarik J. Laser-assisted intracytoplasmic sperm injection. Fertil Steril. 2001;76:1045–7.
49. Nagy ZP, Oliveira SA, Abdelmassih V, Abdelmassih R. Novel use of laser to assist ICSI for patients with fragile oocytes: a case report. Reprod Biomed Online. 2002;4:27–31.
50. Abdelmassih S, Cardoso J, Abdelmassih V, Dias JA, Abdelmassih R, Nagy ZP. Laser-assisted ICSI: a novel approach to obtain higher oocyte survival and embryo quality rat. Hum Reprod. 2002;17:2694–9.
51. Ebner T, Moser M, Yaman C, Sommergruber M, Hartl J, Jesacher K, Tews G. Prospective hatching of embryos developed from oocytes exhibiting difficult oolemma penetration during ICSI. Hum Reprod. 2002;17:1317–20.
52. Schieve LA, Meikle SF, Peterson HB, Jeng G, Burnett NM, Wilcox LS. Does assisted hatching pose a risk for monozygotic twinning in pregnancies conceived through in vitro fertilization? Fertil Steril. 2000;74:288–94.
53. Moser M, Ebner T, Sommergruber M, Gaisswinkler U, Jesacher K, Puchner M, Wiesinger R, Tews G. Laser-assisted zona pellucida thinning prior to routine ICSI. Hum Reprod. 2004;19:573–8.
54. Blake DA, Forsberg AS, Johannson BR, Wikland M. Laser zona pellucida thinning—an alternative approach to assisted hatching. Hum Reprod. 2001;16:1959–64.
55. Moomjy M, Scott Sills E, Rosenwaks Z, Palermo GD. Implications of complete fertilization failure after intracytoplasmic sperm injection for subsequent fertilization and reproductive outcome. Hum Reprod. 1998;13:2212–6.

56. Tesarik J, Rienzi L, Ubaldi F, Mendoza C, Greco E. Use of a modified intracytoplasmic sperm injection technique to overcome sperm-borne and oocyte-borne oocyte activation failures. Fertil Steril. 2002;78:619–24.
57. Ebner T, Moser M, Sommergruber M, Jesacher K, Tews G. Complete oocyte activation failure after ICSI can be overcome by a modified injection technique. Hum Reprod. 2004;19:1837–41.
58. Van Blerkom J, Davis P, Mathwig V, Alexander S. Domains of high polarized and low-polarized mitochondria may occur in mouse and human oocytes and early embryos. Hum Reprod. 2002;17:393–406.
59. Wilding M, Dale B, Marino M, di Matteo L, Alviggi C, Pisaturo ML, Lombardi L, De Placido G. Mitochondrial aggregation patterns and activity in human oocytes and preimplantation embryos. Hum Reprod. 2001;16:909–17.
60. Barritt J, Kokot M, Cohen J, Steuerwald N, Brenner CA. Quantification of human ooplasmic mitochondria. Reprod Biomed Online. 2002;4:243–7.
61. Baltaci V, Ayvaz OU, Unsal E, Aktaş Y, Baltacı A, Turhan F, Ozcan S, Sönmezer M. The effectiveness of intracytoplasmic sperm injection combined with piezoelectric stimulation in infertile couples with total fertilization failure. Fertil Steril. 2010;94(3):900–4.
62. Rybouchkin AV, Van der Straeten F, Quatacker J, et al. Fertilization and pregnancy after assisted oocyte activation and intracytoplasmic sperm injection in a case of round-headed sperm associated with deficient oocyte activation capacity. Fertil Steril. 1997;68:1144–7.
63. Dumoulin JCM, Coonen E, Bras M, et al. Embryo development and chromosomal anomalies after ICSI: effect of the injection procedure. Hum Reprod. 2001;16:306–12.

Chapter 17
Mechanism of Human Oocyte Activation During ICSI and Methodology for Overcoming Low or Failed Fertilization

Dmitri Dozortsev and Mohammad Hossein Nasr-Esfahani

Mechanism of Human Oocyte Activation During Fertilization Using Intracytoplasmic Sperm Injection

The mechanism of fertilization after intracytoplasmic sperm injection (ICSI) is markedly different from that during natural fertilization. Whereas during normal fertilization process, sperm–oocyte fusion is followed by incorporation in the cytoplasm of a demembranated, "naked" sperm nucleus, which immediately becomes accessible for ooplasmic factors, including thiol-reducing agents [1]. Following ICSI, not a "naked" sperm nucleus but the whole sperm cell, enclosed in its membrane, is exposed to the ooplasm [2, 3].

Sperm Plasma Membrane Damage

It has been demonstrated that whole sperm cells behave in a different way than partially demembranated sperm cells in cytoplasmic cell extracts [4]. If an intact spermatozoon injected into the ooplasm, there will be no interaction between the spermatozoon and the oocyte. This is because ooplasm does not have an enzyme to digest sperm plasma membrane to enable interaction (Dozortsev, unpublished). Therefore, sperm plasma membrane has to be damaged prior to the fertilization.

D. Dozortsev, MD, PhD (✉)
Reproductive Laboratories, Advanced Fertility Center of Texas, Houston, TX, USA
e-mail: dmitrid385@hotmail.com

M.H. Nasr-Esfahani, PhD
Royan Institute, Isfahan Fertility and Infertility Center, Isfahan, Iran

Even though sperm cells appear to have distinctive compartments, such as a head, midpiece, and tail, they have only one plasma membrane covering the entire cell. Therefore, sperm plasma membrane can be damaged in any area, in order to enable sperm–egg interaction after injection. Usually, during ICSI, the sperm plasma membrane is damaged by "touching" tail [5], which in reality is pressing the sperm tail with a glass pipette, until the sperm membrane damage becomes sufficient for the membrane to loose its ability to maintain cell integrity, which leads to disabling Na/K pump and loosing membrane potential. To the observer, this event is marked by the sperm ceasing movement. The sperm membrane damage can also be revealed using vital staining technique, such as Eosin B [5] as can be seen on the figure further in the text. Vital staining is based on the intact membrane ability to exclude Eosin B. But once the membrane loses its charge, Eosin B migrates inside of the cell and stains the nucleus.

Effect of PVP

PVP, which is usually present in the culture medium, has the ability to act as a membrane's "band-aid" and prevents the stain migration into the nucleus. The plasma membrane damage induced by "touching" tail does not allow anything from the sperm cell to "leak" into surrounding medium. Indeed, the sperm cells retain full capacity to fertilize an oocyte for several hours following immobilization [6].

Initial Sperm Nucleus Swelling

Within minutes after injection, the sperm nucleus becomes accessible for the thiol-reducing agents (primarily glutathione—GSH) of the ooplasm and swells [7]. It is important to understand that this initial swelling is not under the same control as nuclear decondensation necessary for pronuclei formation. This swelling can also be easily duplicated in vitro using thiol-reducing agent—dithiothreitol (DTT).

The most abundant low-molecular-weight nonprotein thiol exists in two forms: reduced GSH and GSH disulfide (GSSG). It has been clearly shown that GSH is a disulfide bond reducer present in the cytoplasm of oocytes [1, 8]. Oocytes can synthesize GSH (tripeptide-glutamyl-cysteinyl-glycine, GSH) during the first meiosis. Oocyte-derived GSH seems to assure the reduction of disulfide bonds in sperm nucleus. This, in turn, promotes nuclear decondensation for male pronucleus formation during fertilization (reviewed by Sutovsky and Schatten [9]). Thus, GSH provides the reducing power to initiate chromatin decondensation, prior to the male pronucleus formation [10, 11]. Depletion of endogenous GSH by a specific inhibitor of GSH synthesis during bovine oocyte maturation blocks the formation of a male pronucleus and prevents the assembly of sperm aster microtubules [9]. The elevated levels of oocyte GSH can enhance male pronuclear formation after IVF [11]. If an excessive amount of PVP is injected with the sperm cell, for the reasons described above, sperm and egg interaction can be delayed.

Sperm-Associated Oocyte-Activating-Factor Release

The initial swelling of the sperm nucleus ruptures sperm plasma membrane and enables the release of the sperm-associated, oocyte-activating factor—PLC zeta—into the ooplasm. The entire mechanism of fertilization after ICSI can be summarized as the following:

1. Sperm plasma membrane damage is induced by "touching" tail, but the damage is masked as long as PVP is present.
2. Following injection, PVP is diluted and reduced GSH and GSH disulfide (GSSG) enter the sperm nucleus inducing sperm nucleus swelling within a few minutes.
3. The nuclear swelling ruptures sperm plasma membrane, enabling the contact between nucleus-bound PLC zeta and ooplasm, inducing oocyte activation and leading to chromatin decondensation. Most likely, due to the variations in the sperm plasma membrane damage and the amount of PVP injected, there is a large disparity in beginning Ca^{2+} oscillations among oocytes in the same cohort. Unlike during natural fertilization, when oscillations begin almost immediately after fertilization, oscillations after ICSI may begin within minutes or hours after injection.

Experimental and Theoretical Basis for Artificial Activation of Human Oocytes

Mechanisms of Activation Failure

Cases in which all MII oocytes become fertilized following ICSI are not common. In fact, the average fertilization rate after ICSI is usually below 80%. Cytological analysis of oocytes that failed to fertilize usually reveals that spermatozoon was interacting with the ooplasm but failed to trigger the activation [7]. Ovulated human oocytes are extremely resilient to parthenogenetic activation by sham-ICSI [12]. Therefore, even if fertilization rate is very low, it is usually due to the presence of some activating factor in the spermatozoon. Thus, the true deficiency of the activating factor should only be suspected when less than 10% of the oocytes failed to fertilize.

In most cases, failure of fertilization can be forecasted based on sperm morphology. It is very uncommon that a morphologically normal motile (live) spermatozoon fails to activate an oocyte due to activating factor deficiency. If activation fails in such case, the activation problem is most likely due to the oocyte.

At the same time, it is important to understand that morphological assessment of the sperm cells is not predictive of its activating potential. For example, acrosomeless (globospermic) spermatozoa in some cases will successfully activate human oocytes [13, 14], while in others, their injection will result in 100% failure of activation [15]. This may, to certain extent, correlate with acrosin-positive or acrosin-negative status of acrosomeless spermatozoa, which in its own turn seem to correlate with respectively the presence or absence of PLC zeta. Similarly, in the case of Kartagener's syndrome, immotile spermatozoa may still activate an oocyte [16].

Since there are strong evidences that PLC zeta is the sperm-derived activating factor, one could argue that using respective antibodies would provide a discriminating testing. However, due to morphological peculiarities of the sperm cell, in situ antibodies testing may often be nonconclusive. Therefore, functional testing, by injecting spermatozoa in question into the oocytes, seems to be the most feasible assay at this time [15].

Tests for Sperm-Activating Ability

Because sperm-activating factor (PLC zeta) is not species-specific [17–19], mouse, bovine as well as oocytes of other mammal oocytes can be used to test activating ability of human spermatozoa. Hamster eggs usually survive injection better, and they can be purchased frozen. However, they are expensive and may be activated by pricking itself, masking true activation capacity of a spermatozoon (although we were not able to activate by sham-ICSI any of the frozen-thawed hamster's eggs). Also, importantly, there is no clear benchmark activation rate has been established for activating potential of the human spermatozoa using hamster' eggs.

Mouse eggs, on the other hand, do not survive injection as well as hamster eggs, and we were not able to locate the source of frozen mouse eggs. Similarly to hamster, mouse eggs may also be activated by pricking, particularly as they age, and their sensitivity to parthenogenetic stimuli increases. Therefore, it is recommended that for the purpose of sperm activation testing, mice would be sacrificed shortly after expected ovulation time and used within 4 h after expected ovulation.

One clear advantage of mouse eggs is that their activation rate (excluding eggs which are damaged or were not injected correctly) following injection of normal human spermatozoa is 100%. Therefore, any deviation from this benchmark is strongly suggestive of activation factor deficiency. Even though the functional tests are available, their practical significance is not very high because usually the initial ICSI attempt will serve as a test and, as experience demonstrates, the underlying reason of failed fertilization will not affect the subsequent treatment modality.

Artificial Activating Factors

Development can be set in motion by a number of artificial stimuli, although their range is smaller than in mice. For example, ethyl alcohol, a very potent activator of mouse oocytes, is not able to induce activation of human oocytes, even 1-day old (Dozortsev et al., unpublished).

The majority of physical and chemical activating stimuli used for artificial activation in the humans elicit Ca^{2+} release into the cytoplasm, mimicking to different extent Ca^{2+} release taking place during natural fertilization [20]. The end point of activation is a physical destruction of cyclin B, which leads to inactivation of p34 kinase and drop in MPF activity [21]. Even though animal research, and in particular Ozil's work [22], assign the importance to the pattern of the Ca^{2+} oscillations during artificial activation, the relevance of activation pattern for human oocytes injected with the sperm is not certain. This is because in animals, the impact of artificial activation stimuli has been tested largely on parthenogenetic embryos, which do not generally develop well due to imprinting problems. In fact, in mammals, even when an oocyte is activated by sperm, but the male genome does not participate in development (gynogenesis), embryo development is usually poor and rarely survives far past implantation. Cloning experiments, where only a tiny minority of embryos develop to term [23], also illustrate an overwhelming importance of genetic makeup of the embryo over the activation modality.

One of the potent artificial activating agents of human oocytes—puromycin—has to be mentioned separately. This is because it does not cause Ca^{2+} release (Dozortsev, unpublished) and probably acts by suppressing synthesis of the cyclin B and by inhibiting its phosphorylation, rather than by its physical destruction. The point of no return in puromycin-activated oocytes is most likely the initiation of DNA synthesis (Dozortsev, unpublished). This observation has practical importance because it predicts that puromycin will act synergistically with Ca^{2+} engaging activation stimuli.

Indications for Artificial Oocyte Activation

Based on the current experience, fertilization failure of any etiology is an indication for artificial activation. Also, it is important to note that even though oocytes that failed to become fertilized following ICSI can be successfully activated on day 1 and many display two pronuclei and a second polar body, no pregnancy has been reported. Therefore, only fresh cases are the candidates for the procedure. Rescue of failed ICSI is likely to be futile not solely because of oocyte aging, since rescue ICSI following conventional insemination has been reported to result in pregnancy. The confounding factor for rescue activation is probably sperm chromatin deterioration to the extent that it prevents embryonic development.

Protocols Resulted in Live Birth After Artificial Activation

Considerations

As a general rule, activation stimulus has to be applied to the oocytes at the same time or shortly after sperm injection. If activation stimulus is applied before sperm injection, changes in the cytoskeleton and plasma membrane may make oocytes more fragile and prone to damage. On the other hand, in the absence of an activation stimulus, injected sperm chromosomes quickly undergo premature chromosomes condensation, and the significant delay between injection and activation may lead to the loss of sperm chromosomes (accessory micronuclei, along side of the pronuclei may be seen in such case).

Another practical consideration is the timing of ICSI and activation relative to hCG administration. Oocytes generally become more susceptible to parthenogenetic activation as they age. However, it has been shown that optimal fertilization window is between 39 and 42 h after hCG [24]. Therefore, it would seem that the best time for artificial activation would be around 42 h after hCG. It should also be noted that if oocyte deficiency is suspected as an underlying reason of failed fertilization, delaying ICSI and activation until 45–47 h post-hCG may be desirable.

Specific Protocols

Reference: Rybouchkin et al. [25]
Diagnosis: Globozoospermia
Outcome: Ongoing pregnancy
Protocol: Four different procedures for assisted oocyte activation were applied to the donated oocytes:

1. 111 Vigorous aspiration of oocyte cytoplasm during sperm injection [6].
2. 121 Same as above protocol plus ionophore A23187 treatment (5 µM during 7 min) at 30 min after sperm injection.
3. 131 Injection of approximately 5pl of 0.1 M $CaCl_2$ along with a spermatozoon, followed by ionophore treatment at 30 min after ICSI (This procedure has been proposed by this study).
4. 141 The same as above plus with ionophore treatment 30 and 60 min after injection.

Reference: Kim et al. [26]
Diagnosis: Round-headed spermatozoa
Outcome: Fertilization rate, implantation, pregnancy, and delivery [21 of 35, 60%; two pronuclei in 18 of 21; three pronuclei in 3 of 21]
Protocol: Oocyte aspiration was performed with transvaginal ultrasound guidance. After 5 h, all oocytes were denuded enzymatically with 0.1% hyaluronidase (Sigma, St. Louis, MO) for 30–60 s, followed by mechanical denudation. Motile round-headed spermatozoa were injected into oocytes in metaphase II, and assisted oocyte activation was performed with calcium ionophore A23187 (Sigma). At approximately 16–18 h after injection, the presence of 2PN was recorded as a sign of fertilization.

Reference: Eldar-Geva et al. [27]
Diagnosis: Normozoospermic patient with previous repeated failed fertilization after ICSI (case report)

Outcome: Fertilization rates in three cycles were 4/6, 5/16, and 7/20 oocytes. Two pregnancies were achieved; the first ended with second trimester miscarriage due to fetal anomaly and the second with a delivery of three healthy babies.

Protocol: Within 1 h of injection, six oocytes were exposed to 10 μmol/L of ionophore A23187 in IVF-50 medium for 7 min at 37°C in 5% CO_2. The oocytes were then washed free of the ionophore through ten drops of fresh culture medium and incubated further as usual.

Reference: Chi et al. [28]
Diagnosis: Normozoospermic patient (case report)
Outcome: The fertilization rate of oocytes activated (12 of 15, 80.0%) was higher than that of the nonactivated oocytes (4 of 16, 25.0%). Twin pregnancy
Protocol: Thirty minutes after ICSI, the oocytes were exposed to 8 μmol/L calcium ionophore for 8 min and subsequently washed thoroughly in P1 medium

Reference: Dirican et al. [29]
Diagnosis: Two siblings with familial globozoospermia
Outcome: Fertilization rate in case 1 and 2 were 33.3 and 9.1%, respectively. Clinical pregnancies with healthy live births were observed.
Protocol: Oocytes were mechanically activated before ICSI.

Reference: Heindryckx et al. [30]
Diagnosis: Failed or low fertilization in previous ICSI cycles or who had well-known sperm-borne activation deficiencies such as globozoospermia
Outcome: High fertilization and acceptable pregnancy rates
Protocol: Oocytes were kept at 37°C in a 6% CO_2 air atmosphere in Cook Cleavage medium (Cook Ireland Ltd, Limerick, Ireland). For ICSI with AOA, spermatozoa resuspended in HEPES-buffered oocyte wash (Cook Ireland Ltd) and an equal volume of 8% polyvinylpyrrolidone (PVP ICSI-100, VitroLife Sweden AB, Kungsbacka, Sweden) was immobilized by pressing the tail to the bottom of the dish and was drawn up into an injection pipette, and the sperm head was kept at the very tip of the pipette. Then the pipette was moved to a drop of 0.1 mol/L $CaCl_2$, and an amount of $CaCl_2$ was aspirated into the injection pipette, which corresponded to the diameter of the oocyte. Oocytes were conventionally injected with the spermatozoa and $CaCl_2$ and kept in Cook Cleavage medium for 30 min. Injected oocytes were exposed for 10 min in the incubator to 10 μmol/L Ca^{2+} ionophore (Ionomycin, cat. no. 159611; MP Biomedicals) dissolved in Cook Cleavage medium and subsequently washed intensively and put in Cook Cleavage for 30 min in the incubator. Finally, ionophore treatment was repeated during 10 min, and after intensive washing, oocytes were placed in Cook Cleavage medium for culture.

Reference: Nasr-Esfahani et al. [31]
Diagnosis: Severe teratozoospermia
Outcome: Improvement of fertilization and cleavage rates after AOA
Protocol: Oocytes were randomly divided into two groups: control and AOA. The injected oocytes in the control group were cultured in G1. The remaining oocytes were chemically activated by exposure to 10 mM ionomycin for 10 min.

Reference: Kyono et al. [32]
Diagnosis: Oocytes from patients with repeated fertilization failure
Outcome: Live birth
Protocol
Materials

- $SrCl_2 \cdot 6H_2O$: Sigma-Aldrich #255521
- Dolbecco's modified Eagle's medium (DMEM): GIBCO #21068

Method

1. $SrCl_2 \cdot 6H_2O$ stock solution
We prepared 100 mM $SrCl_2$ stock solution in DMEM and stocked at −30°C.

2. The microdroplet of 10 mM $SrCl_2$ solution (in DMEM) was overlaid mineral oil and stored in 6% CO_2, 5% O_2, and 89.9% N_2 air condition overnight.

These oocytes were cultured in Universal IVF medium for 30 min and then activated in $SrCl_2$ (10 mmol/L), 10% synthetic serum supplement, and Dulbecco's modified Eagle's medium (Gibco, USA) 20 μL/drop under 6% CO_2, 5% O_2, and 89% N_2 under humidified conditions for 60 min.

Reference: Ahmady et al. [33]
Diagnosis: Nonviable testicular sperm is used for intracytoplasmic injection (ICSI).
Outcome: Full-term delivery
Protocol: The injected oocyte was incubated in G-Fert (Vitrolife, Englewood, Colo) medium containing 10 mg/mL calcium ionophore A23187 (stock solution 10 mg/mL in dimethyl sulfoxide A23187 (stock solution 10 mg/mL in dimethyl sulfoxide stored at 220°C; Sigma Chemical Co, St Louis, MO) for 10 min.

Reference: Heindryckx et al. [15]
Diagnosis: Patients with previously failed fertilization and globozoospermia
Outcome: After AOA, fertilization rates were 77 and 71% in the sperm- and oocyte-related groups, respectively. Five pregnancies were achieved in the globozoospermia group and three in cases of oocyte-related activation failure.
Protocol: Activation capacity was assessed by 2-cell formation (mouse oocyte activation test, MOAT). When no activation occurred, AOA was done by ICSI with $CaCl_2$ followed by a $CaCl_2$ (0.1 mol/L) ionophore (10 mmol/L ionophore) exposure.

Reference: Juan Chen et al. [34]
Diagnosis: Patients with fertilization failure or low fertilization rates
Outcome: Improve fertilization rates (78.8%) and embryo quality (41.5%) (17/41) in cases with fertilization failure after ICSI
Protocol: Oocytes were activated in calcium-free HTF medium containing 10% (v/v) SSS and 10 mM $SrCl_2$ (Sigma Chemical) for 60 min at 37°C and 5% CO_2 [35].

Acknowledgments To Koichi Kyono, MD, PhD, for his extended activation protocol and to Marzeyeh Tavalaee, MS, for the help in preparation of this manuscript

References

1. Perreault SD, Wolff RA, Zirkin BR. The role of disulfide bond reduction during mammalian sperm nuclear decondensation in vitro. Dev Biol. 1984;101(1):160–7.
2. Palermo G, Joris H, Derde MP, Camus M, Devroey P, Van Steirteghem A. Sperm characteristics and outcome of human assisted fertilization by subzonal insemination and intracytoplasmic sperm injection. Fertil Steril. 1993;59(4):826–35.
3. Van Steirteghem A, Liu J, Nagy Z, Joris H, Tournaye H, Liebaers I, Devroey P. Use of assisted fertilization. Hum Reprod. 1993;8(11):1784–5.
4. Maleszewski M. Decondensation of mouse sperm chromatin in cell-free extracts: a micromethod. MoI Reprod Dev. 1990;27(3):244–8.
5. Dozortsev D, Nagy P, Abdelmassih S, Oliveira F, Brasil A, Abdelmassih V, Diamond M, Abdelmassih R. The optimal time for intracytoplasmic sperm injection in the human is from 37 to 41 hours after administration of human chorionic gonadotropin. Fertil Steril. 2004;82(6):1492–6.
6. Dozortsev D, Rybouchkin A, De Sutter P, Dhont M. Sperm plasma membrane damage prior to intracytoplasmic sperm injection: a necessary condition for the sperm nucleus decondensation. Hum Reprod. 1995;10(11):2960–4.
7. Dozortsev D, De Sutter P, Dhont M. Behaviour of spermatozoa in human oocytes displaying no or one pronucleus after intracytoplasmic sperm injection. Hum Reprod. 1994;9(11):2139–44.
8. Perreault SD, Barbee RR, Elstein KH, Zucker RM, Keefer CL. Interspecies differences in the stability of mammalian sperm nuclei assessed in vivo by sperm microinjection and in vitro by flow cytometry. Biol Reprod. 1988;39(1):157–67.
9. Sutovsky P, Schatten G. Depletion of glutathione during bovine oocyte maturation reversibly blocks the decondensation of the male pronucleus and pronuclear apposition during fertilization. Biol Reprod. 1997;56(6):1503–12.
10. Yoshida M, Ishigaki K, Nagai T, Chikyu M, Pursel VG. Glutathione concentration during maturation and after fertilization in pig oocytes: relevance to the ability of oocytes to form male pronucleus. Biol Reprod. 1993;49(1):89–94.
11. Funahashi H, Cantley TC, Stumpf TT, Terlouw SL, Day BN. Use of low-salt culture medium for in vitro maturation of porcine oocytes is associated with elevated oocyte glutathione levels and enhanced male pronuclear formation after in vitro fertilization. Biol Reprod. 1994;51(4):633–9.
12. Dozortsev D, Rybouchkin A, De Sutter P, Qian C, Dhont M. Human oocyte activation following intracytoplasmic injection: the role of the sperm cell. Hum Reprod. 1995;10(2):403–7.
13. Dirican EK, Isik A, Vicdan K, Sozen E, Suludere Z. Clinical pregnancies and livebirths achieved by intracytoplasmic injection of round headed acrosomeless spermatozoa with and without oocyte activation in familial globozoospermia: case report. Asian J Androl. 2008;10(2):332–6.
14. Stone S, O'Mahony F, Khalaf Y, Taylor A, Braude P. A normal livebirth after intracytoplasmic sperm injection for globozoospermia without assisted oocyte activation: case report. Hum Reprod. 2000;15(1):139–41.
15. Heindryckx B, Van der Elst J, De Sutter P, Dhont M. Treatment option for sperm- or oocyte-related fertilization failure: assisted oocyte activation following diagnostic heterologous ICSI. Hum Reprod. 2005;20(8):2237–41.

16. Matsumoto Y, Goto S, Hashimoto H, Kokeguchi S, Shiotani M, Okada H. A healthy birth after intracytoplasmic sperm injection using ejaculated spermatozoa from a patient with Kartagener's syndrome. Fertil Steril. 2010;93(6):2074.e17–9.
17. Rybouchkin A, Dozortsev D, Pelinck MJ, De Sutter P, Dhont M. Analysis of the oocyte activating capacity and chromosomal complement of round-headed human spermatozoa by their injection into mouse oocytes. Hum Reprod. 1996;11(10):2170–5.
18. Terada Y, Nakamura S, Morita J, Tachibana M, Morito Y, Ito K, Murakami T, Yaegashi N, Okamura K. Use of Mammalian eggs for assessment of human sperm function: molecular and cellular analyses of fertilization by intracytoplasmic sperm injection. Am J Reprod Immunol. 2004;51(4):290–3.
19. Dozortsev D, De Sutter P, Rybouchkin A, Dhont M. Timing of sperm and oocyte nuclear progression after intracytoplasmic sperm injection. Hum Reprod. 1995;10(11):3012–7.
20. Nasr-Esfahani MH, Deemeh MR, Tavalaee M. Artificial oocyte activation and intracytoplasmic sperm injection. Fertil Steril. 2010;94(2):520–6.
21. Hyslop LA, Nixon VL, Levasseur M, Chapman F, Chiba K, McDougall A, Venables JP, Elliott DJ, Jones KT. Ca(2+)-promoted cyclin B1 degradation in mouse oocytes requires the establishment of a metaphase arrest. Dev Biol. 2004;269(1):206–19.
22. Ozil JP. The parthenogenetic development of rabbit oocytes after repetitive pulsatile electrical stimulation. Development. 1990;109(1):117–27.
23. Wakayama T, Yanagimachi R. Mouse cloning with nucleus donor cells of different age and type. Mol Reprod Dev. 2001;58(4):376–83.
24. Dozortsev D, Nagy P, Abdelmassih S, Oliveira F, Brasil A, Abdelmassih V, Diamond M, Abdelmassih R. The optimal time for intracytoplasmic sperm injection in the human is from 37 to 41 hours after administration of human chorionic gonadotropin. Fertil Steril. 2004;82(6):1492–6.
25. Rybouchkin AV, Van der Straeten F, Quatacker J, De Sutter P, Dhont M. Fertilization and pregnancy after assisted oocyte activation and intracytoplasmic sperm injection in a case of round-headed sperm associated with deficient oocyte activation capacity. Fertil Steril. 1997;68(6):1144–7.
26. Kim ST, Cha YB, Park JM, Gye MC. Successful pregnancy and delivery from frozen-thawed embryos after intracytoplasmic sperm injection using round-headed spermatozoa and assisted oocyte activation in a globozoospermic patient with mosaic Down syndrome. Fertil Steril. 2001;75(2):445–7.
27. Eldar-Geva T, Brooks B, Margalioth EJ, Zylber-Haran E, Gal M, Silber SJ. Successful pregnancy and delivery after calcium ionophore oocyte activation in a normozoospermic patient with previous repeated failed fertilization after intracytoplasmic sperm injection. Fertil Steril. 2003;79 Suppl 3:1656–8.
28. Chi HJ, Koo JJ, Song SJ, Lee JY, Chang SS. Successful fertilization and pregnancy after intracytoplasmic sperm injection and oocyte activation with calcium ionophore in a normozoospermic patient with extremely low fertilization rates in intracytoplasmic sperm injection cycles. Fertil Steril. 2004;82(2):475–7.
29. Dirican EK, Isik A, Vicdan K, Sozen E, Suludere Z. Clinical pregnancies and livebirths achieved by intracytoplasmic injection of round headed acrosomeless spermatozoa with and without oocyte activation in familial globozoospermia: case report. Asian J Androl. 2008;10(2):332–6.
30. Heindryckx B, De Gheselle S, Gerris J, Dhont M, De Sutter P. Efficiency of assisted oocyte activation as a solution for failed intracytoplasmic sperm injection. Reprod Biomed Online. 2008;17(5):662–8.
31. Nasr-Esfahani MH, Razavi S, Javdan Z, Tavalaee M. Artificial oocyte activation in severe teratozoospermia undergoing intracytoplasmic sperm injection. Fertil Steril. 2008;90(6):2231–7.

32. Kyono K, Kumagai S, Nishinaka C, Nakajo Y, Uto H, Toya M, Sugawara J, Araki Y. Birth and follow-up of babies born following ICSI using SrCl2 oocyte activation. Reprod Biomed Online. 2008;17(1):53–8.
33. Ahmady A, Michael E. Successful pregnancy and delivery following intracytoplasmic injection of frozen-thawed nonviable testicular sperm and oocyte activation with calcium ionophore. J Androl. 2007;28(1):13–4.
34. Chen J, Qian Y, Tan Y, Mima H. Successful pregnancy following oocyte activation by strontium in normozoospermic patients of unexplained infertility with fertilisation failures during previous intracytoplasmic sperm injection treatment. Reprod Fertil Dev. 2010;22(5):852–5.
35. Yanagida K, Morozumi K, Katayose H, Hayashi S, Sato A. Successful pregnancy after ICSI with strontium oocyte activation in low rates of fertilization. Reprod Biomed Online. 2006;13(6):801–6.

Chapter 18
Livestock Production via Micromanipulation

Akira Onishi and Anthony C.F. Perry

We summarize the use of micromanipulation techniques in the production of livestock mammals, focusing on intracytoplasmic sperm injection (ICSI) and the pig, *Sus scrofa*. ICSI is a powerful method for assisted fertilization. It is typically employed where semen characteristics are insufficient for conventional in vitro fertilization (IVF), in which sperm and eggs are mixed and fuse in culture. Unlike IVF, ICSI mechanically delivers the sperm deep inside the egg cytoplasm by injection through a micropipette.

Mammalian ICSI was first demonstrated in hamster oocytes [1] and subsequently applied to humans to overcome impaired fertility [2]. In livestock, ICSI is also used as a procedure for fertilization, but its purpose is not restricted to impaired male fertility. Although circumstances do not ordinarily justify ICSI for breeding normal livestock, there are clear exceptions. Where sperm-containing ejaculates cannot be obtained, a small number of sperm may be obtained by biopsy, with ICSI as the method of choice for delivery into oocyte. Owing to its technical robustness, ICSI is especially beneficial where the breeding male stock has high genetic merit. These applications are now considered in greater detail.

A. Onishi, PhD (✉)
Transgenic Pig Research Unit, National Institute of Agrobiological Sciences, Tsukuba, Japan
e-mail: onishi@affrc.go.jp

A.C.F. Perry, BSc, PhD
Laboratory of Mammalian Molecular Embryology, Centre for Regenerative Medicine,
University of Bath, Bath, UK

Department of Biology and Biochemistry, University of Bath, Bath, UK

The Application of Intracytoplasmic Sperm Injection

The potential of ICSI in the conservation of genetic resources, transgenesis, and animal production using sex-sorted spermatozoa have all long been recognized [3]. However, ICSI in livestock animals is less widely applied than it is in humans due to the low success rate coupled to the prohibitive costs involved. This low success rate likely reflects the complexity of interactions between gamete components. Some of these interactions are ectopic, since ICSI introduces sperm plasma and outer acrosomal membranes in addition to acrosomal contents—all components that do not enter the oocyte during natural fertilization. The formation of male pronuclei after ICSI is affected by these ectopic components [4], and to address this, a range of methods have been employed that deplete sperm membranes before ICSI (e.g., [3]). Methods include sperm treatment with triton X-100, dithiothreitol (DTT), progesterone, repeated freezing and thawing without cryoprotectant, or piezo-driven pulses. These methods all damage membranes leading to loss of motility, but the use of *living*, motile spermatozoa is not necessary in delivery by ICSI. Methods that set out to damage membranes are not essential in human and mouse ICSI.

In livestock animals, oocytes are usually removed from ovaries collected at the abattoir and matured in vitro (IVM) because direct collection of sufficient oocyte numbers following maturation in vivo is prohibitively time-consuming and costly. For example, porcine ovulation after hormone treatment yields ~35 oocytes (i.e., in vivo-matured oocytes) per animal at a cost of JP ¥40,000–50,000 (US $455–569 as of July 2010), whereas a single ovary obtained from the abattoir for ~JP ¥150 (US $2) yields 10 oocytes after IVM. Although relatively large numbers of oocytes can be stably sourced via IVM, their developmental potential is probably slightly lower than that of oocytes matured in vivo (Table 18.1). Nevertheless, IVM oocytes support development to term at comparable rates, making them considerably more cost-effective.

Overcoming Technical Difficulties

Discrepancies between the developmental potential of oocytes derived in vitro and in vivo may also reflect their respective abilities to support physiological oocyte activation, which includes metaphase II (mII) exit and cell cycle progression [5]. In humans and mice, ICSI using sperm from healthy donors is generally sufficient to induce oocyte activation. In livestock animals, additional artificial activation stimuli (parthenogenetic agents) may be required to induce viable embryonic development (Table 18.1), for reasons that are largely unclear. Activation stimuli include electrical pulses, ethanol, calcium ionophore, or specifically ionomycin combined with the protein kinase inhibitor, 6-dimethylaminopurine (DMAP) (Table 18.1). The necessity of supplemental activation factors after ICSI in livestock presumably reflects one or more deficiencies of IVM oocytes, perhaps caused by the failure of injected sperm to trigger release Ca^{2+}, but this cannot always be the case [6, 7], and

Table 18.1 Experience with micromanipulation techniques in farm animal species

Species	Oocytes	Sperm	Activation	No. embryos transferred (recipients)	No. offspring (pregnancies) [% embryos]	References
Pig (*Sus scrofa*)	In vivo	Fresh	Sperm	69 (3)	3 (1) [4.3]	Martin [21]
Pig	In vivo	Fresh	Ca^{2+} ionophore	84 (4)	1 (1) [1.2]	Kolbe and Holtz [22]
Pig	IVM	Frozen	Electrical	16 (1)	1 (1) [6.3]	Lai et al. [23]
Pig	In vivo	FACS	$CaCl_2$	341 (4)	13 (4) [3.8]	Probst and Rath [24]
Pig	IVM	Frozen	Electrical	598 (7)	3 (2) [0.5]	Nakai et al. [25]
Pig	IVM	Frozen	Sperm	452 (6)	1 (2) [0.2]	Yong et al. [6]
Pig	IVM	Fresh	Sperm	197 (7)	12 (3) [6.1]	Katayama et al. [7]
Cattle (*Bos primigenius*)	IVM	Fresh	Sperm	8 (7)	3 + 1?(4) [50.0]	Wei and Fukui [26]
Cattle	IVM	Fresh	Ethanol	nd (10)	5 (5) [–]	Horiuchi et al. [27]
Cattle	IVM	Frozen	Sperm	11 (6)	1 (2) [9.1]	Galli et al. [28]
Cattle	IVM	Frozen	Ethanol	19 (17)	9 (10) [47.4]	Oikawa et al. [29]
Cattle	IVM	Frozen	Ionomycin + DMAP	11 (8)	1 (1) [9.1]	Oikawa et al. [29]
Cattle	IVM	Fresh	Ethanol	61 (54)	24 (28) [39.3]	Horiuchi [30]
Sheep (*Ovis aries*)	IVM	Fresh	Sperm	38 (17)	9 (6) [23.7]	Gomez et al. [31]
Horse (*Equus ferus*)	In vivo	Fresh	Sperm	31(12)	2 (3) [6.5]	Cochran et al. [32]
Goat (*Capra aegagrus*)	No reports					

there is little direct evidence for it. There are no reports of Ca^{2+} release in pig ICSI, but demembranated pig spermatozoa contain the activating factor, phospholipase C zeta, and readily activate mouse eggs leading to pronuclear formation [8]. This suggests that the failure involves a maternal effect, although porcine oocytes can also be induced to undergo Ca^{2+} release [9]. However, unlike mouse oocytes, those of pigs and some other livestock species (including cattle) do not respond to the parthenogenetic agent, $SrCl_2$, so there may be fundamental differences that are not readily explained by differences in the oocyte maturation protocols (e.g., in vitro vs. in vivo or mouse vs. pig). In cattle, there is a single report that ICSI induces abnormal Ca^{2+} oscillations and activation, with the majority of oocytes unable to undergo any Ca^{2+} oscillations at all [10]. These findings seem germane to the low success rates of ICSI in livestock species to date.

The retrieval of eggs—or ovum pickup (OPU)—is available for the nonsurgical collection of cattle and goat oocytes matured in vivo. However, with the exceptions of pig and horse (Table 18.1), there are few, if any, reports of ICSI in livestock animals using in vivo-matured oocytes. The application of ICSI in livestock animals has gradually increased, notwithstanding that the efficiency remains low—a source of optimism for those who wish to improve the efficiency further.

Using Micromanipulation to Engineer Livestock Genomes

One potential prize for such an improvement is the enhancement of transgenesis (the generation of animals with completely or partially prescribed genome alterations). Microinjection of DNA directly into zygotic pronuclei has been used for several years in livestock animals [11, 12], but zygotes (1-cell embryos) are difficult to obtain and manipulate (those of species such as *S. scrofa* are opaque, due to high lipid content), and the efficiency of integration and transgenerational transmission of the foreign DNA remains low [13]. Relatively recently, this problem has been addressed by somatic cell nuclear transfer (NT) (Fig. 18.1). Broadly, somatic cells—for example, ear punch or embryonic fibroblasts—may be cultured and subjected to genetic modification in vitro by transfection with a suitable DNA construct, prior to their use as nucleus donors. This enables the structure and expression level of the resulting integrant to be determined so that the best can be expanded clonally. In this way, donor cell cultures containing ~100% of the desired integrant can be used for NT, yielding high rates of transgenesis [14].

Perhaps the most powerful application of the transfection-NT approach is in the production of gene-targeted livestock animals [15]. In mice, targeted genomic mutagenesis by homologous recombination is widely achieved using embryonic stem (ES) cells, but widely accepted ES cells have not yet been established from livestock animals. The rate of homologous recombination in most somatic cells is typically lower than that in mouse ES cells, with the notable exception of the chicken cell line, DT40 [16]. However, this relative inefficiency may not hold for acutely isolated embryonic cells; gene targeting is efficient in pig embryonic fibroblasts,

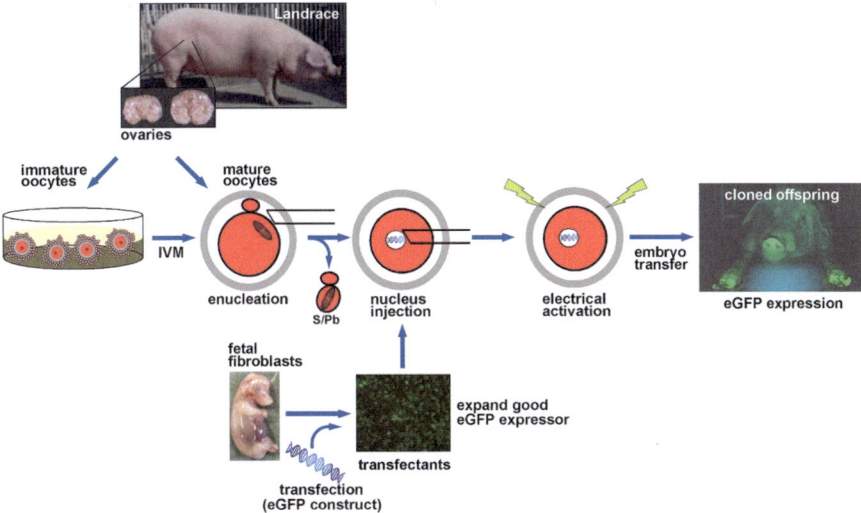

Fig. 18.1 Production of the enhanced green fluorescent protein (eGFP) transgenic pigs by somatic cell nuclear transfer. Fetal fibroblasts were transfected, and cells expressing high levels of eGFP were selected for use as nucleus donors. This method results in cloned pigs that almost always exhibit broad, high-level eGFP expression. *S/Pb* spindle/first polar body

resulting in the production of gene knockout pigs by NT (unpublished data). Thus, the transfection-NT combination holds considerable promise in transgenic livestock production.

ICSI provides an alternative to transfection-NT for the production of transgenic livestock animals, although, so far, not gene-targeted ones. In this method, spermatozoa are incubated with the transgene DNA construct to form a sperm–DNA complex that is injected into the egg; in effect, the sperm acts as a carrier for the transgene, at least in the mouse [17]. This technique is advantageous in the stable incorporation and expression of large (>100 kb) DNA constructs such as yeast artificial chromosomes (YACs) that are not amenable to transfection or viral delivery [18]. The successful production of nontargeted transgenic pigs following both ICSI and NT techniques has been reported, albeit without using artificial chromosomes [19].

ICSI in Large Animal Xenografting

Recently, viable piglets have been produced with spermatozoa from immature testicular tissue xenografted into immunodeficient mice [20]. In these experiments, testes from 6- to 12-day-old piglets (i.e., prepubertal pigs) were minced and grafted into the testes of immunodeficient mice. It was possible to collect porcine spermatozoa from the engrafted host mice 133–280 days later and utilize them for porcine

ICSI. Although only six piglets from two recipients in 23 trials were obtained, all grew normally. The xenograft-ICSI technique has several potential applications. It represents one avenue for the conservation of species and other genetic resources and suggests a new means to sustain lineages—especially genetically modified ones—that otherwise propagate with high rates of male neonatal mortality.

References

1. Uehara T, Yanagimachi R. Microsurgical injection of spermatozoa into hamster eggs with subsequent transformation of sperm nuclei into male pronuclei. Biol Reprod. 1976;15:467–70.
2. Palermo G, Joris H, Devroey P, Van Steirteghem AC. Pregnancies after intracytoplasmic injection of single spermatozoon into an oocyte. Lancet. 1992;340:17–8.
3. Garcia-Roselló E, Garcia-Mengual E, Coy P, Alfonso J, Silvestre MA. Intracytoplasmic sperm injection in livestock species: an update. Reprod Domest Anim. 2009;44:143–51.
4. Morozumi K, Yanagimachi R. Incorporation of the acrosome into the oocyte during intracytoplasmic sperm injection could be potentially hazardous to embryo development. Proc Natl Acad Sci U S A. 2005;102:14209–14.
5. Perry ACF, Verlhac M-H. Second meiotic arrest and exit in frogs and mice. EMBO Rep. 2008;9:246–51.
6. Yong HY, Hao Y, Lai L, Li R, Murphy CN, Rieke A, Wax D, Samuel M, Prather RS. Production of a transgenic piglet by a sperm injection technique in which no chemical or physical treatments were used for oocytes or sperm. Mol Reprod Dev. 2006;73:595–9.
7. Katayama M, Rieke A, Cantley T, Murphy C, Dowell L, Sutovsky P, Day BN. Improved fertilization and embryo development resulting in birth of live piglets after intracytoplasmic sperm injection and in vitro culture in a cysteine-supplemented medium. Theriogenology. 2007;67:835–47.
8. Fujimoto S, Yoshida N, Fukui T, Amanai M, Isobe T, Itagaki C, Izumi T, Perry ACF. Mammalian phospholipase C zeta induces oocyte activation from the sperm perinuclear matrix. Dev Biol. 2004;274:370–83.
9. Macháty Z, Bonk AJ, Kühholzer B, Prather RS. Porcine oocyte activation induced by a cytosolic sperm factor. Mol Reprod Dev. 2000;57:290–5.
10. Malcuit C, Maserati M, Takahashi Y, Page R, Fissore RA. Intracytoplasmic sperm injection in the bovine induces abnormal $[Ca^{2+}]i$ responses and oocyte activation. Reprod Fertil Dev. 2006;18:39–51.
11. Martin MJ, Pinkert CA. Production of transgenic swine by DNA microinjection. In: Pincert CA, editor. Transgenic animal technology: a laboratory handbook. 2nd ed. California: Academic; 2002. p. 307–36.
12. Niemann H, Döpke HH, Hadeler KG. Production of transgenic ruminants by DNA microinjection. In: Pincert CA, editor. Transgenic animal technology: a laboratory handbook. 2nd ed. California: Academic; 2002. p. 337–57.
13. Robl JM, Wang Z, Kasinathan P, Kuroiwa Y. Transgenic animal production and animal biotechnology. Theriogenology. 2007;67:127–33.
14. Yazaki S, Iwamoto M, Onishi A, Miwa Y, Suzuki S, Fuchimoto D, Sembon S, Furusawa T, Hashimoto M, Oishi T, Liu D, Nagasaka T, Kuzuya T, Maruyama S, Ogawa H, Kadomatsu K, Uchida K, Nakao A, Kobayashi T. Successful cross-breeding of cloned pigs expressing endogalactosidase C and human decay accelerating factor. Xenotransplantation. 2009;16:511–21.
15. Laible G, Alonso-González L. Gene targeting from laboratory to livestock: current status and emerging concepts. Biotechnol J. 2009;4:1278–92.

16. Buerstedde JM, Takeda S. Increased ratio of targeted to random integration after transfection of chicken B cell lines. Cell. 1991;67:179–88.
17. Perry ACF, Wakayama T, Kishikawa H, Kasai T, Okabe M, Toyoda Y, Yanagimachi R. Mammalian transgenesis by intracytoplasmic sperm injection. Science. 1999;284:1180–3.
18. Perry ACF, Rothman A, de las Heras JI, Feinstein P, Mombaerts P, Cooke HJ, Wakayama T. Efficient metaphase II transgenesis with different transgene archetypes. Nat Biotechnol. 2001;19:1071–3.
19. Umeyama K, Watanabe M, Saito H, Kurome M, Tohi S, Matsunari H, Miki K, Nagashima H. Dominant-negative mutant hepatocyte nuclear factor 1alpha induces diabetes in transgenic-cloned pigs. Transgenic Res. 2009;18:697–706.
20. Nakai M, Kaneko H, Somfai T, Maedomari N, Ozawa M, Noguchi J, Ito J, Kashiwazaki N, Kikuchi K. Production of viable piglets for the first time using sperm derived from ectopic testicular xenografts. Reproduction. 2010;139:331–5.
21. Martin MJ. Development of in vivo-matured porcine oocytes following intracytoplasmic sperm injection. Biol Reprod. 2000;63:109–12.
22. Kolbe T, Holtz W. Birth of piglet derived from an oocyte fertilized by intracytoplasmic sperm injection (ICSI). Anim Reprod Sci. 2000;64:97–101.
23. Lai L, Sun Q, Wu G, Murpy CN, Kühholzer B, Park KW, Bonk AJ, Day BN, Prather RS. Development of porcine embryos and offspring after intracytoplasmic sperm injection with liposome transfected or non-transfected sperm into in vitro matured oocytes. Zygote. 2001;9:339–46.
24. Probst S, Rath D. Production of piglets using intracytoplasmic sperm injection (ICSI) with flowcytometrically sorted boar semen and artificially activated oocytes. Theriogenology. 2003;59:961–73.
25. Nakai M, Kashiwazaki N, Takizawa A, Hayashi Y, Nakatsukasa E, Fuchimoto D, Noguchi J, Kaneko H, Shino M, Kikuchi K. Viable piglets generated from porcine oocytes matured in vitro and fertilized by intracytoplasmic sperm head injection. Biol Reprod. 2003;68:1003–8.
26. Wei H, Fukui Y. Births of calves derived from embryos produced by intracytoplasmic sperm injection without exogenous oocyte activation. Zygote. 2002;10:149–53.
27. Horiuchi T, Emuta C, Yamauchi Y, Oikawa T, Numabe T, Yanagimachi R. Birth of normal calves after intracytoplasmic sperm injection of bovine oocytes: a methodological approach. Theriogenology. 2002;57:1013–24.
28. Galli C, Vassiliev I, Lagutina I, Galli A, Lazzari G. Bovine embryo development following ICSI: effect of activation, sperm capacitation and pre-treatment with dithiothreitol. Theriogenology. 2003;60:1467–80.
29. Oikawa T, Takada N, Kikuchi T, Numabe T, Takenaka M, Horiuchi T. Evaluation of activation treatments for blastocyst production and birth of viable calves following bovine intracytoplasmic sperm injection. Anim Reprod Sci. 2005;86:187–94.
30. Horiuchi T. Application study of intracytoplasmic sperm injection for golden hamster and cattle production. J Reprod Dev. 2006;52:13–21.
31. Gòmez MC, Catt JW, Evans G, Maxwell WMC. Cleavage, development and competence of sheep embryos fertilized by intracytoplasmic sperm injection and in vitro fertilization. Theriogenology. 1998;49:1143–54.
32. Cochran R, Meintjes M, Reggio B, Hylan D, Carter J, Pinto C, Paccamonti D, Godke RA. Live foals produced from sperm-injected oocytes derived from pregnant mares. J Equine Vet Sci. 1998;11:736–40.

Chapter 19
Assisted Hatching in IVF

Itziar Belil and Anna Veiga

The Zona Pellucida and Embryo Hatching

Zona Pellucida

The zona pellucida (ZP) of mammalian eggs and embryos is an acellular matrix composed of sulfated glycoproteins with different roles during fertilization and embryo development [1]. Three distinct glycoproteins have been described both in mice and in humans (ZP1, ZP2, and ZP3) [2]. Acrosome-reacted spermatozoa bind to ZP receptors, and biochemical changes have been observed after fertilization [3] responsible for the prevention of polyspermic fertilization.

The main function of the ZP after fertilization is the protection of the embryo and the maintenance of its integrity [4]. It has been postulated that blastomeres may be weakly connected and that the ZP is needed during the migration of embryos through the reproductive tract to maintain the embryo structure. Implantation has been observed after replacement of zona-free mouse morulas or blastocysts, while the transfer of zona-free precompacted embryos results in the adherence of transferred embryos to the oviductal walls or to one another. A possible protective role against hostile uterine factors has also been described [4]. Degeneration of sheep eggs after complete or partial ZP removal that could be ascribed to an immune response was described by Trounson and Moore [5].

I. Belil, BSc (✉) • A. Veiga, PhD
Department of Obstetrics, Gynecology, and Reproduction, Reproductive Medicine Service, Institut Universitari Dexeus, Gran Via Carles III, 71-75, 08029 Barcelona, Spain
e-mail: itzbcl@dexeus.com; aveiga@cmrb.eu

Hatching

Embryo hatching involves a spontaneous rupture of the ZP. Once in the uterus, the blastocysts must get out of the ZP to allow interaction between trophectoderm and endometrial cells so that implantation can occur. The loss of the ZP in the uterus is the result of embryonic and uterine events. Expansion and ZP thinning occurs in mammalian blastocysts prior to hatching. As a result of several cycles of contraction and expansion and because of its elasticity, the ZP thins. Lysins of embryonic and/or uterine origin are also involved in ZP thinning and hatching. It seems that hatching is predominantly the result of zona lysis, whereas physical expansion of the blastocyst, even though involved in hatching, does not seem to be the primary mechanism [6, 7]. Contraction-expansion cycles as well as cytoplasmic extensions of trophectoderm (trophectoderm projections, TEPs) have been documented by time-lapse video recording in human blastocysts [8]. It is not clear whether TEPs are needed in vivo for ZP hatching, but they seem to have a role in attachment, implantation, and possibly embryo locomotion [9]. Mouse embryo hatching in vitro seems to be dependent on a sufficient number of blastomeres constituting the embryo. Hatching in vivo must be different from that in vitro, the difference possibly involving uterine and/or uterine-induced trophectoderm lytic factors [10].

Assisted Hatching

Definition

Failure of implantation after IVF may result from the inability of the blastocyst to hatch out of the ZP. Artificial disruption of the ZP by micromanipulation techniques to enhance the ability of embryo to hatch is known as assisted hatching (AH) and has been proposed as a method for improving the success of IVF. The first report of the use of AH in human embryos was published by Cohen et al. in 1990 [11]. These authors documented an important increase of implantation rates with mechanical AH in embryos from unselected IVF patients.

Indications for Assisted Hatching

Human embryos resulting from superovulation develop more slowly in vitro compared to embryos in vivo, manifest a relatively high degree of genetic abnormalities, undergo cell fragmentation, and only a small proportion achieve blastocyst stage development [12]. Cultured embryos also hatch and implant at lower rates than natural [13, 14]. It is unclear whether this is due to hardening of the zona pellucida as a result of cross-linking of its constituent glycoproteins (ZP1, ZP2, ZP3) in an in vitro environment[4], but it is believed that ZP hardening may be exacerbated at any stage of embryo development after long-term in vitro culture and cryopreservation [15]. Zona thickness appears to be influenced by woman's age and proliferative phase follicle-stimulating hormone (FSH) profile, and correlates negatively with embryo implantation rates [16].

Under these considerations, AH can be performed in the following cases:

- Recurrent failure of embryo implantation after embryo transfer (three or more embryo transfers without a pregnancy)
- Embryos exhibiting thick zona pellucida
- Advanced maternal age (over 37 years)
- Women with elevated FSH levels
- Cryopreservation cycles

How to Perform Assisted Hatching

Embryo implantation seems to occur earlier after AH, possibly by allowing earlier embryo–endometrium contact [17]. Partial ZP drilling, ZP thinning, and total ZP removal are different ways to perform embryo AH using various micromanipulation techniques. It is very important to minimize the time that the embryo is out of the incubator and to optimize methodologies to reduce pH and temperature variations that can be detrimental for embryo development, during embryo manipulation. To reduce environmental variations, AH has to be performed in microdrops of HEPES-buffered medium (to minimize pH changes during the procedure) covered with oil, under an inverted microscope with Nomarski or Hoffman optics, on a heated microscope stage, at 37°C. Microtools for AH can be made by means of a pipette puller and microforge, but are also commercially available. Micropipettes are mounted on micromanipulators. A 30-min culture period seems to be sufficient before the transfer of the manipulated embryos. Embryo transfer to the uterus has to be performed as atraumatically as possible to avoid damage of ZP-manipulated embryos.

Partial Zona Drilling

An artificial gap drilling completely the ZP can be made using micromanipulation techniques. It is important that the size of the hole created in the zona is large enough to avoid trapping of the embryo during hatching, but not so large that it permits blastomere loss. The adequate size of the hole seems to be ~30 μm. Zona drilling can be achieved by mechanical, enzymatic, chemical, or thermolytic effect [18].

Zona Pellucida Thinning

The human zona is bilayered, with a less dense, thick, easily digestible outer layer, and a more compact but resilient inner layer [19]. The aim of ZP thinning is to thin the outer layer of the ZP without complete lysis and perforation of the inner layer. It involves the thinning of about 50% of the zona thickness of a cross-shaped area (partial zona thinning) or of the complete surface (circumferential zona thinning) of the ZP of the embryo [18]. Care has to be taken not to rupture the ZP completely. By not breaching the zona, the potential risk of blastomere loss and embryonic infection is minimized. Zona-thinned embryos show higher implantation rate and seem to be more physiological than total ZP drilling when embryo transfer is performed on day 3 of embryo culture [20].

Zona pellucida thinning has been described using chemical or enzymatic action or with laser methodology.

Zona Pellucida Removal

Total ZP removal before embryo transfer has been expected to bring about closer contact and communication of the trophectoderm of the blastocyst with the endometrium thereby improving implantation. Full ZP removal has shown to improve the outcome of blastocyst transfer in patients showing repeated implantation failure [21] as well as of blastocyst transfer after vitrification [22]. Total ZP removal at the cleavage stage may have adverse effects such as loss of blastomeres and an increased risk of monozygotic multiple gestation. The ZP can be totally removed by chemical or enzymatical methods or by using laser and mechanical pipetting.

Methods of Assisted Hatching

The AH procedure to breach or thin the ZP can be performed using various methods.

Mechanical Partial Zona Dissection

AH following mechanical opening of the ZP and showing an increased implantation rate was first reported in 1990 [11]. The method of partial zona dissection (PZD) used was similar to that described for oocytes, to assist oocyte zona pellucida penetration by spermatozoa [23] with no preincubation of the embryos in sucrose.

Embryos denuded of corona cells are micromanipulated in microdrops of HEPES-buffered medium under paraffin oil. The procedure is performed at 37°C, under an inverted microscope. The embryo is held with a holding pipette, and the ZP is tangentially pierced with a microneedle from the 1 to the 11 o'clock position. The embryo is released from the holding pipette, and the part of the ZP between the two points is rubbed against the holding pipette until a slit is made in the ZP. The embryo is washed twice in fresh culture medium and placed in the transfer dish. Three-dimensional-PZD (3D-PZD) in the shape of a cross has also been described [24]. The procedure starts as conventional PZD, and a second cut is made in the ZP under the first slit. A cross-shaped cut can be seen on the surface of the ZP. This method allows the creation of larger openings while permitting protection of the embryo by the ZP flaps during embryo transfer. A new technique called "controlled zona dissection" (CDZ) has been described as a variation of PZD [25]. The embryo is held at 8 o'clock position by a beveled opened holding pipette and a thin angled hatching needle with a blunted tip pierce the ZP at 5 o'clock position. The hatching needle is inserted deeply into the holding pipette until the embryo is pushed to the angle of the hatching needle. The curve of the needle is then pressed against the bottom of the dish to cut the pierced ZP. A large slit (two thirds of embryo's diameter) created by CDZ enhances significantly the rate of complete in vitro hatching of blastocysts compared to 3D-PZD.

Chemical Zona Drilling

The human ZP can be dissolved in a low-pH solution as the acid Tyrode's solution (AT solution: pH of 2.2–2.6). AT solution can be prepared in the laboratory with the protocol of Hogan et al. [26] and adjusted to a pH of 2.5 or can be purchased commercially.

Selective AH to promote blastocyst hatching involving chemical opening of the zona with AT was first reported in 1992 [27]. One advantage of AT drilling compared with PZD is the possibility of increasing the size of the hole in the ZP. Large holes have proved to be more efficient for enhancing hatching and avoiding embryo entrapment. In order to perform chemical zona drilling, the embryo is held with a holding pipette in such a way that the micropipette containing AT (internal diameter 3–5 μm) and located at the 3 o'clock position faces a large perivitelline space or an area with cytoplasmic fragments of the embryo. The acid solution is gently delivered with the help of a microinjector over a small area of the ZP, with the tip of the pipette positioned very close to the zona. Accumulation of AT in a single area must be avoided. As soon as a hole in the ZP is created, suction is applied to avoid excess AT entering the perivitelline space. If the inner region of the ZP is difficult to breach, creation of the hole can be facilitated by pushing the AT micropipette against the ZP. Extracellular fragments can also be removed by aspiration during the procedure [27]. It is necessary to rinse the embryo several times in fresh culture medium immediately after the AT hatching procedure, prior to returning it back into the culture dish, to avoid detrimental effects of the acid solution on the blastomeres.

The ZP can also be chemically removed from embryos reaching the blastocyst stage on day 5 of in vitro culture. Embryos are placed into a 30 μL drop of prewarmed AT solution under mineral oil for approximately 10 s, followed by careful washing in five drops fresh culture medium.

Enzymatic Zona Digestion

Blastocyst transfer after enzymatic treatment with pronase of the ZP, to either soften or remove totally the zona before transfer, has shown high pregnancy and implantation rates in patients with previous repeated implantation failure [21]. The first delivery of a healthy baby after an enzymatically treated zona-free blastocyst transfer was reported on 1997 [28].

The ZP can be softened or totally dissolved after treatment with pronase at concentrations of 10 IU/mL in medium under oil in a 5–6% CO_2 in air atmosphere and at 37°C for exposure periods of no longer than 1.5 min. Embryos have to be washed several times in fresh medium after the AH procedure. There are some evidence that pronase treatment in blastocysts for longer periods may cause adverse effects on the trophectoderm and inner cell mass [29].

Laser Technologies

The application of a laser on the ZP for AH results in photoablation of the zona pellucida. For fast and efficient clinical use of laser systems in AH, it is important that the laser is accurately controlled and produces precise ZP openings without thermal or mutagenic effects [18].

The first use of a laser for ZP drilling was reported in 1991 with an ArF excimer laser (ultraviolet (UV) region, 193 nm wavelength) [30]. This laser system is a contact mode laser and makes necessary to touch the ZP with the laser-delivering pipette. Another contact mode laser, the erbium:yttrium–aluminum–garnet (Er:YAG) laser (2,940 nm radiation), has also been used for ZP drilling and thinning, and its safety and efficacy have been demonstrated in clinical practice [31]. No degenerative alterations on the ZP and membrane of embryos were observed using light and scanning electron microscopy after ZP drilling with such a system [32]. But the necessity of sterile micropipettes and optical fibers to deliver the laser beam to the target is the main disadvantage of contact mode lasers.

Noncontact laser systems allow microscope objective-delivered accessibility of laser light to the target. Laser propagation is made through water, and as it avoids the UV absorption peak of DNA, no mutagenic effect on the oocyte or embryo is expected [18]. Several noncontact laser systems have proved to be useful for ZP drilling in the mouse model [33, 34]. Rink et al. introduced an InGaAsP noncontact diode laser that use infrared light at 1.48 μm wavelength [35]. Its high absorption in water causes rapid and precisely localized heating of the target region. The drilling mechanism is explained by a thermal effect induced at the focal point by absorption of the laser energy by water and/or ZP macromolecules, leading to thermolysis of the ZP. Laser absorption by the culture dish and medium is minimal. The effect on the ZP is greatly localized, and the holes obtained are cylindrical and precise. Exposure time (1–20 ms) can be minimized. The system is compact and easily adapted to all kinds of microscopes. The size of the hole is related to the laser exposure time. The safety and usefulness of the system has been demonstrated in mice and human [36, 37].

This is actually the laser system preferred to drill the ZP of human embryos since it is simple, quick, and easy to use.

AH may be performed a few hours or immediately prior to ET. A culture dish with several 10 µL drops of HEPES-buffered culture medium and overlaid with prewarmed mineral oil has to be prepared shortly before the procedure. Embryos selected for transfer are placed individually in separate drops, and the dish is placed on the heated stage of the inverted microscope equipped with the laser technology. It is recommended to stabilize the embryo with a holding micropipette. An area between two blastomeres with a large perivitelline space has to be chosen for laser drilling.

Routinely, a single opening of ~30 µm (about 10% of the ZP circumference) is created by dissecting the full thickness of the ZP (Fig. 19.1). Thinning the ZP can be done focusing the laser shoots to the outer layer of the zona. Several pulses (2–8 pulses) are necessary to complete the cut through the ZP or to thin a quarter of the embryo circumference.

It has to be taken in account that diode laser beam produces superheated water approaching 200°C on the beam axis. The action of the laser must be strictly limited to the targeted region of the ZP, since focused laser irradiation on a specific cell would cause damage and would probably be lethal to that cell. Following irradiation, the heat is conducted away from the target and is dissipated into the surrounding medium. The potential to damage blastomeres adjacent to the hole created by the laser is minimized by using short pulse durations (≤ 5 ms)and mild laser power (~100 mW) at a safe distance from the blastomeres [38–40].

At the end of the procedure, the embryo is immediately washed, replaced in the culture media, and returned to the incubator.

Embryo Stage to Perform Assisted Hatching

AH can be performed at different stages of embryo development, but the first results published were obtained after performing AH to early stage developing embryos, [11, 27] probably because embryo transfer was routinely performed on day 2 or 3 of culture.

Early Embryo Stage

At day 3 of development, normal embryos should have 6–8 noncompacted blastomeres. AH, thought to be the best method currently available to overcome the ZP barrier in unexplained implantation failure in fresh embryo transfer, is usually

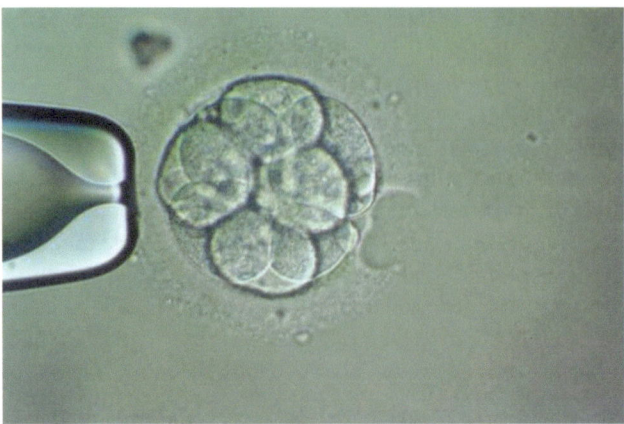

Fig. 19.1 Laser-assisted hatching. The zona pellucida (ZP) of an eight-cell embryo drilled through photoablation by laser technology: a single opening of ~30 µm is created by dissecting the full thickness of the ZP. (From Veiga et al. [18], with permission)

performed on day 3. AH prior to transfer, by total disruption or by thinning of the ZP, seems to enhance pregnancy and implantation rates in some selected groups of patients.

Fragment Removal

Embryo development is sometimes associated with a certain degree of cytoplasmic fragmentation. The potential of fragmented embryos for implantation is determined partly by the distribution of fragments. The use of microsurgical fragment removal may alter the course of development for some embryos and can improve their implantation potential [41].

Embryo fragmentation can be reduced by mechanical aspiration after AH prior to embryo replacement. Embryo denuded of corona cells is micromanipulated in microdrops of HEPES-buffered medium under paraffin oil. As mentioned above, the procedure is performed at 37°C, under an inverted microscope with micromanipulation system. The embryos stabilized with a holding pipette held at the 9 o'clock position. AH can be performed mechanically, chemically, or with laser. A 10-µm micropipette is oriented at the 3 o'clock position adjacent to the area with cytoplasmic fragments of the embryo where the hole has been created. Cytoplasmic fragments are removed by gentle aspiration. The embryo is then rinsed several times and returned to the standard culture media to the incubator until transfer.

Blastocyst Stage

Although AH is usually performed on early cleavage stage embryos, it seems to be more physiologically feasible to assist this process in vitro at the blastocyst stage as in vivo hatching occurs at that stage just prior to implantation.

AH performed at the blastocyst stage seems to enhance embryo implantation [21, 22]. It is preferable to apply AH to day 5 blastocysts (initial blastocysts) than to expanded blastocysts to avoid harmful effects on trophectoderm cells.

As mentioned above, to perform partial zona drilling or zona thinning, the procedure is performed in microdrops of HEPES-buffered medium under paraffin oil, at 37°C, under an inverted microscope with micromanipulation system. The blastocyst is stabilized with a holding pipette held at the 9 o'clock position. AH can be performed to the blastocyst mechanically, chemically, or with laser. The embryo is then rinsed several times and returned to the incubator until transfer.

Full ZP removal has shown to improve the outcome of blastocyst transfer after vitrification [22]. It has been observed that human blastocysts completely hatched in vitro do not stick to the surface of the culture dishes or the inner surface of embryo replacement catheter. Therefore, these blastocysts can be handled like intact blastocysts [18]. Total ZP removal of blastocyst can be done enzymatically or chemically as described above.

Frozen–Thawed Embryos

Elasticity and thinning of the ZP can be adversely influenced by the freezing–thawing process. The stress induced by the freeze–thaw process may lead to zona hardening, impairing the ability of blastocysts to hatch. AH in frozen–thawed cycles has been shown to increase pregnancy and implantation rates both in early cleavage stage embryos [42, 43] and blastocysts [22].

Frozen–vitrified–thawed early stage developed embryos or blastocysts can undergo AH by the different methods described above.

Necrotic Material Removal

The implantation rate of embryos partially surviving cryopreservation seems to be impaired. It can be speculated that the lysed blastomeres are producing factors as they degrade that are detrimental or toxic to the other cells in the embryo or that may disrupt cell-to-cell communication. There is evidence of possible benefits of the removal of lysed cells from frozen–thawed embryos [44, 45] with no clear explanation about such benefits.

Day 2 or day 3 frozen embryos are thawed 1 day before embryo transfer. AH of frozen–thawed embryos is usually performed shortly before embryo transfer. However, removal of lysed material is easier when AH is performed soon after the embryo thawing process. The frozen–thawed embryo, placed in a dish with microdrops of HEPES-buffered medium under mineral oil, at 37°C, under an inverted microscope with micromanipulation system, is stabilized with a holding pipette held at the 9 o'clock position. AH is performed as usually by creating an opening in the zona pellucida using AT or laser system. The AH micropipette (10 µm) has to be oriented to the necrotic material area of the embryo where the hole has been created. Lysed blastomeres are removed by gentle aspiration. Embryo is then washed several times in fresh medium and returned to the incubator for further culture till transfer.

Potential Adverse Effects

Patients whose embryos are hatched are often treated with antibiotics and steroids before and after embryo transfer, exposing them to the potential risks and side effects of such treatments.

Embryo Damage

The AH procedure may be associated with specific complications independent of the IVF procedure itself, including lethal damage to the embryo and damage to individual blastomeres with reduction of embryo viability, probably as an adverse effect of embryo micromanipulation.

Risk of Increased Monozygotic Twinning

Artificial manipulation of the ZP has been associated with an increased risk of monozygotic twinning [46, 47]. Artificially induced damage to the ZP may be related with inner cell mass splitting during hatching and thus may result in monozygotic twinning. The size of the hole performed by ZP micromanipulation could be a conditional factor. However, a recent systematic review found insufficient data to assess the impact of AH on monozygotic twinning [48].

Commentary

It is questionable whether different methods of AH yield similar outcomes. Mechanical hatching by PZD is limited by the difficulty of creating a hole of consistent size. The use of AT for zona drilling can carry potential problems due to its variability and possible embryotoxicity. Enzymatic methods to dissolve or thin the zona seem to be effective and safe. Although the equipment may be expensive, the use of a 1.48-μm diode infrared noncontact laser system for zona drilling appears to be the most suitable method for AH in the IVF laboratory: it offers a low potential risk and is quick and relatively simple to perform with high consistency between operators.

Key Issues

Higher clinical pregnancy and implantation rates have been reported after AH, but a recently published Cochrane meta-analysis concluded that, although live birth should be considered the primary outcome, there is insufficient evidence to determine any effect of AH on live birth rates [48]. Thereby, the conclusions concerning AH benefits and taking in account the variability in methods and studies performed are as follows:

1. AH does not enhance the outcome in patients undergoing their first IVF attempt.
2. AH increases the pregnancy rate in patients with previous implantation failures or poor prognosis in both fresh and frozen embryo transfer.
3. It is not clear whether AH is beneficial for patients of advanced age, embryos with a thick ZP, or for frozen–thawed embryos.
4. More robust trials with adequate methodological quality and power to investigate the role of assisted hatching in different groups with live birth reports and multiple pregnancy data are needed.
5. Currently, there is insufficient evidence to recommend assisted hatching as a routine technique in patients undergoing ART.

References

1. Dean J. Biology of mammalian fertilization: the role of the zona pellucida. J Clin Invest. 1992;89:1055–9.
2. Shabanowitz RB, O'Rand MG. Characterization of the human zona pellucida from fertilized and unfertilized eggs. J Reprod Fertil. 1988;82:151–61.
3. Ducibella T, Kurasawa S, Ramgarajan S, et al. Precocious loss of cortical granules during oocyte meiotic maturation and correlation with an egg-induced modification of the zona pellucida. Dev Biol. 1990;137:46–55.
4. Cohen J. Assisted hatching of human embryos. J In Vitro Fertil Embryo Transf. 1991;8:179–90.
5. Trounson AO, Moore NW. The survival and development of sheep eggs following complete or partial removal of the zona pellucida. J Reprod Fert. 1974;41:97–105.
6. Gordon J, Dupont UP. A new mouse model for embryos with a hatching deficiency and its use to elucidate the mechanism of blastocyst hatching. Fertil Steril. 1993;59:1296–301.
7. Schiewe MC, Hazeleger NL, Sclimenti C, et al. Physiological characterization of blastocyst hatching mechanisms by use of a mouse antihatching model. Fertil Steril. 1995;63:288–94.
8. Gonsales D, Bavister B. Zona pellucida escape by hamster blastocysts in vitro is delayed and morphologically different compared with zona escape in vivo. Biol Reprod. 1995;52:470–80.

9. Gonsales DS, Jones JM, Pinyopumintr P, et al. Trophectoderm projections: a potential means for locomotion, attachment and implantation of bovine, equine and human blastocysts. Hum Reprod. 1996;11:2739–45.
10. Montag M, Koll B, Holmes P, et al. Significance of the number of embryonic cells and the state of the zona pellucida for hatching of mouse blastocysts in vitro versus in vivo. Biol Reprod. 2000;62:1738–44.
11. Cohen J, Elsner C, Kort H, et al. Impairment of the hatching process following IVF in the human and improvement of implantation by assisted hatching using micromanipulation. Hum Reprod. 1990;5:7–13.
12. Hsu MI, Mayer J, Aronshon M, et al. Embryo implantation in in vitro fertilization and intracytoplasmic sperm injection: impact of cleavage status, morphology grade, and number of embryos transferred. Fertil Steril. 1999;72(4):679–85.
13. Harlow GM, Quinn P. Development of preimplantation mouse embryos in vitro and in vivo. Aust J Biol Sci. 1982;35:187–93.
14. Mercader A, Simon C, Galan A, et al. An analysis of spontaneous hatching in a human endometrial epithelial coculture system: is assisted hatching justified? J Assist Reprod Genet. 2001;18(6): 315–9.
15. Ludwig M, Al-Hasani S, Felderbaum DK. New aspects of cryopreservation of oocytes and embryos in assisted reproduction and future perspectives. Hum Reprod. 1999;14 Suppl 1:162–85.
16. Loret De Mola JR, Garside WT, Bucci J, et al. Analysis of the human zona pellucida during culture: correlation with diagnosis and the preovulatory hormonal environment. J Assist Reprod Genet 1997;14:332–7.
17. Liu HC, Cohen J, Alikani M, et al. Assisted hatching facilitates earlier implantation. Fertil Steril. 1993;60:871–5.
18. Veiga A, Boiso I, Belil I. Assisted hatching. In: Gardner DK, Weissman A, Howles CM, Shoham Z, editors. Textbook of assisted reproductive technologies. 3rd ed. London: Informa Healthcare; 2009. p. 181–90.
19. Tucker MJ, Biol MI, Wicker SR, et al. Embryonal zona pellucida thinning and uterine transfer. Assist Reprod Rev. 1993;3: 168–71.
20. Mantoudis E, Podsiadly BT, Gorgy A, et al. A comparison between quarter, partial and total laser assisted hatching in selected infertility patients. Hum Reprod. 2001;16:2182–96.
21. Fong CY, Bongso A, Ng SC, et al. Blastocyst transfer after enzymatic treatment of the zona pellucida: improving in-vitro fertilization and understanding implantation. Hum Reprod. 1998;13: 2926–32.
22. Hiraoka K, Fuchiwaki M, Hiraoka K, et al. Zona pellucida removal and vitrified blastocyst transfer outcome: a preliminary study. Reprod Biomed Online. 2007;15(1):68–75.
23. Malter HE, Cohen J. Partial zona dissection of the human oocyte: a non traumatic method using micromanipulation to assist zona pellucida penetration. Fertil Steril. 1989;51:139–48.
24. Cieslak J, Ivakhnenko V, Wolf G, et al. Three dimensional partial zona dissection for preimplantation genetic diagnosis and assisted hatching. Fertil Steril. 1999;71:308–13.
25. Lyu QF, Wu LQ, Li YP, et al. An improved mechanical technique for assisted hatching. Hum Reprod. 2005;20:1619–23.
26. Hogan B, Constantini F, Lacy E. Manipulating the Mouse Embryo: a Laboratory Manual. New York: Cold Spring Harbor Laboratory Press; 1986.
27. Cohen J, Alikani M, Trowbridge J, et al. Implantation enhancement by selective assisted hatching using zona drilling of human embryos with poor prognosis. Hum Reprod. 1992;7:685–91.
28. Fong CY, Bongso A, Ng SC, et al. Ongoing normal pregnancy after transfer of zona-free blastocysts: implications for embryo transfer in the human. Hum Reprod. 1997;12:557–60.
29. Fong CY, Bongso A, Sathananthan H, et al. Ultrastructural observations of enzymatically treated human blastocyst: zona-free blastocyst transfer and rescue of blastocyst with hatching difficulties. Hum Reprod. 2001;16:540–6.

30. Palanker D, Ohad S, Lewis A, et al. Technique for cellular microsurgery using the 193 nm excimer laser. Laser Surg Med. 1991;11:586–9.
31. Obruca A, Strohmer H, Sakkas D, et al. Use of lasers in assisted fertilization and hatching. Hum Reprod. 1994;9:1723–6.
32. Obruca A, Strohmer H, Blaschitz A, et al. Ultrastructural observations in human oocytes and preimplantation embryos after zona opening using an Er:YAG laser. Hum Reprod. 1997;12:2242–5.
33. Blanchet GB, Russell JB, Fincher CR, et al. Laser micromanipulation in the mouse embryo: a novel approach to zona drilling. Fertil Steril. 1992;57:1337–41.
34. Neev J, Schiewe M, Sung VW, et al. Assisted hatching in mouse embryos using a noncontact Ho:YSGG laser system. J Assist Reprod Genet. 1995;12:288–93.
35. Rink K, Delacretaz G, Salathe RP, et al. Non-contact microdrilling of mouse zona pellucida with an objective-delivered 1.48 μm diode laser. Laser Surg Med. 1996;18:52–62.
36. Germond M, Nocera D, Senn A, et al. Improved fertilization and implantation rates after non touch zona pellucida microdrilling of mouse oocytes with a 1.48μm diode laser beam. Hum Reprod. 1996;11:1043–8.
37. Baruffi R, Mauri AL, Petersen C, et al. Assisted hatching with a laser diode in patients <37 years old with no previous failure of implantation: a prospective randomized study. Hum Reprod 1999;14 (abstr book 1) [Abstracts of the 15th Annual meeting of the ESHRE, Tours, France].
38. Douglas-Hamilton DH, Conia J. Thermal effects in laser-assisted pre-embryo zona drilling. J Biomed Opt. 2001;6:205–13.
39. Chatzimeletiou K, Picton HM, Handyside AH. Use of a non-contact, infrared laser for zona drilling of mouse embryos: assessment of immediate effects on blastomere viability. Reprod Biomed Online. 2001;2:178–87.
40. Tinney GM, Windt ML, Kruger TF, et al. Use of a zona laser treatment system in assisted hatching: optimal laser utilization parameters. Fertil Steril. 2005;84:1737–41.
41. Alikani M, Cohen J, Tomkin G, et al. Human embryo fragmentation in vitro and its implications for pregnancy and implantation. Fertil Steril. 1999;71:836–42.
42. Check J, Hoover L, Nazari A, et al. The effect of assisted hatching on pregnancy rates after frozen embryo transfer. Fertil Steril. 1996;65:254–7.
43. Balaban B, Urman B, Yakin K, et al. Laser-assisted hatching increases pregnancy and implantation rates in cryopreserved embryos that were allowed to cleave in vitro after thawing: a prospective randomized study. Hum Reprod. 2006;21:2136–40.
44. Nagy ZP, Taylor T, Elliott T, et al. Removal of lysed blastomeres from frozen–thawed embryos improves implantation and pregnancy rates in frozen embryo transfer cycles. Fertil Steril. 2005;84:1606–12.
45. Rienzi L, Nagy ZP, Ubaldi F, et al. Laser-assisted removal of necrotic blastomeres from cryopreserved embryos that were partially damaged. Fertil Steril. 2002;77:1196–201.
46. Hershlag A, Paine T, Cooper GW, et al. Monozygotic twinning associated with mechanical assisted hatching. Fertil Steril. 1999;71:144–6.
47. Schieve LA, Meikle SF, Peterson HB, et al. Does assisted hatching pose a risk for monozygotic twinning in pregnancies conceived through in vitro fertilization? Fertil Steril. 2000;74:288–94.
48. Das S, Blake D, Farquhar C, Seif MMW. Assisted hatching on assisted conception (IVF and ICSI). Cochrane review. The Cochrane Library 2009(4)

Part IV
Biopsy Procedures on Oocytes and Embryos

Chapter 20
Polar Body Biopsy

Markus Montag, Maria Köster, K. van der Ven, and Hans van der Ven

Polar body biopsy was first proposed in 1990 by Verlinsky and collaborators [1]. Since then, several groups have applied polar body biopsy to a variety of diagnostic applications like detection of single gene disorders [2–4], translocation analysis [5], HLA typing [6] and detection of X-linked disorders [7]. However, to date, most cases of polar body diagnosis are performed for aneuploidy screening [8–11].

Polar bodies are by-products of the meiotic division. Removal of the first and/or second polar body is an indirect approach allowing the genetic status of the oocyte to be inferred from that of the polar body. The first polar body is not required for successful fertilization or normal embryonic development. The second polar body which is extruded from the oocyte after initiation of the fertilization cascade by the spermatozoa is similarly not required for subsequent embryo development. Therefore, removal of both polar bodies for the purposes of genetic diagnosis should have no deleterious effect on the developing embryo.

Technical Aspects of Polar Body Biopsy

The most relevant parts of polar body biopsy are the timing of biopsy, the atraumatic opening of the zona pellucida and the removal of the polar bodies.

M. Montag, PhD (✉)
Department of Gynecological Endocrinology and Fertility Disorders
University of Heidelberg, Voßstr. 9, 69115 Heidelberg, Germany
e-mail: markus.montag@med.uni-heidelberg.de

M. Köster, DVSc • K. van der Ven • H. van der Ven, MD
Department of Gynecological Endocrinology and Reproductive Medicine,
University of Bonn, Bonn, Germany

Timing

An oocyte presenting a first polar body is usually considered to be in metaphase II. However, recent investigations using polarization microscopy have shown that some oocytes may be still in telophase I due to the presence of a connective spindle strand between the first polar body and the oocyte [12]. Such a spindle bridge is a remnant of the meiotic division and is only present for a limited time period of 1–2 h after extrusion of either the first or the second polar body. Therefore, it is important not to biopsy polar bodies within a too short time period after their formation, because chromosomal material from the oocyte may still be attached to these spindle fibres and pulled out during biopsy.

In view of this, removal of the first and second polar bodies can be done at separate time points or at the same time point. Simultaneous biopsy of the first and second polar bodies is best accomplished in a time window of 6–14 h after fertilization. Too early biopsy bears the risk of spindle remnants in the second polar body, and too late biopsy may result in a first polar body which already started disintegration or degeneration. The latter problem is especially important if the analysis is based on fluorescence in situ hybridization (FISH) as it may contribute to diagnostic failures [8]. Simultaneous biopsy requires only one manipulation and helps to reduce stress to the oocyte.

Zona Opening

Various methods have been proposed for the opening of the zona pellucida and subsequent removal of polar bodies: chemical, mechanical and laser-assisted opening.

Chemical Opening

Acidic tyrode solution was the first method ever used for opening of the zona pellucida by chemical means [13]. Although acidic tyrode can be applied at the embryo stage, there was an inhibitory effect on embryonic development when oocytes were exposed to acid tyrodes [14]. Therefore, since both the oocyte and polar body are sensitive to the effects of acid, zona drilling by acidic tyrode solution is unsuitable for polar body biopsy.

Mechanical Opening

A very efficient mechanical technique was elaborated by Cieslak et al. [15] and is based on 3D zona dissection and subsequent biopsy. For this procedure, the oocyte is affixed to the holding capillary. Using a sharp needle, a slit is made close to the area where the polar bodies are located. After turning the oocytes by 90°, a second slit is made creating a cross-like incision in the zona which allows accessing the polar bodies. This method can be performed with simple glass tools; however, multiple steps including dissection, release and rotation of the oocyte are needed. Therefore, this procedure is technically difficult and requires extensive experience.

Another approach is the use of a bevelled micropipette (12–15 µm in diameter) which due to its sharpness will assist in opening the zona. For this technique, the oocyte is oriented so that the polar body is located at the 12 o'clock position. The bevelled micropipette is passed through the zona and into the perivitelline space tangentially towards the polar body which can then be aspirated into the pipette. This method works very well if only one polar body is biopsied; however, it is more tedious if the first and second polar bodies need to be biopsied and if both are not lying close to each other. Naturally, this method bears a certain risk of damaging the oocyte due to the sharpness of the needle.

Laser-Assisted Opening

The ultimate way of opening the zona pellucida is by a laser beam. Lasers were initially used to assist fertilization in cases of severe male factor infertility. The introduction of laser-assisted zona opening [16] has entered the field of polar body [11, 17] and embryo biopsy [18] and has helped in reducing the rate of biopsy damages as well as the time required [19].

Biopsy Procedure

The whole procedure of laser-assisted polar body biopsy is illustrated in Fig. 20.1.

Laser-assisted polar body biopsy is best accomplished when the oocyte is affixed to the holding capillary with the first polar body at the 12 o'clock position and the second polar body located right of the first one but in the same focal plane. An opening of 18–25 µm is drilled at 2–3 o'clock, and by pushing the biopsy capillary into the perivitelline space, both polar bodies can be removed simultaneously. The positioning of the second polar body next to the aspiration capillary allows pushing the second polar body far to the left side towards the holding capillary, and this stretching movement usually is sufficient to break the cytoplasmic bridge between the second polar body and the oocyte. Due to the use of a blunt-ended capillary, even manipulation in direct vicinity to the oolemma does not damage the oocyte.

In general, the size of the drilled opening is usually in the range of 18–25 µm, but it can be easily adjusted to the diameter of the aspiration capillary. As the capillary can be introduced through the laser-drilled opening, there is no need for a sharp aspiration needle. This allows the use of flame-polished, blunt-ended aspiration needles and greatly reduces the risk of damaging the polar body or the remaining oocyte. The procedure is accurate, reproducible and safe, and it also reduces the

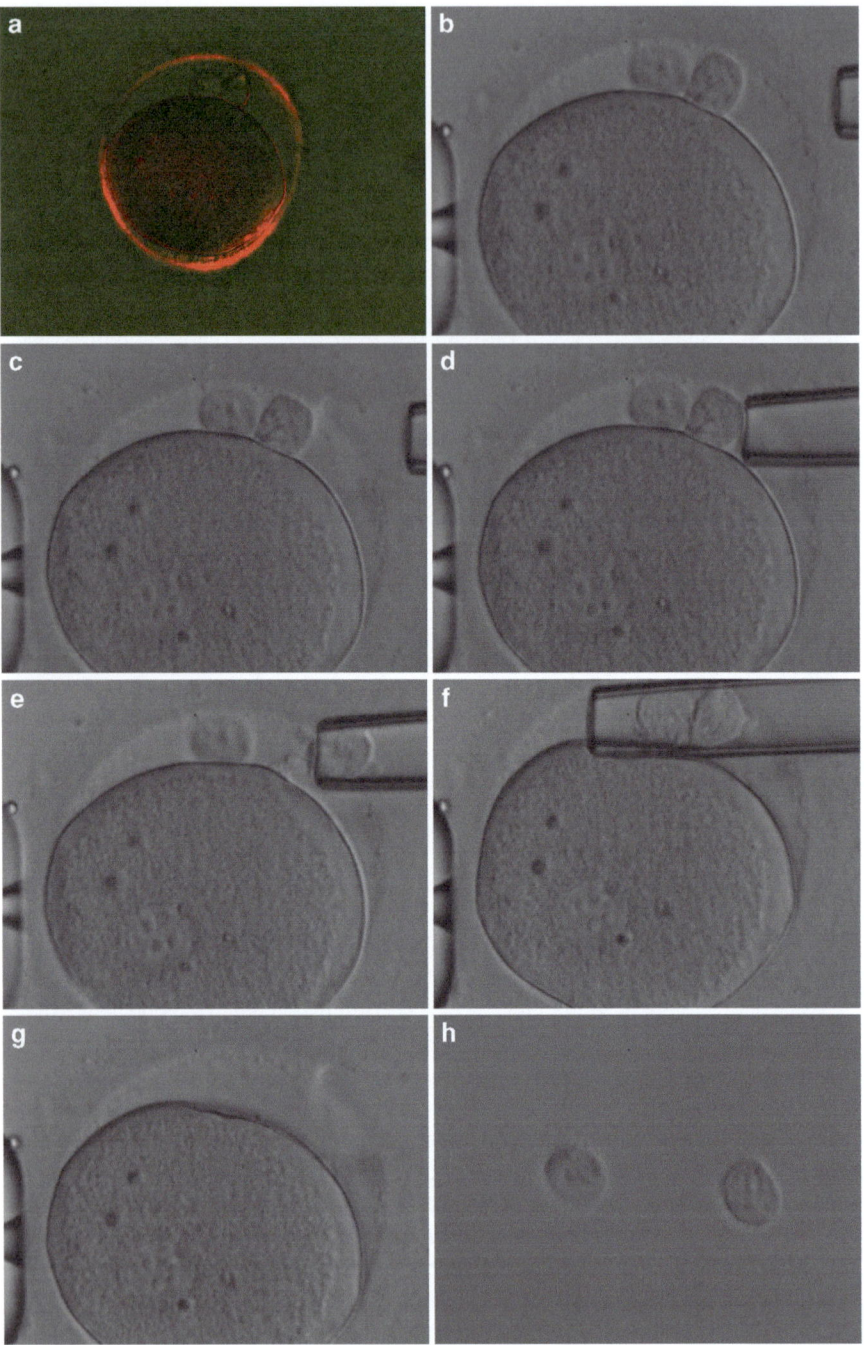

Fig. 20.1 Polar body biopsy following polarization microscopy. Prior to biopsy of the first polar body, the presence of a connective spindle bridge between one of the polar bodies and the oocytes was excluded by polarization microscopy (**a**). For biopsy, the first and second polar bodies were aligned with a holding capillary so that the second PB faced to the biopsy capillary (**b**). Using a non-contact 1.48-μm diode laser, an opening was introduced into the zona pellucida using 2–3 laser

number of cells which cannot be reliably diagnosed as a result of technical problems during the biopsy procedure [20]. Another benefit is that laser drilling and subsequent biopsy can be performed without changing the culture dish or the capillaries in contrast to zona drilling using acidic tyrode solution. This may help to prevent contamination of samples to be diagnosed by sensitive techniques such as polymerase chain reaction (PCR).

Pitfalls

The different approaches to generate an opening in the zona pellucida do result in different characteristics of the shape of the openings as well as the behaviour of the corresponding oocytes and embryos. To date, only the effect of laser drilling has been studied intensively.

Although the use of the laser seems to be easy and straightforward, it is still essential that the technique is trained properly in order to avoid possible pitfalls [21]. Laser opening of the zona can be done at very high precision and giving reproducible results. Consequently, it was shown that laser-assisted biopsy does not interfere with further development of mouse embryos [17] as long as the laser is used in a proper way [21] and a few examples will be given below.

Laser-drilled openings will stay permanently in the zona, and therefore, gentle handling during subsequent transfer of oocytes to other media droplets and even during the embryo transfer is strongly recommended.

Dependent on the size and position of laser openings, inappropriate hatching may occur at the blastocyst stage [21]. If the biopsy of both polar bodies is done at different time points, one should avoid drilling another opening. If polar bodies were retrieved through separate openings, problems may arise at the time of hatching because the embryo could hatch through both openings simultaneously and therefore may get trapped within the zona [21].

While introducing an opening in the zona, care should be taken to generate a sufficiently large opening which allows consecutive hatching at the blastocyst stage because smaller openings (<15 μm) may also cause trapping of the embryo followed by degeneration [21].

Fig. 20.1 (continued) shots (**c**) through which the biopsy capillary could be easily introduced (**d**). The second polar body is usually connected to the oolemma via a cytoplasmic strand (**e**). In order to remove the second polar body without damaging the oocyte, it is *not* recommended to suck the second PB into the capillary, as shown in (**e**). Instead the capillary is pushed slowly over the second PB and towards the first PB (**f**). Once the first PB enters the capillary, the strand between the second PB and the oolemma will break due to shear stress, and both polar bodies can be easily removed (**f**) leaving the oocyte without any damage (**g**). Polar bodies should be placed in one droplet for further processing for FISH analysis (**h**) or in two different droplets if a PCR-based analysis will be performed

Independent of the method used for biopsy, it is extremely important to note the shape of the polar body. Especially a fragmented polar body must be classified as that because this does require special care during later transfer for further evaluation. If fragments are lost, one will get an incomplete diagnosis or even a misdiagnosis.

Isolation of Polar Bodies

Once polar bodies are biopsied, they need to be transferred for further analysis by FISH or PCR. This transfer is a crucial step as it bears the risk of loss of material or even of contamination.

Transfer for FISH

Immediately after biopsy of an oocyte, the corresponding polar bodies are placed in a neighbouring droplet of medium until all oocytes are biopsied. For FISH, it is not essential to place the first and second polar bodies in different droplets, as they can be visually distinguished during fluorescence evaluation. Due to the small cytoplasmic content of polar bodies, a special pretreatment like hypo-osmotic swelling or proteinase/pronase treatment prior FISH is not necessary. For transfer onto the glass slide, polar bodies of one oocyte are removed from their drop and transferred into a tiny drop (0.2 µL) of water placed on a clean glass slide. The small volume guarantees that the polar body will attach to the slide within a small area and that the fluid will dry out very fast, which reduces the risk of a dislocation of the polar body on the slide. It is recommended to use for this transfer the biopsy capillary and to perform the complete procedure under visual control at the microscope. Placing the polar bodies directly at the bottom of the slide will prevent floating and rupture of the polar bodies. The drying process must be observed under a stereomicroscope, and the final location of the polar body after air-drying should be marked on top of the slide by encircling with a diamond marker. With some experience, polar bodies from 6 to 10 oocytes can be placed within a round area of 10 mm, each encircled with a diamond marker. Subsequent fixation can be performed with 2–3 drops of 10 µL methanol/acetic acid (3:1, ice-cold −20°C) followed by another fixation after air-drying using methanol at room temperature for 5 min [22].

Transfer for PCR

In contrast to the isolation for FISH, the differentiation of the first and second polar bodies is crucial for any PCR-based evaluation, either for monogenetic diseases or for array-CGH. Therefore, the first and second polar bodies are released after biopsy in different droplets with medium in a dish covered with mineral oil. These droplets should be rather large (approx. 10 µL) as this will facilitate to aspirate the polar bodies without sucking up some mineral oil. For PCR, the polar bodies need to be transferred into a PCR tube. This can be easily done by preloading the PCR tube with 1.6 µL buffer (PBS or cell extraction buffer). Using a low-volume pipette (0.2–2.0 µL), one polar body is aspirated in a total of 0.4 µL medium and released into the buffer in the PCR tube by pipetting several times up and down. This process must be done in a clean environment, preferably a lamina flow bench, in order to avoid any contamination with other cells or genetic material.

Summary

Polar body biopsy is the initial step prior to investigation of the first and second polar bodies regarding genetic dispositions or structural and/or numerical chromosomal disorders. Polar body diagnosis allows concluding on the genetic/chromosomal constitution of the oocyte. The most frequently used biopsy methods are mechanical by 3D zona dissections or by laser. Isolation of polar bodies depends on the methods used for diagnosis. For FISH analysis, both polar bodies can be simply placed in a water droplet on a glass slide, whereas any PCR-based approach requires separate processing of the first and second polar bodies under sterile conditions.

Accurate timing and technique of biopsy are important for optimal results and reduction of oocyte trauma. Differences in techniques may explain differences in previous studies on the success of polar body diagnosis for PGS. Proper training as well as future improvements and refinements may help to optimize polar body biopsy and subsequent diagnosis in the daily laboratory work. Although FISH and PGS were and probably still are the predominant applications of polar body-based diagnosis, recent advances in array-CGH will change the field of polar body biopsy and boost PCR-based diagnosis [23].

References

1. Verlinsky Y, Ginsberg N, Lifchez A, et al. Analysis of the first polar body: preconception genetic diagnosis. Hum Reprod. 1990;5:826–9.
2. Verlinsky Y, Rechitsky S, Cieslak J, et al. Preimplantation diagnosis of single gene disorders by two-step oocyte genetic analysis using first and second polar body. Biochem Mol Med. 1997;62:182–7.
3. Strom CM, Ginsberg N, Rechitsky S, et al. Three births after preimplantation genetic diagnosis for cystic fibrosis with sequential first and second polar body analysis. Am J Obstet Gynecol. 1998;178:1298–306.
4. Kuliev A, Rechitsky S, Verlinsky O, et al. Birth of healthy children after preimplantation diagnosis of thalassemias. J Assist Reprod Genet. 1999;16:207–11.
5. Munné S, Fung J, Cassel MJ, et al. Preimplantation genetic analysis of translocations: case-specific probes for interphase cell analysis. Hum Genet. 1998;102:663–74.
6. Verlinsky Y, Rechitsky S, Schoolcraft W, et al. Preimplantation diagnosis for Fanconi anemia combined with HLA matching. JAMA. 2001;285:3130–3.

7. Verlinsky Y, Rechitsky S, Verlinsky O, et al. Polar body-based preimplantation diagnosis for x-linked disorders. Reprod Biomed Online. 2002;4:38–42.
8. Munné S, Dailey T, Sultan KM, et al. The use of first polar bodies for preimplantation diagnosis of aneuploidy. Hum Reprod. 1995;10:1015–21.
9. Verlinsky Y, Cieslak J, Freidine M, et al. Pregnancies following pre-conception diagnosis of common aneuploidies by fluorescent in-situ hybridization. Hum Reprod. 1995;10:1923–7.
10. Verlinsky Y, Tur-Kaspa I, Cieslak J, et al. Preimplantation testing for chromosomal disorders improves reproductive outcome of poor-prognosis patients. Reprod Biomed Online. 2005;11:219–25.
11. Montag M, van der Ven K, Dorn C, van der Ven H. Outcome of laser-assisted polar body biopsy. Reprod Biomed Online. 2004;9:425–9.
12. Montag M, Schimming T, van der Ven H. Spindle imaging in human oocytes: the impact of the meiotic cell cycle. Reprod Biomed Online. 2006;12:442–6.
13. Gordon JW, Talansky BE. Assisted fertilization by zona drilling: a mouse model for correction of oligospermia. J Exp Zool. 1987;239:347–81.
14. Malter HE, Cohen J. Blastocyst formation and hatching in vitro following zona drilling of mouse and human embryos. Gamete Res. 1989;24:67–80.
15. Cieslak J, Ivakhenko V, Wolf G, et al. Three-dimensional partial zona dissection for preimplantation genetic diagnosis and assisted hatching. Fertil Steril. 1999;71:308–13.
16. Rink K, Delacrétaz G, Salathé RP, et al. 1.48 μm diode laser microdissection of the zona pellucida of mouse zygotes. Proc Soc Photo Opt Instrum Eng. 1994;213A:412–22.
17. Montag M, van der Ven K, Delacrétaz G, et al. Laser assisted microdissection of zona pellucida facilitates polar body biopsy. Fertil Steril. 1998;69:539–42.
18. Boada M, Carrera M, De La Iglesia C, et al. Successful use of a laser for human embryo biopsy in preimplantation genetic diagnosis: report of two cases. J Assist Reprod Genet. 1997;15:301–5.
19. Joris H, De Vos A, Janssens R, et al. Comparison of the results of human embryo biopsy and outcome of PGD after zona drilling using acid Tyrode medium or a laser. Hum Reprod. 2003;18:1896–902.
20. Montag M, van der Ven K, van der Ven H. Erste klinische Erfahrungen mit der Polkörperdiagnostik in Deutschland. J Fertil Reprod. 2002;4:7–12.
21. Montag M, van der Ven H. Laser-assisted hatching in assisted reproduction. Croat Med J. 1999;40:398–403.
22. Montag M, van der Ven K, van der Ven H. Polar body biopsy. In: Gardner D, Weissman A, Howles C, Shoham Z, editors. Textbook of assisted reproductive techniques: laboratory and clinical perspectives. 3rd ed. New York: Informa Healthcare; 2009. p. 357–70.
23. Geraedts J, Collins J, Gianaroli L, et al. What next for preimplantation genetic screening? A polar body approach! Hum Reprod. 2010;3:575–7.

Chapter 21
Cleavage-Stage Embryo Biopsy

Alan R. Thornhill

The first PGD cycles were carried out in late 1989 in a series of couples at risk of X-linked disease and involved cleavage-stage embryo biopsy [1]. Theoretically, PGD can be accomplished at any developmental stage between the mature oocyte and blastocyst, but to date, only three discrete stages have been proposed: polar body, cleavage-stage, and blastocyst. Clearly, each of these stages is biologically different, and thus, the strategic considerations have both advantages and disadvantages [2] (Table 21.1). However, cleavage-stage biopsy has remained the most widely practiced form of embryo biopsy worldwide (according to the ESHRE PGD Consortium) accounting for approximately 90% of all reported PGD cycles to date [3]. Currently, this embryo biopsy strategy requires the removal of one or more cells from each embryo, making it comparable to amniocentesis or CVS at fetal stages since the primary aim is the removal of sufficient embryonic tissue to allow diagnosis. Cleavage-stage embryo biopsy is a two-step micromanipulation process involving the penetration or removal of part of the zona pellucida surrounding the oocyte or embryo followed by removal of one or more cells. Many of the biopsy techniques currently in use for human embryos [4] were pioneered in animal models, notably the mouse [5–7]. While the total number of human embryos biopsied in clinical cases is vast, relatively little work has been published to define the relative merits of different biopsy methods and their safety and efficacy in clinical application (Table 21.2). This chapter focuses on cleavage-stage embryo biopsy since the majority of PGD centers and clinical cases reported have employed this technique [3].

A.R. Thornhill, PhD, HCLD (✉)
The London Bridge Fertility, Gynaecology and Genetics Centre,
1 St. Thomas Street, London SE1 9RY, UK
e-mail: athornhill@thebridgecentre.co.uk

Table 21.1 Advantages and disadvantages of cleavage-stage embryo biopsy

Stage	Advantages	Disadvantages
Cleavage-stage accuracy (blastomeres)	Diagnosis of maternally and paternally inherited disease	Chromosomal mosaicism compromises accuracy
	Gender determination possible	Choice of blastomere is critical
	Large body of clinical data available	Time for analysis may be limited
	1–3 cells available for analysis	Most cells in interphase (no karyotypic data)
	Biopsied embryos develop into normal blastocysts	Single-cell-sensitive analysis required
		Reduced embryo implantation potential post-biopsy
2–4 cell	95% Embryo cohort available for analysis	Detrimental effects of acid/reduced cell mass
		Possible selected cell allocation to TE/ICM
6–10 cell	1 or 2 cell removal still results in viable development	Reduced embryo cohort on day of biopsy
		Possible selected cell allocation to TE/ICM

Penetration of the Zona Pellucida

Until the advent of noncontact lasers for use in micromanipulation (see below), two basic methods were employed for zona pellucida penetration. Both methods were pursued initially as a means to enhance fertilization rates with oligozoospermic men and have now been superseded for this purpose by intracytoplasmic sperm injection (ICSI).

Mechanical Zona Penetration

The first approach, partial zona dissection (PZD), employs a fine needle to penetrate the zona at two separate points around the circumference. The oocyte or embryo is then detached from the holding pipette as it is effectively held on the needle and a gentle rubbing action against the side of the holding pipette used to make a slit between the two apertures generated by the needle taking care to avoid damage to the oocyte or embryo [8]. Although a narrow-diameter micropipette can be pushed through such a slit, it is difficult to use one large enough to aspirate cleavage-stage blastomeres, and with the human embryo, pressure on the zona can lead to lysis of

Table 21.2 Cleavage-stage embryo biopsy methods—benefits, limitations, and factors critical to success

Zona penetration method	Benefits	Limitations	Factors critical to success
Mechanical	Least invasive to embryo (safer) Improved survival after freeze–thaw? Inexpensive	Difficult to learn Operator dependent Time-consuming	Operator skill essential Appropriate microtools needed
Chemical (Acidified Tyrode's solution)	Relatively inexpensive Widespread clinical experience	Operator dependent Difficult to limit aperture size Effect on cryopreservation? Double tool holder optimal	Acidified Tyrode's pH 2.2–2.4 Sensitive control of acid Rinse acid from embryos
Laser (1.48 μm noncontact diode)	Rapid and reproducible Simple to use Documentation/measurement software	Capital cost (30–60,000 US dollars) Not all systems portable Invisible thermal damage/stress	Laser alignment and calibration Pulse duration and number Distance between laser and zona
Cell removal method			
Aspiration	Ability to select cell	Cell lysis during aspiration	Appropriate microtools needed Sensitive suction device
Fluid displacement	Aspiration pipette does not contact cells	Limited ability to select cell	Operator skill essential
Mechanical displacement	Aspiration pipette does not contact cells	Limited ability to select cell Damage to non-biopsied cells?	Operator skill essential

blastomeres and/or, where a slit has been made, force blastomeres out through the slit. The latter approach is used for embryo biopsy in some centers but requires highly skilled micromanipulation, can be difficult to control, does not allow precise selection of blastomeres, and the risk of lysis can be high. A modification is to make two slits to create a "flap" or "cross" in the zona that can be flipped open, allowing more flexibility in the size of the opening created. This method is effective for both blastomere and polar body biopsy [9].

Chemical Zona Penetration

In general, mechanical methods for zona penetration are time-consuming and require skillful micromanipulation, possibly making them inaccessible to some IVF laboratories. As an alternative, zona drilling using acidified Tyrode's solution (pH 2.2–2.4) to dissolve the zona glycoproteins has been extensively used and is commercially available from most culture medium manufacturers. This method developed in the mouse embryo model, with the aim of improving fertilization rates with low sperm densities [10], was of limited value when using human oocytes, as an increased fertilization rate was offset against developmental arrest in the zygote, presumably consequent to changes in intracellular pH [11]. With zona drilling, the effect of the acidified Tyrode's is localized to a small area of the zona (generally between 20 and 30 µm) using a fine micropipette, with an inner diameter of 5–10 µm. The pipette is placed very close to or in direct contact with the zona pellucida at the desired position and the acidified solution gently expelled from the pipette until the zona thins, and an aperture is drilled (in some cases, the zona can be seen to "pop" as an aperture is made). The flow, facilitated via oil-filled syringe (hydraulic), air-filled syringe (pneumatic), or by using a mouth pipette, must be carefully directed and controlled to limit the size of the zona breach. The human zona is bilayered, and the zona drilling process must be carefully monitored as the outer layer dissolves more rapidly than the inner layer. Moreover, there is great variation in zonae pellucidae both between and within cohorts of human oocytes and embryos. The final diameter of the aperture made will be determined by a combination of the above factors. An excessively large aperture may result in the unwanted loss of blastomeres but, more significantly, may indicate that the blastomeres were exposed to potentially damaging quantities of acid which could compromise further development. Physiologic pH of the medium was originally maintained by employing phosphate-buffered saline but is now routinely maintained using modified culture medium buffered with either 4-morpholinepropanesulfonic acid (MOPS) or 4-(2-hydroxyethyl)-1-piperazineethanesulfonic acid (HEPES). When the drilling is complete, the micropipette is immediately withdrawn and, if necessary, excess acidified Tyrode's aspirated from the biopsy drop.

Non-contact Laser (Thermal Ablation of the Zona)

Since the first PGD cycles reported by the ESHRE PGD Consortium, there has been a marked shift across centers worldwide from zona drilling using predominantly acidified Tyrode's [12] to laser ablation of the zona pellucida with the laser now accounting for more than 70% cleavage-stage embryo biopsies [3]. This shift may be more to do with ease of use and the elimination of the need for a double tool holder and batch testing of acidified Tyrode's solutions rather than any measurable improvement in safety or efficacy.

The preferred model of laser is the near infrared (NIR) solid-state compact diode 1.48 μm laser. The advantage of using light as a cutting tool is that it obviates the need for a double tool holder and either disposable or reusable cutting tools. It is extremely precise and, if used appropriately, provides consistent, reproducible, and rapid results. Furthermore, the likelihood of introducing contamination or pH changes in the medium surrounding the embryo is greatly reduced as neither microtools nor reagents are required to dissect the zona. The 1.48-μm diode laser is small but, at the appropriate pulse duration, can emit light at power levels sufficient to cause selective thermal disruption of the zona pellucida glycoproteins and is not absorbed by water. This noncontact laser can be inserted into the body of the microscope on which the manipulations take place or be integrated in a special objective and the beam delivered to the target through the dish.

Since the laser beam travels up through an objective which lies below the sample, localized heating causes denaturation of the zona proteins in a cylindrical spot where the laser beam is focused, and the size of the aperture created is controlled by adjusting the laser pulse duration. The thermal energy created produces a groove in the zona perpendicular to the microscope stage, rather than a circular aperture. However, an "aperture" is produced in the zona at the point at which the zona is perpendicular to the microscope stage (Fig. 21.1). The size of the aperture (or more accurately, the

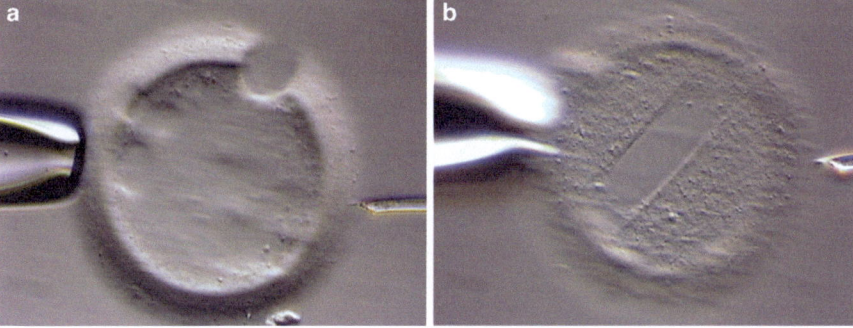

Fig. 21.1 Empty human zona pellucida after thermal ablation using noncontact laser. (**a**) Cross-sectional view as used during biopsy procedure indicating aperture through which biopsy aspiration pipette is passed. (**b**) The same zona pellucida rotated through 90° to show the path of the laser

width of the groove at its widest point) created in the zona ranges from 5 to 20 μm and is governed by the pulse irradiation time (ranging from 3 to 100 ms) or the accumulation of pulses along the length of the zona margin. The precision of the laser is illustrated by the fact that drilled mouse and human embryos show no sign of extraneous thermal damage under light or scanning microscopy [13].

Clearly, such equipment may be used for assisted hatching as well as PGD [14], and if used appropriately, there appears to be no detrimental effect of the laser itself on development to the blastocyst stage or pregnancy rates in animal and human studies [3, 15–17]. However, studies of the immediate effects at the blastomere level in a mouse model [18] and following assisted hatching in a clinical program [19] have shown that the laser can cause damage if used inappropriately. Certainly, if the laser beam is fired in an area in direct contact with a blastomere, its viability is always compromised. However, as the pulse length and therefore localized heating is increased, the distance between the laser beam and blastomere required to avoid damage increases [18]. Hence, care is required to drill the zona away from underlying blastomeres and from as far away as possible and also to use minimum pulse lengths to restrict any damaging effects. Several practical guidelines have emerged to ensure safe and effective use of the laser for human embryo biopsy as follows. Wherever possible, a single aperture only should be made for cellular aspiration. Double or multiple apertures may cause problems during embryo hatching as the embryo will attempt to hatch out of multiple openings which could compromise further inner cell mass (ICM) development or lead to increased monozygotic twinning. To generate the desired aperture, several pulses of short duration are preferable to a single pulse of long duration (with higher energy) which could cause thermal damage. During laser use, it is imperative to maintain the oocyte or embryo as close to the bottom of the biopsy dish as possible to allow a focused beam to ablate the zona pellucida. As the embryo is raised above the dish surface, the beam energy is diffused and can create localized heating or simply prevent effective ablation of the zona. The use of the laser is deceptively simple, and it is imperative that the operator is constantly aware of the possible detrimental effects to the embryo of unnecessary or misplaced ablations.

Blastomere Removal

Having created an aperture large enough for the safe passage of one or more blastomeres, the operator must select a method for cell removal. The most frequently used method of blastomere removal is aspiration, but other methods have been described and used clinically, although no studies have been conducted to compare their relative safety and efficacy.

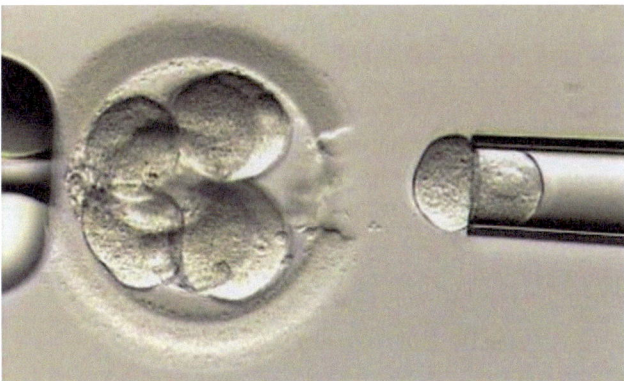

Fig. 21.2 Human cleavage-stage embryo from which a single blastomere with a single visible interphase nucleus is being removed by micromanipulation after laser ablation of the zona pellucida

Aspiration

If performing aspiration in conjunction with zona drilling using acidified Tyrode's, it is easier to use a double tool holder containing a second aspiration micropipette (internal diameter of 30–40 µm depending on the cell size) filled with biopsy medium [2] rather than changing the micropipette in a single tool holder for each biopsy procedure. A single micropipette may be used for both drilling and subsequent aspiration, but care is needed to prevent overexposure to acid [20, 21]. Any advantage accrued in terms of speed of the procedure may be offset by potential damage as a result of overexposure to acid.

A typical procedure for cleavage-stage biopsy using laser and blastomere aspiration is illustrated in Fig. 21.2. Briefly, following laser ablation of the zona pellucida adjacent to the blastomere selected for analysis, the blastomere is aspirated by gentle suction using a finely polished "sampling" pipette. The aperture may be sited adjacent to either a selected blastomere or a sub-zonal space between blastomeres. The pipette is placed through the aperture, close to the blastomere to be aspirated. By gentle suction, the blastomere is drawn into the pipette while the pipette is withdrawn from the aperture. The aperture of the sampling pipette is critical for successful biopsy. If the internal diameter is too large for the cell being removed, the pipette will have little purchase on that cell and may result in unwanted suction on non-biopsied cells. Conversely, an undersized pipette will cause the biopsied cell to be squeezed unnecessarily, resulting in blebbing on the cell membrane and ultimately lysis, which will likely reduce the chances of a successful diagnosis in that embryo.

Similarly, use of a holding pipette with an internal diameter of 30 μm (i.e., larger than a regular ICSI holding pipette) ensures safe and reliable suction on the zona particularly during difficult biopsies.

Once the blastomere is free of the embryo, it is gently expelled from the sampling pipette. Following biopsy, the embryo should be rinsed in culture medium at least twice to remove residual embryo biopsy medium before returning to culture. The blastomere should be washed extensively in handling medium before proceeding to the analysis.

Alternative Methods of Blastomere Removal

In the extrusion method, after zona pellucida drilling, the blastomere is extruded through the aperture by pushing against the zona at another site (usually at 90° to the aperture) using a blunt pipette [6]. The slit in the zona pellucida can be introduced using mechanical means, chemical (acidified Tyrode's) exposure, or laser ablation as described above.

Another variation in the method of cell removal involves fluid displacement whereby culture medium surrounding the embryo is used to displace individual cells following a zona breach. This method was pioneered in mouse embryos by introducing a slit in the zona with a sharpened needle and, through a second puncture site, injecting medium to dislodge the blastomere through the first puncture site [7]. This method requires the production of two separate apertures and considerable skill to displace the blastomere of choice but has been successfully modified for clinical application [22]. A challenge common to both of these methods is to ensure that only the selected cell or cells are removed.

Practical Considerations for Embryo Biopsy

Preparation Prior to Biopsy

ICSI is still recommended for all PGD cases involving DNA amplification to reduce the chance of paternal contamination from extraneous sperm attached to the zona pellucida or non-decondensed sperm within blastomeres [23]. Similarly, as far as is practically and safely possible, all cumulus cells should be removed before biopsy as these cells can contaminate both fluorescence in situ hybridization (FISH) and polymerase chain reaction (PCR)-based diagnoses. Embryo and blastomere identity (individual drops or dishes) should be checked throughout the procedure so that diagnostic results can be reliably linked to specific embryos [23–26]. The use of standard IVF culture medium during biopsy is acceptable, but its effectiveness may be highly dependent upon the developmental stage of the embryo biopsied with compacting eight-cell embryos proving more difficult to biopsy. Commercially produced calcium- and magnesium-free (Ca^{2+}/Mg^{2+}-free) medium which temporarily reverses calcium-dependent cell–cell adhesion [27] is widely available and is used by many centers for routine clinical biopsy with the benefit of reducing the frequency of cell lysis [23] combined with a shorter time needed to perform the biopsy procedure.

Timing of Biopsy

Most cleavage-stage biopsy takes place on the third morning following insemination, although the exact timing varies according to timings of procedures in different laboratories and may be patient-specific or even cohort-specific for particular patients. One variation, allowing more time for genetic analysis, is to alter the timing of ICSI to allow cleavage-stage biopsy at the same embryonic stage, but late on day 2 since biopsy at earlier cleavage-stages on day 2 may adversely affect embryo development [28]. In cases where retarded development is observed, the possibility of delaying the biopsy procedure to allow diagnosis of a larger proportion of the embryo cohort should be considered. The use of Ca^{2+}/Mg^{2+}-free medium has also facilitated later biopsy (i.e., beyond eight-cell stage) making the laboratory timings more flexible. Furthermore, the increased use of sequential media and blastocyst culture and transfer has led to the routine delay of transfer until day 4 or more commonly day 5. This extended culture period allows additional time for diagnostic analysis and allows more opportunity to preferentially select the most developed embryos for transfer with the aim of improving pregnancy and implantation rates during a fresh transfer cycle and facilitating elective single embryo transfer to reduce multiple pregnancy rates [29].

Most laboratories exclude very poor quality embryos or those not reaching a predefined cell stage from the embryo biopsy procedure. Of the centers surveyed, most will consider only embryos at the five-cell stage and beyond only for biopsy [12]. Biopsy at the four-cell stage in mouse results in a distorted allocation of cells to ICM and trophectoderm and abnormal postimplantation development [30], while human embryos biopsied on day 2 show cleavage rate retardation and smaller blastocysts [28]. Conversely, four-cell stage human embryos surviving freeze–thaw procedures with the loss of one or more blastomeres can develop, implant, and result in live birth, albeit at a reduced rate compared with nonfrozen embryos [31, 32]. Stringent biopsy policies have the benefits that fewer embryos need to be biopsied and fewer cells prepared and tested with only developmentally competent embryos considered with relatively little loss in pregnancy potential for that cycle. On the down side, an opportunity to identify genotypes on a full cohort of embryos may be lost.

Number of Cells to Remove During Cleavage-Stage Biopsy

In deciding how many cells to biopsy from cleavage-stage embryos, it is axiomatic to balance diagnostic accuracy with potential to implant and develop, which is progressively compromised as a greater proportion of the embryo is removed [33].

There is no consensus on the number of blastomeres that can be safely removed during cleavage-stage embryo biopsy. In many centers, a second blastomere is removed from embryos having seven or more cells regardless of the type of analysis involved, but this approach has been criticized as compromising the implantation potential of the biopsied embryo based on extrapolation from frozen–thaw embryo implantation rates [32]. The decision to remove one or two cells is based on many factors including the embryo cell number and the accuracy and reliability of the diagnostic test used. Removal of two cells should only be considered on embryos with six or more cells [34]. While removal of two blastomeres decreases the likelihood of blastocyst formation, compared with removal of one blastomere, day 3 in vitro developmental stage is a stronger predictor for day 5 developmental potential than the removal of one or two cells. The biopsy of only one cell significantly lowers the efficiency of a PCR-based diagnosis, whereas the efficiency of the FISH PGD procedure remains similar whether one or two cells are removed [35]. However, a recent trial demonstrated that live birth rate was compromised at a level of one birth for every 33 cycles of two-cell embryo biopsy suggesting that, ideally, one cell biopsy should always be performed unless the diagnostic test is suboptimal [36].

In the case of lost or anucleate blastomeres and failed diagnosis, rebiopsy of embryos is possible, but embryo cell number and timing of rebiopsy should be considered to avoid excessive harm to the embryo. Although technically challenging, the original zona breach site should be accessed to prevent later problems, including monozygotic twinning, possibly the result of embryos hatching via multiple sites. No specific recommendations for time limits for embryos out of the incubator are available, but ideally, biopsy should be performed as quickly as possible (certainly less than 5 min in total and, ideally, 1–2 min per embryo) to ensure pH, temperature, and osmolality are maintained. A documented record for biopsy timings should be maintained for quality assurance purposes [26, 27].

Success Rates After Biopsy

The reliability of cleavage-stage biopsy has now been established in many centers, and in a recent ESHRE PGD Consortium report, the efficiency of successful embryo biopsy is 98% in over 150,000 cleavage-stage embryos in clinical PGD cycles [3]. Pregnancy rates after PGD are notoriously difficult to assess between different indications and centers. Nevertheless, in the largest series analyzed in detail to date, mostly following cleavage-stage biopsy, pregnancy rates are only 22% per oocyte retrieval and 30% per embryo transfer on average [3]. The reasons for the apparently low success rates are many fold but unsurprising considering that a proportion of embryos cannot be transferred because they are diagnosed as affected, and in many countries, the number of embryos transferred is limited to a maximum of two. To demonstrate the possible detrimental effects of embryo biopsy alone, one would need to conduct a clinical trial involving biopsied and non-biopsied embryos which would be transferred after selection on purely morphological grounds post-biopsy (i.e., without any genetic selection). Such a trial could be considered unethical. However, data from a recent trial provides some insight into the possible detrimental effects of biopsy with a reduction in implantation potential evident in undiagnosed biopsied embryos compared with non-biopsied control embryos [37, 38].

It is well established in mammalian embryos that as an increasing proportion of the embryo is removed or destroyed before transfer, implantation and fetal development rates decline, suggesting a lower limit of embryo mass compatible with implantation and development [39]. Reduction of 50% or more of the cell mass frequently results in cell proliferation in the absence of normal differentiation; thus, it is important to minimize the cellular mass removed at biopsy. However, cell reduction within this limit is compatible with normal embryo metabolism, blastocyst development, and fetal growth, while cell numbers in the trophectoderm (TE) and ICM of blastocysts were in proportion to the cellular mass removed at biopsy, making cleavage-stage biopsy for PGD a viable option [40]. Hence, human cleavage-stage biopsy is delayed until just before the beginning of compaction, the process of intercellular adhesion, and junction formation, which progressively makes removal of blastomeres more difficult and eventually impossible without causing damage to the embryo. Generally, cells identified as having completed the third cleavage division (on the basis of their size) are selected for biopsy. Theoretically, therefore, each blastomere removes only one-eighth of the cellular mass of the embryo. As zona drilling for assisted hatching may be beneficial for some indications [41], it is also possible that the hatching process itself offsets to some extent the adverse effects of reducing the cell mass of the embryo.

In frozen embryo transfer (FET) cases, viable pregnancies are routinely achieved, albeit at a reduced rate compared with fresh transfer cycles. Moreover, no increase in fetal abnormalities has been reported following transfer of cryopreserved embryos in which some cells have been destroyed by freezing and subsequent thawing of cleavage-stage embryos [42, 43]. Indeed, estimates of the loss of implantation potential have been made based on outcomes following FET involving cleavage-stage embryos with one or more nonviable cells after thawing [31, 32], although it is clear that the growth rate of viable cells may be more important than the loss of cells per se [31, 42]. It is now apparent that cleavage-stage biopsy should be considered a "cost" to the embryo, and this must always be weighed against the potential benefit to the embryo of any diagnostic testing.

Selection of Cells in the Cleavage-Stage Embryo

Biopsy at cleavage-stages is based on the principle that at these stages, the blastomeres remain totipotent and equivalent such that the removal of a single blastomere will (a) provide a representative sample of the entire embryo and (b) compromise the embryo only to the extent of one-eighth of the embryo mass rather than removal of a developmentally crucial blastomere. The importance of selecting a blastomere with a single visible interphase nucleus cannot be stressed enough (Fig. 21.2). Aside from the increased diagnostic efficiency observed in mononucleated blastomeres

[44], mononucleation is a marker for and directly correlates with implantation potential [45]. Nevertheless, embryos containing blastomeres, all of which have no visible nucleus, should still be considered for biopsy as nuclear material is likely to be present and should yield results in molecular tests [44]. After micromanipulation skills, blastomere selection is probably the most challenging aspect of effective cleavage-stage biopsy. Time spent in careful examination of the embryo and orientation to selectively remove specific blastomeres is essential to attain the high diagnostic efficiencies required for clinical effectiveness. The reasons for this are that, first, an interphase nucleus is essential for FISH analysis since the nucleus is prepared on a slide by a process of cell lysis in which individual chromosomes from a metaphase plate may not be visible and are likely to be lost during cell preparation [46]. Second, post-zygotic chromosomal mosaicism arising during cleavage is known to be associated with nuclear abnormalities [47]. The exception is binucleate blastomeres, in which there are two normal-sized nuclei. In most cases, these are generated through failure of cytokinesis, and both nuclei contain the normal diploid chromosomal complement for that embryo [48]. In general, multinucleate cells should not be selected at biopsy if FISH analysis for aneuploidy detection follows, and the removal of mononucleate cells only is recommended [23]. The dilemma with this selection procedure is that in a chromosomally mosaic embryo (which contains significant proportions of both normal diploid and aneuploid cells), removal of only mononucleate cells (which are more likely to be chromosomally normal) may result in only the chromosomally abnormal multinucleated cells remaining in the embryo. For accuracy during FISH-based diagnosis, it is advisable to only use bi- or multinucleated cells as a last resort in the absence of mononucleated cells. This may be less critical for PCR-based testing in which presence or absence of a specific parental chromosome is important rather than copy number per se. However, even with careful blastomere selection, diagnostic efficiency is not 100%, and aneuploid results are common even in mononucleate blastomeres primarily as a result of chromosomal loss and mitotic nondisjunction, leading to chromosomal mosaicism [48]. Biopsy of two nucleated blastomeres is only possible in good-quality embryos at a sufficiently advanced stage, such that even with a two-cell biopsy policy, a mixture of embryos with one or two blastomeres for analysis is common [34]. Where possible, one of the smaller blastomeres should be selected to minimize the reduction in mass, and the relative sizes of cells may provide an indication of recent mitosis. This may also reduce the risk that a cell in metaphase will be taken; the chromosomes of which could be lost during the fixation process.

Safety of Cleavage-Stage Embryo Biopsy

As with any micromanipulation procedure involving human gametes or embryos, every reasonable precaution should be taken to minimize cellular damage and stress during the procedure. General precautions include the correct installation, calibration, and maintenance of all micromanipulation equipment (particularly the laser).

In advance of all clinical procedures, one should ensure that all appropriate reagents and micromanipulation tools are available, sterile, and within their expiration date. Biopsy and cell preparation should be performed by a suitably qualified and trained person. Regular reviews of key performance indicators [26, 27] such as the rate of biopsied cell lysis, post-biopsy survival, morphology, and cell numbers of untransferred embryos provide an indication of the possible harm as a result of biopsy as do pregnancy rates after biopsy—particularly those not progressing beyond the biochemical stage. Clearly, effects on postimplantation development should also be closely monitored as any increase in fetal malformations or congenital abnormalities would be unacceptable. To date, studies of pregnancies and children born after PGD have identified no significant increase in abnormalities above the rate seen in routine IVF [3, 49–51]. The main problem in terms of diagnostic efficiency with cleavage-stage biopsy is the presence of chromosomal mosaicism which is reported to occur in up to 80% cleavage-stage embryos [52–54]. A full discussion of the impact of chromosomal mosaicism on the accuracy of PGD is beyond the scope of this review, but its impact on both diagnostic accuracy and clinical effectiveness of PGD can be significant. Mosaicism is thought to be the primary reason for the high rate of false positives depleting the pool of chromosomally "normal" embryos for transfer and hence significantly lowering the chance of live birth following preimplantation genetic diagnosis of chromosomal aneuploidy (PGS) compared with controls in a recent randomized controlled trial [37]. However, the impact of mosaicism on the misdiagnosis rate when performing PGD by PCR analysis appears to be less significant [55]. While polar body biopsy appears to offer a solution to the problem of mosaicism by focusing on maternal mutations and/or meiotic errors— acknowledged to be the main source of aneuploidy in human IVF—the approach does not address either paternal mutations, meiotic errors, or post-zygotic errors arising in the embryo [2]. Blastocyst biopsy has been proposed as a solution to the problem of cleavage-stage mosaicism and has been used successfully in the clinical setting [56–59]. While its use is becoming more widespread, it is still unclear whether or not any residual mosaicism reduces diagnostic accuracy and hence clinical effectiveness at this developmental stage, although its use in aneuploidy detection appears to be superior to that of cleavage-stage biopsy and analysis [59]. Since blastocyst biopsy focuses on only the most developmentally competent embryos within a cohort, diagnostic costs may be lower, and the outcomes per biopsied embryo improved; however, a comprehensive diagnosis of the embryo cohort is not possible.

As an alternative to blastocyst biopsy, it is possible to coculture blastomeres biopsied at cleavage-stages with the biopsied embryo [60]. Over a period of 3 days, division and development of the biopsied blastomere mirrors the behavior of the parent embryo. Hence, if the embryo reached the blastocyst stage, in most cases, the blastomere divided and developed into a small TE vesicle. On average, those blastomeres that divided and formed these vesicles divided two or three times, resulting in an average of 5.6 ± 0.6 ($n = 13$) cells for single eight-cell-stage blastomeres and 9.1 ± 1.1 ($n = 11$) cells where two blastomeres were biopsied and encouraged to form a single morula. In this approach, the behavior of the cleavage-stage biopsy in vitro could predict the potential for the biopsied embryo [61], thereby avoiding the difficulties and damage of biopsy at the blastocyst stage itself and the possibility of having no embryos to biopsy if one elected for blastocyst biopsy alone.

Cryopreservation of Embryos Following Cleavage-Stage Biopsy

A major challenge at present is to develop an effective standardized method for cryopreservation of biopsied embryos. Attempts to use established protocols either in the mouse model or in humans have shown extensive damage after thawing, presumably because of the loss of protection from ice crystals in the medium provided by an intact zona pellucida [62, 63]. However, recently, several improved slow-freezing protocols for biopsied cleavage-stage embryos have been reported in which damage is much reduced [64, 65]. However, following successful application in animal models, vitrification looks set to replace slow freezing for both cleavage- and blastocyst-stage embryos after polar body or embryo biopsy [59, 66–68]. With the high rate of multiple pregnancies reported after PGD, it is imperative to develop effective methods of cryopreservation that will (1) allow storage of unaffected embryos for later transfer so that the numbers transferred can be limited to two or even single embryo transfers and (2) provide additional time to perform more extensive diagnostic tests.

Future Developments

With the introduction of quality management systems and accreditation in IVF laboratories [25–27], safer and more effective biopsy should be achieved through agreed definitions of successful and safe biopsy, standardized training and procedures, and validation of new techniques as well as calibration of new and existing instruments such as the laser. It has become clear that embryo biopsy, as with any form of invasive testing or manipulation, exacts a cost to the embryo in the form of cellular depletion and metabolic stress. Thus, it is imperative to assess the potential benefit to the embryo itself in terms of improved selection or disease-free status before performing embryo biopsy. However, in the future, it may be possible to diagnose inherited diseases or chromosomal imbalance in early human embryos by noninvasive analysis of the secretome or metabolome in spent culture medium, an advance which would shift the cost–benefit ratio heavily toward potential benefit. At present, noninvasive analyses are likely to be used as an adjunct to assess embryo quality and viability with the genetic test requiring biopsied cellular material [69]. For the time being, it is critical that the diagnostic laboratory optimizes the use of each single biopsied blastomere. Whole genome amplification is one such optimization allowing testing of multiple loci, repeat testing, sample sharing for external quality assessment, and archiving for later assessment of additional loci.

A sufficiently large amount of DNA is generated following this process such that microarray-based testing is possible from a single cell for detection of either chromosome, single gene, or a combination of both [70].

In conclusion, blastomere biopsy of human cleavage-stage embryos remains the most commonly performed form of biopsy for genetic diagnosis of the early embryo. The various techniques used appear to be largely safe in terms of pregnancy outcomes and health of children, but it is clear that biopsy of even a single blastomere has some degree of cost to that embryo, manifested as reduced implantation potential. For this reason, the benefit of the possible diagnosis should always be weighed against the "cost" of the embryo biopsy. The noncontact laser has largely overtaken other methods for breaching the zona pellucida and has made embryo biopsy techniques accessible to any embryology laboratory with micromanipulation capabilities. The comparative ease with which the laser may be used should be carefully considered to avoid any inadvertent damage to embryos through misuse. The combined introduction of the laser and large diagnostic laboratories providing PGD services on a satellite basis to embryology laboratories worldwide has greatly improved access for patients to PGD services. The biggest change in practice in future is a shift away from cleavage-stage biopsy, in which chromosomal mosaicism is an occupational and biological "hazard," toward more trophectoderm biopsy from blastocysts in which greater accuracy and diagnostic reliability is predicted.

References

1. Handyside AH, Kontogianni EH, Hardy K, Winston RM. Pregnancies from biopsied human preimplantation embryos sexed by Y-specific DNA amplification. Nature (London). 1990;344: 768–70.
2. Handyside AH, Thornhill AR. Human embryo biopsy procedures. In: Gardner DK, Howles CM, Weissman A, Shoham Z, editors. Textbook of assisted reproductive technologies. 3rd ed. London: Informa Healthcare; 2009. p. 191–206.
3. Harper JC, Coonen E, De Rycke M, Harton G, Moutou C, Pehlivan T, Traeger-Synodinos J, Van Rij MC, Goossens V. ESHRE PGD Consortium data collection X: cycles from January to December 2007 with pregnancy follow-up to October 2008. Hum Reprod. 2010;25(11):2685–707.
4. Tarin JJ, Handyside AH. Embryo biopsy strategies for preimplantation diagnosis. Fertil Steril. 1993;59:943–52.
5. Wilton LJ, Shaw JM, Trounson AO. Successful single-cell biopsy and cryopreservation of preimplantation mouse embryos. Fertil Steril. 1989;51(3):513–7.
6. Roudebush WE, Kim JG, Minhas BS, Dodson MG. Survival and cell acquisition rates after preimplantation embryo biopsy: use of two mechanical techniques and two mouse strains. Am J Obstet Gynecol. 1990;162(4):1084–90.
7. Pierce KE, Michalopoulos J, Kiessling AA, Seibel MM, Zilberstein M. Preimplantation development of mouse and human embryos biopsied at cleavage-stages using a modified displacement technique. Hum Reprod. 1997;12(2):351–6.
8. Cohen J, Malter H, Wright G, Kort H, Massey J, Mitchell D. Partial zona dissection of human oocytes when failure of zona pellucida penetration is anticipated. Hum Reprod. 1989;4:435–42.
9. Cieslak J, Ivakhnenko V, Wolf G, Sheleg S, Verlinsky Y. Three-dimensional partial zona dissection for preimplantation genetic diagnosis and assisted hatching. Fertil Steril. 1999;71:308–13.

10. Gordon JW, Talansky BE. Assisted fertilization by zona drilling: a mouse model for correction of oligospermia. J Exp Zool. 1986;239:347–54.
11. Malter HE, Cohen J. Partial zona dissection of the human oocyte: a nontraumatic method using micromanipulation to assist zona pellucida penetration. Fertil Steril. 1989;51:139–48.
12. Geraedts J, Handyside A, Harper J, Liebaers I, Sermon K, Staesse C, et al. ESHRE Preimplantation Genetic Diagnosis (PGD) Consortium: preliminary assessment of data from January 1997 to September 1998. ESHRE PGD Consortium Steering Committee. Hum Reprod. 1999;14(12):3138–48.
13. Germond M, Nocera D, Senn A, Rink K, Delacrétaz G, Fakan S. Microdissection of mouse and human zona pellucida using a 1.48-microns diode laser beam: efficacy and safety of the procedure. Fertil Steril. 1995;64(3):604–11.
14. Park S, Kim EY, Yoon SH, Chung KS, Lim JH. Enhanced hatching rate of bovine IVM/IVF/IVC blastocysts using a 1.48-micron diode laser beam. J Assist Reprod Genet. 1999;16:97–101.
15. Boada M, Carrera M, De La Iglesia C, Sandalinas M, Barri PN, Veiga A. Successful use of a laser for human embryo biopsy in preimplantation genetic diagnosis: report of two cases. J Assist Reprod Genet. 1998;15:302–7.
16. Han TS, Sagoskin AW, Graham JR, Tucker MJ, Liebermann J. Laser-assisted human embryo biopsy on the third day of development for preimplantation genetic diagnosis: two successful case reports. Fertil Steril. 2003;80:453–5.
17. Joris H, De Vos A, Janssens R, Devroey P, Liebaers I, Van Steirteghem A. Comparison of the results of human embryo biopsy and outcome of PGD after zona drilling using acid Tyrode medium or a laser. Hum Reprod. 2003;18:1896–902.
18. Chatzimeletiou K, Picton HM, Handyside AH. Use of a non-contact, infrared laser for zona drilling of mouse embryos: assessment of immediate effects on blastomere viability. Reprod Biomed Online. 2001;2:178–87.
19. Venkat G, Thornhill A, Wensvoort S, Craft I. Does laser assisted hatching using partial zona thinning (LAH) improve outcome in frozen embryo transfer (FET) cycles? J Clin Embryol. 2008;11(4): 17–30.
20. Chen SU, Chao KH, Wu MY, Chen CD, Ho HN, Yang YS. A simplified two-pipette technique is more efficient than the conventional three-pipette method for blastomere biopsy in human embryos. Fertil Steril. 1998;69:569–75.
21. Inzunza J, Iwarsson E, Fridstrom M, et al. Application of single-needle blastomere biopsy in human preimplantation genetic diagnosis. Prenat Diagn. 1998;8(13):1381–8.
22. Levinson G, Fields RA, Harton GL, Palmer FT, Maddalena A, Fugger EF, et al. Reliable gender screening for human preimplantation embryos, using multiple DNA target-sequences. Hum Reprod. 1992;7(9):1304–13.
23. Harton GL, Magli MC, Lundin K, Montag M, Lemmen J, Harper JC. ESHRE PGD Consortium/Embryology Special Interest Group—best practice guidelines for polar body and embryo biopsy for preimplantation genetic diagnosis/screening (PGD/PGS). Hum Reprod. 2011;26(1):41–6.
24. Preimplantation Genetic Diagnosis International Society (PGDIS). Guidelines for good practice in PGD: programme requirements and laboratory quality assurance. Reprod Biomed Online. 2008;16(1): 134–47.
25. Harper JC, SenGupta S, Vesela K, Thornhill A, Dequeker E, Coonen E, Morris MA. Accreditation of the PGD laboratory. Hum Reprod. 2010;25(4):1051–65.
26. Thornhill A, Repping S. Quality control and quality assurance in preimplantation genetic diagnosis. In: Harper J, editor. Preimplantation genetic diagnosis. New Jersey: Wiley and Sons; 2008.
27. Dumoulin JC, Bras M, Coonen E, Dreesen J, Geraedts JP, Evers JL. Effect of Ca^{2+}/Mg^{2+}-free medium on the biopsy procedure for preimplantation genetic diagnosis and further development of human embryos. Hum Reprod. 1998;13:2880–3.
28. Tarin JJ, Conaghan J, Winston RM, Handyside AH. Human embryo biopsy on the 2nd day after insemination for preimplantation diagnosis: removal of a quarter of embryo retards cleavage. Fertil Steril. 1992;58:970–6.

29. Blake DA, Farquhar CM, Johnson N, Proctor M. Cleavage-stage versus blastocyst stage embryo transfer in assisted conception. Cochrane Database Syst Rev. 2007;4:CD002118.
30. Tsunoda Y, McLaren A. Effect of various procedures on the viability of mouse embryos containing half the normal number of blastomeres. J Reprod Fertil. 1983;69:315–22.
31. Tang R, Catt J, Howlett D. Towards defining parameters for a successful single embryo transfer in frozen cycles. Hum Reprod. 2006;21(5):1179–83.
32. Cohen J, Wells D, Munne S. Removal of 2 cells from cleavage-stage embryos is likely to reduce the efficacy of chromosomal tests that are used to enhance implantation rates. Fertil Steril. 2007;87(3):496–503.
33. Liu J, Van den Abbeel E, Van Steirteghem A. The in-vitro and in-vivo developmental potential of frozen and non-frozen biopsied 8-cell mouse embryos. Hum Reprod. 1993;8(9):1481–6.
34. Van de Velde H, De Vos A, Sermon K, Staessen C, De Rycke M, Van Assche E, et al. Embryo implantation after biopsy of one or two cells from cleavage-stage embryos with a view to preimplantation genetic diagnosis. Prenat Diagn. 2000;20(13):1030–7.
35. Goossens V, De Rycke M, De Vos A, Staessen C, Michiels A, Verpoest W, et al. Diagnostic efficiency, embryonic development and clinical outcome after the biopsy of one or two blastomeres for preimplantation genetic diagnosis. Hum Reprod. 2008;23(3):481–92.
36. De Vos A, Staessen C, De Rycke M, Verpoest W, Haentjens P, Devroey P, Liebaers I, Van de Velde H. Impact of cleavage-stage embryo biopsy in view of PGD on human blastocyst implantation: a prospective cohort of single embryo transfers. Hum Reprod. 2009;24(12):2988–96.
37. Mastenbroek S, Twisk M, van Echten-Arends J, Sikkema-Raddatz B, Korevaar JC, Verhoeve HR, et al. In vitro fertilization with preimplantation genetic screening. N Engl J Med. 2007;357(1):9–17.
38. Cohen J, Grifo J. Multicentre trial of preimplantation genetic screening reported in the New England Journal of Medicine: an in-depth look at the findings. Reprod Biomed Online. 2007;15(4):365–6.
39. Rossant J. Postimplantation development of blastomeres isolated from 4- and 8-cell mouse eggs. J Embryol Exp Morphol. 1976;36:283–90.
40. Hardy K, Martin KL, Leese HJ, Winston RML, Handyside AH. Human preimplantation development in vitro is not adversely affected by biopsy at the 8-cell stage. Hum Reprod. 1990;5:708–14.
41. Das S, Blake D, Farquhar C, Seif MM. Assisted hatching on assisted conception (IVF and ICSI). Cochrane Database Syst Rev. 2009(2):CD001894 (review).
42. Sutcliffe AG, D'Souza SW, Cadman J, Richards B, McKinlay IA, Lieberman B. Outcome in children from cryopreserved embryos. Arch Dis Child. 1995;72(4):290–3.
43. Edgar DH, Archer J, McBain J, Bourne H. Embryonic factors affecting outcome from single cryopreserved embryo transfer. Reprod Biomed Online. 2007;14(6):718–23.
44. Cui KH, Matthews CD. Nuclear structural conditions and PCR amplification in human preimplantation diagnosis. Mol Hum Reprod. 1996;2(1):63–71.
45. Ziebe S, Lundin K, Janssens R, Helmgaard L, Arce JC, MERIT (Menotrophin vs Recombinant FSH in vitro Fertilisation Trial) Group. Influence of ovarian stimulation with HP-hMG or recombinant FSH on embryo quality parameters in patients undergoing IVF. Hum Reprod. 2007;22(9):2404–13.
46. Harper JC, Coonen E, Ramaekers FC, et al. Identification of the sex of human preimplantation embryos in two hours using an improved spreading method and fluorescent *in situ* hybridization (FISH) using directly labelled probes. Hum Reprod. 1994;9:721–4.
47. Munné S, Cohen J. Unsuitability of multinucleated human blastomeres for preimplantation genetic diagnosis. Hum Reprod. 1993;8:1120–5.
48. Kuo HC, Ogilvie CM, Handyside AH. Chromosomal mosaicism in cleavage-stage human embryos and the accuracy of single-cell genetic analysis. J Assist Reprod Genet. 1998;15:276–80.
49. Strom CM, Levin R, Strom S, Masciangelo C, Kuliev A, Verlinsky Y. Neonatal outcome of preimplantation genetic diagnosis by polar body removal: the first 109 infants. Pediatrics. 2000;106(4): 650–3.
50. Banerjee I, Shevlin M, Taranissi M, Thornhill A, Abdalla H, Ozturk O, Barnes J, Sutcliffe A. Health of children conceived after preimplantation genetic diagnosis: a preliminary outcome study. Reprod Biomed Online. 2008;16(3):376–81.

51. Liebaers I, Desmyttere S, Verpoest W, De Rycke M, Staessen C, Sermon K, Devroey P, Haentjens P, Bonduelle M. Report on a consecutive series of 581 children born after blastomere biopsy for preimplantation genetic diagnosis. Hum Reprod. 2010;25(1): 275–82.
52. Harper JC, Coonen E, Handyside AH, Winston RM, Hopman AH, Delhanty JD. Mosaicism of autosomes and sex chromosomes in morphologically normal, monospermic preimplantation human embryos. Prenat Diagn. 1995;15(1):41–9.
53. Magli MC, Jones GM, Gras L, Gianaroli L, Korman I, Trounson AO. Chromosome mosaicism in day 3 aneuploid embryos that develop to morphologically normal blastocysts in vitro. Hum Reprod. 2000;15(8):1781–6.
54. Bielanska M, Tan SL, Ao A. Chromosomal mosaicism throughout human preimplantation development in vitro: incidence, type, and relevance to embryo outcome. Hum Reprod. 2002;17(2):413–9.
55. Dreesen J, Drüsedau M, Smeets H, de Die-Smulders C, Coonen E, Dumoulin J, Gielen M, Evers J, Herbergs J, Geraedts J. Validation of preimplantation genetic diagnosis by PCR analysis: genotype comparison of the blastomere and corresponding embryo, implications for clinical practice. Mol Hum Reprod. 2008;14(10):573–9.
56. Veiga A, Sandalinas M, Benkhalifa M, Boada M, Carrera M, Santalo J, et al. Laser blastocyst biopsy for preimplantation diagnosis in the human. Zygote. 1997;5(4):351–4.
57. Papanikolaou EG, Kolibianakis EM, Tournaye H, Venetis CA, Fatemi H, Tarlatzis B, et al. Live birth rates after transfer of equal number of blastocysts or cleavage-stage embryos in IVF. A systematic review and meta-analysis. Hum Reprod. 2008;23(1): 91–9.
58. Kokkali G, Traeger-Synodinos J, Vrettou C, Stavrou D, Jones GM, Cram DS, et al. Blastocyst biopsy versus cleavage-stage biopsy and blastocyst transfer for preimplantation genetic diagnosis of beta-thalassaemia: a pilot study. Hum Reprod. 2007;22(5):1443–9.
59. Schoolcraft WB, Fragouli E, Stevens J, Munne S, Katz-Jaffe MG, Wells D. Clinical application of comprehensive chromosomal screening at the blastocyst stage. Fertil Steril. 2010;94(5):1700–6.
60. Geber S, Winston RM, Handyside AH. Proliferation of blastomeres from biopsied cleavage-stage human embryos in vitro: an alternative to blastocyst biopsy for preimplantation diagnosis. Hum Reprod. 1995;10:1492–6.
61. Geber S, Sampaio M. Blastomere development after embryo biopsy: a new model to predict embryo development and to select for transfer. Hum Reprod. 1999;14:782–6.
62. Joris H, Van den Abbeel E, Vos AD, Van Steirteghem A. Reduced survival after human embryo biopsy and subsequent cryopreservation. Hum Reprod. 1999;14:2833–7.
63. Magli MC, Gianaroli L, Fortini D, Ferraretti AP, Munné S. Impact of blastomere biopsy and cryopreservation techniques on human embryo viability. Hum Reprod. 1999;14:770–3.
64. Jericho H, Wilton L, Gook DA, Edgar DH. A modified cryopreservation method increases the survival of human biopsied cleavage-stage embryos. Hum Reprod. 2003;18:568–71.
65. Stachecki JJ, Cohen J, Munne S. Cryopreservation of biopsied cleavage-stage human embryos. Reprod Biomed Online. 2005;11(6): 711–5.
66. Agca Y, Monson RL, Northey DL, Peschel DE, Schaefer DM, Rutledge JJ. Normal calves from transfer of biopsied, sexed and vitrified IVP bovine embryos. Theriogenology. 1998;50(1):129–45.
67. Baranyai B, Bodo S, Dinnyes A, Gocza E. Vitrification of biopsied mouse embryos. Acta Vet Hung. 2005;53(1):103–12.
68. Parriego M, Sole M, Aurell R, Barri PN, Veiga A. Birth after transfer of frozen-thawed vitrified biopsied blastocysts. J Assist Reprod Genet. 2007;24(4):147–9.
69. Edwards R, Hollands P. New advances in human embryology: implications of the preimplantation diagnosis of genetic disease. Hum Reprod. 1988;3(4):549–56.
70. Handyside AH, Harton GL, Mariani B, Thornhill AR, Affara N, Shaw MA, Griffin DK. Karyomapping: a universal method for genome wide analysis of genetic disease based on mapping crossovers between parental haplotypes. J Med Genet. 2009;47: 651–8.

Chapter 22
Embryo Biopsy for PGD: Current Perspective

Steven J. McArthur, Don Leigh, Maria Traversa, James Marshall, and Robert P.S. Jansen

This chapter sets out to examine the major recent advances in embryo biopsy, specifically blastocyst-stage biopsy and preimplantation genetic testing and diagnosis (together *PGD*) which are transforming singleton live birth rates in families at risk of passing on monogenic diseases or chromosomal translocations.

The Development of Embryo Biopsy

Embryo biopsies for clinical PGD generally were performed at day 3, when the embryo typically was at the 6- to 8-cell stage, and involved the removal of one or two blastomeres. The zona was breached by dissolving the protein with acid Tyrode's solution. The embryo was incubated in a calcium-/magnesium-free medium to reduce cell–cell interactions and make the removal of cells easier. There has been debate about the impact of removing multiple cells, and in general it was considered that two-cell removal was more detrimental than removing just a single cell and should not be performed—although the reliability of amplification of two cells was considered less prone to allele dropout. An alternative biopsy approach involved the removal of either the first and second polar bodies—either sequentially on day 0 and day 1, or both at day 1. PCR analysis of blastomeres or polar bodies involves amplification of a single allelic copy of the target. Similarly, analysis by FISH is a single-cell test. Biopsy at the blastocyst stage, when embryos typically comprise upward of 100 cells, enables the removal of 3–5 trophectoderm cells

---

S.J. McArthur, BSc (✉) • D. Leigh, PhD (UNSW) • M. Traversa, BSc, Msc, (Med)
J. Marshall, BAppSc (UTS) • R.P.S. Jansen, MD CREI
Sydney IVF, Sydney, Australia
e-mail: Steve.mcarthur@sydneyivf.com

without significant cell mass depletion. Putting several cells into a PCR reaction should decrease the likelihood of amplification failure (allele dropout, or ADO) and, with FISH analyses, should provide an opportunity to confirm signal patterns.

During the early 2000s, Genea (formerly Sydney IVF)moved comprehensively to blastocyst culture and blastocyst-stage transfers and cryostorage and experienced a corresponding increase in take-home baby rates, substantial reductions in multiple pregnancies, and reduced rates of miscarriage [1–7]. In 2004, we described the first clinical application of blastocyst biopsy to routine PGD practice [1]. Embryos were "hatched" on day 3 using a Hamilton Thorne Zilos Tk near-infrared laser and were then incubated for another 2 days to enable blastocoel expansion and herniation of trophectoderm cells through the opened zona for biopsy [1, 6]. Suitable embryos were placed in 5 μL drops of standard medium under oil. A holding pipette, the same as used in ICSI practice, was employed to immobilize the embryo, while a 30-μL biopsy pipette was used to collapse the blastocyst cavity and hold the tissue sample. Several pulses with the laser set at low level loosened cell–cell interactions 3–5, permitting a small piece of tissue to be teased off the exposed trophectoderm. The embryo was then removed and placed into fresh medium for further incubation (until the results were known and the embryo was transferred, cryostored, or disposed of). The tissue piece was washed and placed into PCR tubes or fixed to glass slides for analysis using FISH.

The advantage of moving from cleavage-stage to blastocyst-stage PGD was demonstrated by comparison of embryo biopsies performed (a) at the day 3 cleavage stage and followed by the transfer of embryos that went on to blastulate successfully, with (b) embryo biopsies taken *at* the blastocyst stage (day 5–6) and followed by almost immediate transfer [7]. This study, in other words, *examined the efficacy of day 3 biopsy vs. day 5 or 6 on the embryo, while controlling for the embryo's ability to blastulate*; patients in this trial had PGD not for infertility or miscarriages but to prevent further propagation of a serious monogenic family disease. The outcome (Table 22.1) implies that, in comparison with the biopsy of blastocysts, day 3 cleavage-stage PGD reduces the implantation potential of at least some embryos. (The same could still also be true of blastocyst biopsy, but appears to be to a much lesser extent.)

Table 22.1 shows the technical outcome data for the embryos biopsied (595 for day 3; 656 for days 5–6), with an average of 6.5 embryos biopsied and tested per retrieval at cleavage, compared with an average of 3.7 embryos biopsied and tested per retrieval when the blastocyst stage was awaited before performing PGD. The proportion of embryos with a conclusive test and with a normal result, thus suitable for transfer, was still approximately 50% in each series, which means that taking the biopsy later in embryo development conferred appreciable laboratory and clinical efficiency through not having to test embryos whose development was compromised. The late-biopsied blastocysts had almost twice the chance of implanting than did the blastocysts that had been biopsied on day 3.

Table 22.2 shows the outcomes of the embryo transfer procedures. In spite of a lower average number of embryos transferred (1.1 vs. 1.5 per transfer procedure), and without taking into account later further pregnancies from cryostored biopsied

Table 22.1 Embryos available for testing for monogenic disease mutations by biopsy on day 3[a] and on day 5–6

	Egg retrievals	Embryos biopsied	Inconclusive test result	Conclusive, favorable test	Embryos transferred fresh	Tested embryos cryostored
Day 3 biopsy + day 5–6 transfer[a]	91	595 av. 6.5 embryos	61 (10.3%)	261 (43.8%)	103	158 (60.5%)
Day 5–6 biopsy + day 5–6 transfer	177	655 av. 3.7 embryos	46 (7.0%)	305 (46.5%)	121	184 (60.3%)

See McArthur et al. [7] for more detailed interpretation of the data
[a]All embryos were developed to blastocysts before transfer

embryos, the day 5–6 biopsy transfers resulted in fewer miscarriages and a higher absolute ongoing pregnancy rate, as well as the expected lower rate of multiple pregnancy. There was one obvious monozygotic twinning event, involving an embryo biopsied on day 3. In about 60% of cases in each series, additional embryos that had tested normally were cryostored for further attempts at pregnancy.

Preimplantation Screening for Aneuploidy

It has been known for more than 15 years that IVF embryos show a high rate of chromosome aneuploidy [8]. It has also been understood for many more years that a chance acquisition of an abnormal number of chromosomes is a frequent event in human conception and, in particular, is the commonest cause for pregnancies to miscarry. It might therefore be expected that screening IVF embryos for aneuploidies before selecting an embryo to transfer should materially improve the chance of pregnancy, reduce the risk of miscarriage, and (by enabling embryos to be transferred efficiently and efficaciously one at a time) greatly reduce the multiple pregnancy rate, thus lessening perinatal morbidity and mortality. The target—improved live birth rates from IVF and less costs for community—is worthy and logical.

Aneuploidy Risk

Several authors have reported that the age of the woman undergoing IVF has a significant bearing on the extent of aneuploidy in the resulting embryos. Studies on the origin of the nondisjunction chromosome anomalies have suggested that most of the abnormalities originate predominantly from female meiosis, especially meiosis I, although analysis of preimplantation embryo polar bodies with FISH has indicated that meiosis II errors could be similar in number [9]. Analysis of later-stage

Table 22.2 Clinical outcomes following biopsy at the cleavage-stage vs. biopsy at the stage of blastocyst, each with transfer of embryos fresh on day 5 or 6

	Embryos transferred n	Transfer procedures n	Pregnancy per retrieval	Implantation per embryo[a]	Miscarriage	Live birth or ongoing pregnancy	Multiple at confinement Single	Twin	Triple
Day 3 biopsy + day 5–6 transferred n = 91 retrievals	1	38	11	11	4	7	7		
	2	28	12	15	1	10	7	2	
	3	3	1	1	0	1	1		
	All av. 1.5	69 (75.8%)	24/91 (26.4%)	27/103 (26.2%)	5/91 (20.1%)	18/91 (19.8%)	15		3 Multiples (16.7%)
Day 5–6 biopsy + day 5–6 transferred n = 177 retrievals	1	105	54	54	8	46	46		
	2	8	4	5	1	3	2	1	
	3	0							
	All av. 1.1	113 (63.8%)	58/177 (32.8%)	59/121 (48.8%)	9/58 (15.5%)	49/177 (27.7%)	48		1 Multiple (2%)

Data from McArthur et al. [7]

[a]The implantation rate for blastocysts biopsied from the trophectoderm as blastocysts (48.8%) was highly significantly better than the implantation rate for blastocysts biopsied using a single cell removed at the day 3 cleavage stage (26.2%, $P < 0.01$)

embryos would therefore be able to identify both meiosis I and meiosis II errors (as well as revealing aneuploidies brought by the fertilizing sperm). Generally, a predisposition to aneuploidy beyond maternal age effect has been hampered by the fact that few studies have looked for or been able to identify genetic causes; rare recessive genetic states that interfere with meiosis have been described [10]. While not extensive, there have been a number of reports suggesting that among women undergoing IVF and experiencing subsequent implantation failure, the chromosome abnormality rate in their embryos is quite high compared to the other IVF cohorts [11–13]. Screening embryos for aneuploidy could reduce the number of embryos subsequently needed to initiate a successful and continuing pregnancy [14]. The efficacy of the screening process must obviously take into account any detrimental aspects of the biopsy and culture processes to be considered truly beneficial for the patient's progress.

Aneuploidy Screening in IVF Programs

Examination of a restricted number of chromosomes using FISH for aneuploidy screening as a routine may not be helpful in all cases and in fact can be harmful if biopsy procedures are not efficient. Mastenbroek et al. showed that biopsy of day 3 (cleavage-stage) embryos for limited PGS—screening for aneuploidy of chromosomes 13, 16, 17, 18, 21, X, and Y—can reduce the chance of an ongoing pregnancy in women aged 35–41 having in vitro fertilization (IVF) [15]. Our considerations above (Tables 22.1 and 22.2) suggest that interfering with an early embryo might lie behind this detrimental result, but other factors could also be important. For the Mastenbroek study, these included such straightforward concerns as the time the embryos spent being manipulated in potentially altered culture conditions across the variety of IVF clinics where the biopsies were performed. They also include more complex issues, such as the inadvertent exclusion from transfer of mosaic embryos in which the biopsied cell happened to be the only cell with the trisomy (a situation that can follow a mitotic nondisjunction event) [9].

Between August 2004 and November 2006, we studied the impact of screening for aneuploidy in younger infertile women (<38 years, median 33.5 years), employing biopsies of blastocysts [5]. All women were in their first or second attempt at IVF. Agreement to have one embryo transferred (eSET) was a precondition for entry. Patients were withdrawn from the study if there were fewer than eight ovarian follicles over 1 cm diameter at 8–10 days of stimulation, fewer than four embryos with seven or more cells on day 3 of culture, or fewer than three blastocysts for biopsy on day 5 or 6; no women had cycles canceled because of a poor response. The biopsies consisted of 2–9 trophectoderm cells and were tested by at least 5-color fluorescent in situ hybridization for, at minimum, chromosomes 13, 18, 21, X, and Y. We compared outcomes between the screened group (Group A, normal ≥5-color pattern in all the removed trophectoderm cells for the transferred embryo) and the

Table 22.3 Pregnancy rates after preimplantation genetic screening for aneuploidy from biopsy of blastocysts on day 5 or 6 of development using 5- or 7-color FISH

Group A. Biopsy				Group B. No biopsy (control)			
n	P	NP	%P	n	P	NP	%P
56	25	30	45.5%	48	26	20	56.5%
Group C. Poor response, withdrawn				Group D. Eligible, nonparticipating			
n	P	NP	%P	n	P	NP	%P
107	36	71	33.6%	1,194	564	630	47.2%

From Jansen et al. [5], with permission
P pregnant; *NP* not pregnant

principal control group (Group B, with zona opening but no biopsy); we also made comparisons with the women who were withdrawn from the study before randomization because of suboptimal responses to stimulation (Group C) and with women who were eligible but elected not to take part in the study (Group D). Table 22.3 gives the results up to the time the trial was suspended. Pregnancies are clinical pregnancies with a normal fetal heart rate on ultrasound scanning in the first trimester. The clinical pregnancy rate (pregnancies with a normal fetal heart rate at 6 weeks' gestation) was high (46.4% of egg retrieval procedures overall), irrespective of whether PGS was performed or not, and is consistent with results we [2, 6] and others [16] have reported previously for elective single blastocyst transfers.

Among the women who underwent biopsy for aneuploidy screening (Group A), the pregnancy rate at 45.5% was insignificantly less than among women who were eligible for the trial but did not take part (Group D, 47.2%) and was trending to be higher than among women who were withdrawn from the trial prior to randomization because of a suboptimal response (Group C, 33.6%; $\chi^2 = 1.7, P < 0.1$, 1-tailed). We could thus find no evidence of clinically important detriment from blastocyst biopsy in women of normal reproductive age. The pregnancy rate compares favorably, with the 25% clinical pregnancy rate reported by Mastenbroek et al.

Unexpectedly, Group B, the embryos subjected to zona opening by near-infrared laser, a standard preparatory step for biopsy and performed on day 3 or 4 (see above), produced the highest clinical pregnancy rate of the groups (56.5%), which while not statistically significantly different from either the biopsied embryos (Group A, $\chi^2 = 0.8$) or the eligible but nonparticipant women's embryos (Group D, $\chi^2 = 1.2$), the trend was opposite to that required to disprove the null hypothesis, and the clinical trial was stopped.

The reason for the strong performance of the embryos in the principal control group, if it is true, is not clear. Assisted hatching by opening of the zona, while advocated from time to time for the embryos of older women to facilitate hatching and implantation, has not been shown to be beneficial among women under 40 or with good blastocyst development. More likely, a too strict set of criteria for assumed meiotic nondisjunction led to overinterpretation and rejection of some blastocysts that would, if left unscreened, have developed normally and contributed to the total number of embryos suitable for transfer.

Testing for Chromosomal Translocations

Reciprocal translocations occur in about 1 in 625 newborns and usually result from the exchange of two terminal segments from different chromosomes, ordinarily resulting in a genome that is balanced. Exchanges can also take place close to the centromeres of two acrocentric chromosomes; these Robertsonian translocations, which occur in about 1 in 900 newborns, also ordinarily provide a balanced genome and bring the overall prevalence of balanced translocations among newborns to about 1:380 [17]. When diploid germ cells with these karyotypes eventually undergo meiosis, however, the chromosomes involved segregate abnormally and yield a varying but significantly high level of unbalanced haploid states among oocytes and spermatozoa—an unbalanced state that is continued into the embryo and which results in implantation failure, miscarriage, stillbirth, or abnormalities at birth. Balanced translocations are ten times more common among couples presenting for treatment with IVF [18].

With *reciprocal translocations*, homologous pairing during meiosis 1 produces a tetravalent structure instead of the usual bivalent. Subsequent segregation to respective daughter cell spindles takes one of three modes: *2:2 alternate segregation* (producing alternately a normal or a balanced abnormal complement, the latter perpetuating the familial condition but both with a balanced genome); *adjacent 1 and 2 segregations* (producing segmental monosomies and trisomies); and comparatively rarely, *3:1 segregations* (involving nondisjunction of a whole chromosome and producing more complete monosomies and trisomies) [19]. Overall, 75% of embryos from a parent with a balanced reciprocal translocation show partially or fully aneuploid chromosome complements (14 different unbalanced combinations compared to two balanced combinations), considerably reducing the number of otherwise healthy appearing embryos available for transfer after PGD.

In *Robertsonian translocations*, a trivalent structure is formed during meiosis 1, with three main segregation modes possible (and nine different chromosome combinations), namely, *alternate* (which returns dosage to its balanced state), *2:1 segregations* (producing complementary monosomies and trisomies), and *3:0 segregation* (produce double trisomy or double monosomy).

Traditional PGD for translocations involves FISH, utilizing either breakpoint-spanning probes (which require access to extensive probe libraries and complicated workups) or (much more simply) combinations of commercially available, quality-controlled centromeric, locus-specific, and subtelomeric probes attached to standard fluorochromes. The use of PGD to screen balanced from unbalanced chromosome sets in the embryos then significantly reduces the failure rate for implantation and should result in fewer miscarriages among the embryos available for transfer [13, 20]. Again, to be truly beneficial, the process of biopsy must do the least amount of harm to the embryo's continued development and to its ability to implant. Table 22.4 shows our experience with cleavage- and blastocyst-stage biopsies among couples with recurrent miscarriage attributable to a balanced reciprocal translocation in one of them. The live baby results have been lower

Table 22.4 Clinical outcomes of PGD for balanced translocation using FISH and from using STR-based PCR

	Reciprocal translocations		Robertsonian translocations	
	FISH	STR-PCR	FISH	STR-PCR
Patients	54	22	17	7
Mean age	35.2	33.1	36.0	33.3
Cycles with egg retrieval	112	22	51	6
Cycles with embryo biopsy	73	22	31	6
Biopsied embryos	320	61	142	17
Actionable PGD result	304	60	136	17
Embryos for transfer	74 (23%)	20 (33%)	44 (31%)	13 (76%)
Embryo transfer cycles	54	13	27	5
Embryos transferred	1.2	1	1.2	1
Total embryos transferred	62	13	32	5
Positive pregnancy test	20	7	14	3
Implantation rate/embryo (%)	32	54	44	60
FH-positive pregnancy rate per transfer	15 (24%)	6 (46%)	12 (38%)	2 (40%)
FH-positive pregnancy rate per egg retrieval (%)	13	27	24	33

Data from McArthur et al. [7] and Traversa et al. [22]
All embryos were biopsied and transferred at the blastocyst stage. Results do not include pregnancies from the embryos cryostored

compared to those we obtain after testing for monogenic disease (Table 22.2), possibly reflecting the large decrement in transferable embryos seen with reciprocal translocations following the demonstration of unbalanced cells by FISH-based PGD. These apparent unbalanced outcomes can be of biological origin but can also be false, due to inherent error rates observed with FISH-based protocols [21] or reflective of a benign mosaic state, but in either case contributing to false positive interpretation of FISH signals and leading to the exclusion of otherwise normal embryos.

In our published series for translocations using FISH [7], 95 egg retrievals were performed and led to biopsy and testing among couples with a *balanced reciprocal translocation*; there were 10 pregnancies among 26 patients who had day 3 biopsies, seven of which went to term—a miscarriage rate of 33%. Of the 12 pregnancies among 21 couples for whom biopsy was performed on day 5–6, eight miscarried (38%). Twenty-three egg retrievals among 15 couples with a *Robertsonian translocation* led to biopsies and testing; there were 3 pregnancies among 7 couples with day 3 biopsies, each of which went to term, and 8 pregnancies among 7 couples with day 5–6 biopsies, one of which miscarried and one of which was an ongoing monozygotic twin pregnancy. Combining day 3 with day 5–6 biopsies, the miscarriage rate after PGD for Robertsonian translocation exclusion was 18%, whereas PGD for excluding unbalanced reciprocal translocations was followed by a miscarriage rate of 45%.

Monogenic Diseases

Monogenic diseases considered appropriate for PGD are those uncommon or rare, fatal, or chronically disabling familial conditions that occur as a result of mutations in a single gene. The location of the mutation can be in an exon, a splice point, or within the control regions and affects the functioning of the specific gene. Inheritance is Mendelian, and classically there are three major classes of phenotypic expression:

1. *Dominant inheritance*, where every individual who inherits the single gene change is likely to be affected by the disorder and will carry a 50% chance of passing on the affected gene to offspring. An example is Huntington's disease. PGD analysis for such mutations must be reliable in detecting a mutation change in a background of normal DNA sequence.
2. *Recessive inheritance*, where carriers of mutations themselves are not affected by the disorder but who partner with another carrier for a mutation in the same gene then produce a reproductive risk for their offspring of 25% for an affected child and 50% for a carrier child. An example is cystic fibrosis. Mutation analysis for these conditions needs to address the ability to analyze for a mutation in a homozygote state or often in a compound heterozygous state.
3. *X-linked inheritance* where, essentially, mutations on the X chromosome typically result in female carriers who have a 25% risk of producing affected male offspring and a 25% risk of reproducing the carrier state in female offspring. An example of a recessive X-linked gene disorder is hemophilia A. An example of an incompletely dominant X-linked disorder is fragile-X syndrome, which causes severe mental retardation in males but which also has a heterozygous female phenotype that includes premature ovarian failure. Analysis must be reliable but, unlike other recessive diseases, or the dominant diseases, there is no normal background DNA sequence for males. Female carriers contribute a nonmutated X chromosome, so confidence with the analysis must be the same as for the autosome mutations.

The starting point for PCR in the case of a single cell from a day 3 biopsy is usually just a single copy of DNA (there is obviously more DNA available with multicellular trophectoderm biopsies). In principle—and regrettably sometimes also in practice—failure of the mutated DNA to amplify (ADO) produces a false-negative result, leading to an incorrect conclusion of a normal state. Any biopsy testing process must be as reliable as possible to avoid any miscalls.

The Near Future for Translocation Testing

STR-Based Molecular Strategies

Our experience, above, revealed no obvious advantage for blastocyst-stage biopsies compared with day 3 cleavage-stage biopsies when FISH is used to infer balanced chromosomal patterns for either reciprocal or Robertsonian translocations. In each case, miscarriage rates remain particularly high for apparently balanced reciprocal translations. We have since reported a molecular strategy utilizing PCR for PGD in translocation carriers that examines highly polymorphic short tandem repeat sequences (STRs), application of which has significantly improved outcomes after biopsies at the blastocyst stage [22].

Using STR profiling to identify chromosomal segments on either side of the known breakpoints, in conjunction with standard cytogenetic segregation tables to predict each unbalanced state, we directly identify the monoallelic and triallelic states that are the direct cause of the phenotypic abnormality and reproductive loss which results from these malsegregants and, in turn, is the immediate pathogenic mechanism behind the reason PGD is offered to translocation carriers. The method requires extensive screening of chromosome-specific STRs to define those markers for which the carrier is heterozygous and where alleles are not shared with the partner. To make this PCR-based test efficient, chosen markers are multiplexed to obtain results within primary or secondary amplifications. The method also lends itself to other PCR-based PGD objectives conducted simultaneously, such as monogenic disease exclusion. Verification of the method has come from the rebiopsy of embryos diagnosed as unbalanced: in each of six cases in which samples were assessed for segmental chromosomal gains and losses using conventional CGH (see below), the predicted malsegregations were confirmed.

Conclusive results in our hands rose to 99% using STR profiling, compared with 93% with blastocyst-based FISH. Any apparent mosaicism seen in the trophectoderm sample has the potential to complicate the interpretation of the translocation state, especially when using FISH, where any visible abnormality tends to disqualify the embryo for transfer, on the subjective basis that failure of a chromosome to hybridize or to hybridize ambiguously is always possible. STR profiling, on the other hand, encompasses multiple loci on each side of the translocation point, reducing ADO-based errors (false monoallelic states from diploid alleles, false biallelic states for trisomic alleles).

Table 22.4 compares our FISH-based blastocyst biopsy experience with our STR-PCR experience. Patients with reciprocal translocations still show the expected predominantly unbalanced segregation patterns predicted by theory, but fewer embryos are falsely disqualified from transfer. Patients with Robertsonian translocations also fare better. Robertsonian translocation carriers can be prone to uniparental disomy, especially when chromosomes 14 and 15 are involved (see [22]); STR-PCR, unlike FISH, enables biparental inheritance to be looked for and to be confirmed or excluded. Finally, the time needed for actionable results with STR-PCR is just 4–5 h, compared with the 6–16 h required for FISH hybridization and interpretation.

The Near Future for Aneuploidy Screening

The majority of aneuploidies arise during female meiosis. The minority are brought to the embryonic genome by the fertilizing sperm and are equally pathogenic. A small number take origin in the first few cleavage divisions through mitotic nondisjunction. The latter lead to mosaic states in the embryo: clearly, the later this happens, the smaller the proportion of triploid cells and the more patchy the distribution among inner cell mass and trophectoderm derivatives. There is a large body of published knowledge on the recognized outcomes, such as confined placental mosaicism. In the embryo proper, trisomic cells will be at a disadvantage compared with their euploid neighbors as tissues and organs develop. Our experience with karyotyping 82 cell lines derived from inner cell masses of slow and stalled embryos, assumed to disproportionally display aneuploidies, provides an indication of this process (Bradley et al., manuscript under review). Sixty-nine (84%) displayed only a normal, diploid karyotype, indicating likely self-correction of mitotic nondisjunction-based mosaic states; a limited number tested showed no cases of loss of heterozygosity, which would indicate uniparental disomy as a consequence of self-correction of meiotic errors. The 13 cellular outgrowths that were cytogenetically abnormal included six single trisomies, a double trisomy, a monosomy, three triploidies, a triploidy with an additional chromosome 22, and a balanced reciprocal translocation. In each of the trisomies, meiotic nondisjunction was confirmed by demonstrating triallelic states for STRs on the affected chromosome. There were no mosaic cell lines.

Thus, for reasons of both relative numbers (mitotic trisomies are from the start mosaic states, whereas meiotic trisomies are pure) and, possibly, a qualitative difference between independent aneuploid states compared with diploid states, the key objective of screening for aneuploidy should be less to count chromosomes than it is to recognize dominant original parent of origin states for any of the 24 chromosomes.

Fluorescent In Situ Hybridization

Specific staining of embryo chromosomes with FISH has been the preferred method to identify the chromosome copy number in a fixed cell preparation. The probes bind to defined regions on the usually interphase cell chromosomes immobilized on a standard microscope slide, usually at interphase. Generally, the probes are purified cloned regions of the specific chromosome, subtracted for repetitive sequences. These probes are labeled with a unique fluorophore which can be visualized with fluorescence microscopy. The preparation and quality control of such material generally means that a commercial supply of the probes is the preferred choice for routine clinical use.

There are limitations to commercially available probe sets. The number of fluorophore colors falls far short of the minimum of 24 required. The fluor needs to be chemically active to attach to the DNA probe and also stable enough to remain attached during the hybridization process. Once hybridized, the color must be able to be visualized using, typically, UV excitation and filtered emission. High-energy wavelength excitation can result in rapid photo bleaching of the fluorophore and hence insufficient time to enumerate the hybridization pattern. The number of fluorophore colors falls far short of the minimum of 24 required. The commercial suppliers have limited their probe labels to a very small set that meet manufacturing standards and the exacting requirements for clinical use. These fluors must be spectrally separable using specific but simple microscope filters. In practice, this means that only 5–7 or so chromosomes can be checked in one hybridization event. Consequently, the number of chromosomes that are there to be counted using FISH means that multiple cycles of hybridization, enumeration, probe stripping, and rehybridization are needed. Each cycle runs the risk of target loss and/or degraded target sites, either of which can result in incorrect chromosome enumeration and thus a misreading of chromosome number—technical considerations that preclude more than 2 or 3 rounds of hybridization. Temporally, adding more than a very few hybridizations would take too much time to permit the transfer of IVF embryos fresh.

Single blastomere biopsy from day 3 embryos gives a single, simple answer: a normal chromosome complement or an abnormal complement. The problems of mosaicism and technical difficulties discussed above, however, still lead to embryos being incorrectly classified and then being excluded from transfer. Biopsy at the blastocyst stage does not resolve these problems but does offer an opportunity to see multiple hybridization signals for a set of cells. Nonetheless, a conservative reading of those signals has meant that observation of mosaic states in multicell biopsies has resulted in the exclusion of embryos that are likely to be substantially normal and suitable for transfer. The policy of disqualifying an embryo for transfer on the basis of 1 or 2 aberrant cells might need to be reexamined.

All other current karyotyping methods applicable to extremely low copy numbers of chromosomes, including analyses of single cells with day 3 embryo biopsies and of typically fewer than ten cells with blastocyst trophectoderm biopsies requires preliminary amplification of DNA copy number.

The first way to satisfy this challenge is to greatly increase the number of chromosome targets to be amplified, enabling any genomic shortcomings in genome-wide amplifications to be overcome by averaging. Over the last few (very few) years, advances in whole genome amplification has advanced the place of the technique of *comparative genomic hybridization* (CGH) by increasing its resolving power within chromosomes as well as improving its quantitative reliability in estimating preamplification DNA copy number.

Comparative Genomic Hybridization

Developed as a chromosomal screen to analyze genomic changes in cancers almost 20 years ago [23], CGH reveals copy amounts of all 22 autosomes and the two sex chromosomes to a resolution of ten million base pairs or so. The technique uses a combination of molecular and cytogenetic approaches to evaluate chromosome complements. Testing cancers with CGH is simpler than testing embryos, however, because generally with cancer samples there is no shortage of extracted DNA to be tested, whereas embryo biopsy specimens are much more limited.

Wells and Delhanty reported CGH analysis of individual cells from human day 3 embryos a decade ago [24]. Wilton and others reported the first reported successful clinical preimplantation use of CGH technique a year later [25]. While the use of CGH promised to deliver a total chromosome aneuploidy screen and the possibility of identifying any chromosome imbalance in an embryo, its labor intensity and its time-consuming nature (which required the embryos to be frozen while testing proceeded over periods of many days) precluded transfer of embryos during the biopsy cycle. There were only a few further reports over the ensuing 6 years [26–28]. Often, what was observed were relatively complex chromosome combinations; these then were given causal roles to explain implantation failure, but screening out aneuploid embryos did not improve embryo implantation rates. In spite of its promise, CGH has not been reported to be in routine use by any group. Recently, however, a report from Wells et al. has reported high implantation rates for blastocysts biopsied and analyzed with CGH after improved whole genome amplification [29]. The embryos were transferred after vitrification and later thawing, and produced an impressive thawed blastocyst implantation rate of 67%—which would warrant routine use, at least in selected patients.

The use of classical CGH on metaphase chromosomes demands high levels of skill, many days of analysis, and the freezing of biopsied embryos until the karyotype is known. One approach to minimizing labor requirements and shortening the testing time has been to employ DNA microarrays [30]. On the one hand, the timing suits polar body analyses and day 3 cleavage-stage biopsies, but both of these sample types offer only a single-cell genome for amplification and analysis, whereas blastocyst biopsy offers several cells to average out the amplification biases more effectively. On the other hand, the additional expense of CGH, however performed, is coming to be more generally appreciated as another reason for identifying embryos that can blastulate before biopsy and testing, in effect providing a self-screening process that reduces the costs of the testing for the individual patient. A pilot study looking at the analysis of polar bodies for aneuploid detection of female origin has been commenced by a consortium from the European Society for Human Reproduction. Implantation rates and pregnancy outcome data are still to be collected. Recent advances combining blastocyst-stage biopsy, micro-array CGH and vitrification have produced high embryo implantation rates and clinical pregnancy outcomes allowing a viable clinical service to be offered [31].

To date, therefore, it is blastocyst-stage biopsy that has given valuable improvement in implantation rates, and it waits to be seen whether the still prevalent day 3 biopsies and day 0–1 biopsies of polar bodies can achieve the same outcomes. With the use of a DNA amplification-based approach, the interpretation problems associated with low-level somatic mosaicism common in embryos and seen with FISH are partially overcome. The tissue sample, typically consisting of 3–5 cells, is analyzed as a whole (and is taken to represent the embryo as a whole), thus producing an averaging effect for the constitutional chromosomes under investigation.

References

1. de Boer KA, Catt JW, Jansen RPS, Leigh D, McArthur S. Moving to blastocyst biopsy for preimplantation genetic diagnosis and single embryo transfer at Sydney IVF. Fertil Steril. 2004;82(2):295–8.
2. Henman M, Catt JW, Wood T, Bowman MC, de Boer KA, Jansen RPS. Elective transfer of single fresh blastocysts and later transfer of cryostored blastocysts reduces the twin pregnancy rate and can improve the in vitro fertilization live birth rate in younger women. Fertil Steril. 2005;84(6):1620–7.
3. Jansen RPS. Female age and the chance of a baby from one in-vitro fertilisation treatment. Med J Aust. 2003;178:258–61.
4. Jansen RPS. Benefits and challenges brought by improved results from in vitro fertilization. Intern Med J. 2005;35(2):108–17.
5. Jansen RPS, Bowman MC, de Boer KA, Leigh DA, Lieberman DB, McArthur SJ. What next for preimplantation genetic screening (PGS)? Experience with blastocyst biopsy and testing for aneuploidy. Hum Reprod. 2008;23(7):1476–8.
6. McArthur SJ, Leigh D, Marshall JT, de Boer KA, Jansen RPS. Pregnancies and live births after trophectoderm biopsy and preimplantation genetic testing of human blastocysts. Fertil Steril. 2005;84(6):1628–36.
7. McArthur SJ, Leigh D, Marshall JT, Gee AT, de Boer KA, Jansen RPS. Blastocyst trophectoderm biopsy and preimplantation genetic diagnosis for familial monogenic disorders and chromosomal translocations. Prenat Diagn. 2008;28(5):434–42.
8. Munné S, Lee A, Rosenwaks Z, Grifo J, Cohen J. Diagnosis of major chromosome aneuploidies in human preimplantation embryos. Hum Reprod. 1993;8(12):2185–91.
9. Kuliev A, Verlinsky Y. Meiotic and mitotic nondisjunction: lessons from preimplantation genetic diagnosis. Hum Reprod Update. 2004;10:401–7.
10. Bolor H, Mori T, Nishiyama S, et al. Mutations of the SYCP3 gene in women with recurrent pregnancy loss. Am J Hum Genet. 2009;84(1):14–20.
11. Landwehr C, Montag M, Van der Ven K, Weber RG. Rapid comparative genomic hybridization protocol for prenatal diagnosis and its application to aneuploidy screening of human polar bodies. Fertil Steril. 2008;90(3):488–96.
12. Vialard F, Hammoud I, Molina-Gomes D, et al. Gamete cytogenetic study in couples with implantation failure: aneuploidy rate is increased in both couple members. J Assist Reprod Genet. 2008;25(11–12):539–45.
13. Voullaire L, Collins V, Callaghan T, McBain J, Williamson R, Wilton L. High incidence of complex chromosome abnormality in cleavage embryos from patients with repeated implantation failure. Fertil Steril. 2007;87(5):1053–8.
14. Schoolcraft WB, Katz-Jaffe MG, Stevens J, Rawlins M, Munne S. Preimplantation aneuploidy testing for infertile patients of advanced maternal age: a randomized prospective trial. Fertil Steril. 2009;92(1):157–62.
15. Mastenbroek S, Twisk M, van Echten-Arends J, et al. In vitro fertilization with preimplantation genetic screening. N Engl J Med. 2007;357(1):9–17.
16. Milki AA, Hinckley MD, Westphal LM, Behr B. Elective single blastocyst transfer. Fertil Steril. 2004;81(6):1697–8.
17. Van Dyke DL, Weiss L, Robertson JR, Babu VR. The frequency and mutation rate of balanced autosomal rearrangements in man estimated from prenatal genetic studies for advanced maternal age. Am J Hum Genet. 1983;35:301–8.
18. Stern C, Pertile M, Norris H, Hale L, Baker H. Chromosome translocations in couples with in-vitro fertilization implantation failure. Hum Reprod. 1999;14:2097–101.
19. Wilton L. Preimplantation genetic diagnosis for aneuploidy screening in early human embryos: a review. Prenat Diagn. 2002;22(6):512–8.
20. Otani T, Roche M, Mizuike M, Colls P, Escudero T, Munne S. Preimplantation genetic diagnosis significantly improves the pregnancy outcome of translocation carriers with a history of

recurrent miscarriage and unsuccessful pregnancies. Reprod Biomed Online. 2006;13(6): 869–74.
21. Munné S, Sandalinas M, Escudero T, Fung J, Gianaroli L, Cohen J. Outcome of preimplantation genetic diagnosis of translocations. Fertil Steril. 2000;73:1209–18.
22. Traversa MV, Carey L, Leigh D. A molecular strategy for routine preimplantation genetic diagnosis in both reciprocal and Robertsonian translocation carriers. Mol Hum Reprod. 2010;16(5):329–37.
23. Kallioniemi A, Kallioniemi OP, Sudar D, et al. Comparative genomic hybridization for molecular cytogenetic analysis of solid tumors. Science. 1992;258(5083):818–21.
24. Wells D, Escudero T, Levy B, Hirschhorn K, Delhanty JD, Munné S. First clinical application of comparative genomic hybridization and polar body testing for preimplantation genetic diagnosis of aneuploidy. Fertil Steril. 2002;78(3):543–9.
25. Wilton L, Williamson R, McBain J, Edgar D, Voullaire L. Birth of a healthy infant after preimplantation confirmation of euploidy by comparative genomic hybridization. N Engl J Med. 2001;345(21):1537–41.
26. Gutiérrez-Mateo C, Gadea L, Benet J, Wells D, Munné S, Navarro J. Aneuploidy 12 in a Robertsonian (13;14) carrier: case report. Hum Reprod. 2005;20(5):1256–60.
27. Obradors A, Fernandez E, Oliver-Bonet M, et al. Birth of a healthy boy after a double factor PGD in a couple carrying a genetic disease and at risk for aneuploidy: case report. Hum Reprod. 2008;23(8):1949–56.
28. Peng W, Takabayashi H, Ikawa K. Whole genome amplification from single cells in preimplantation genetic diagnosis and prenatal diagnosis. Eur J Obstet Gynecol Reprod Biol. 2007;131(1):13–20.
29. Wells D, Fragouli E, Stevens J, Munné S, Schoolcraft WB, Katz-Jaffe MG. Fertil Steril. 2010; 90:s80.
30. Hu DG, Webb G, Hussey N. Aneuploidy detection in single cells using DNA array-based comparative genomic hybridization. Mol Hum Reprod. 2004;10(4):283–9.
31. Traversa MV, Marshall J, McArthur S, Leigh D. The genetic screening of preimplantation embryos by comparative geneome hybridisation. Reprod Biol. 2011;10 (Supp 3):51–60.

Chapter 23
Microarrays and CGH for PGD of Chromosome Abnormalities and Gene Defects

Gary Harton and Santiago Munné

Fish and Array-Based Testing

More than 50% of cleavage-stage embryos produced in vitro are chromosomally abnormal, increasing to up to 80% in women over 42 years of age [1–4]. Although some abnormal embryos arrest during extended culture, most do not, and even at the blastocyst stage, more than half of all embryos are abnormal (mean maternal age 38 years) [5]. The majority of numerical chromosome abnormalities detected in embryos are not compatible with implantation or birth which negatively affects the success of assisted reproductive treatments. The detrimental effect of aneuploidy is illustrated by the high prevalence of chromosome abnormalities detected in spontaneous abortions, exceeding 70% in some studies [6–11]. It has been hypothesized that selection of embryos for transfer based on chromosome normalcy (euploidy) could improve success rates in assisted reproductive procedures [12]. This process is known as preimplantation genetic diagnosis (PGD) of aneuploidy or preimplantation genetic screening (PGS). For a glossary of terms (see Glossary).

Shortcomings of Pre-Array Technologies

The first PGD strategies to be described employed fluorescence in situ hybridization (FISH) analysis of cells biopsied from day-3 embryos [12–16], trophectoderm cells biopsied from blastocyst-stage embryos [17], or polar bodies biopsied from oocytes or zygotes [18–21]. The FISH methods allowed analysis of 5–12 chromosomes in

G. Harton, BS, TS (ABB) • S. Munné, PhD (✉)
Department of Molecular Genetics, Reprogenetics, LLC, 3 Regent Street, Suite 301, Livingston, NJ 07039, USA
e-mail: munne@reprogenetics.com

each oocyte or embryo but were unable to provide a full evaluation of the chromosome complement. Nevertheless, that was enough to detect more than 80% of chromosomally abnormal embryos detected by array technology [22].

Some studies utilizing FISH-based strategies reported an improvement in implantation rates, reduction in spontaneous abortions, and/or an increase in take-home-baby rates [15, 21, 23–32]. However, these studies were not randomized. Other studies, some performed in a randomized fashion, did not produce significant improvements or showed a detrimental effect of PGD for aneuploidy [33–36]. Several reasons for these conflicting results have been advanced.

The biological argument, which does not explain differences in reports, but attempts to understand why some studies observed a negative effect on outcome, argues that cleavage-stage embryos have such high rates of chromosomal mosaicism that any analysis based upon a single cell is unreliable. Although it is true that mosaicism is common in cleavage-stage embryos (about 30% according to FISH analyses) [1–4], the majority of these embryos display chromosome abnormalities in every cell. In such cases, the biopsied cell may not be chromosomally identical to the remaining cells of the embryo, they may contain errors affecting different chromosomes, but the clinical diagnosis of "abnormal" is still valid. Large follow-up studies of preimplantation embryos diagnosed using FISH estimate only a 5–7% error caused by mosaicism [15, 37] when embryos are reanalyzed in all their cells by FISH. Even less, only 2% when analyzed by array CGH [38], thus mosaicism is unlikely to be the primary cause of poor outcomes following PGD.

The most probable cause of intercenter differences in PGD results are variations in the biopsy and genetic technologies employed. These encompass all aspects of the process and have been previously reviewed [39]. Here we will discuss briefly only a few of the key factors. Probably the most important variable in PGD is the embryo biopsy itself. One of the studies showing no difference in IVF outcome following PGD involved biopsy of two cells from each cleavage-stage embryo [33]. However, the same group later reported that two-cell biopsy, in contrast to single-cell biopsy, is detrimental to embryo development [40].

Even biopsying one cell in suboptimal conditions could be extremely damaging to embryo potential. A study conducted by Mastenbroek et al. [35] reported an astonishingly high rate of diagnostic failure (20%), resulting in many embryos being transferred without a diagnosis. The implantation rate of these undiagnosed embryos was 59% lower than the control. In this case, the only difference between the control and test groups appears to have been the biopsy, suggesting that embryo viability was drastically reduced by the biopsy procedures used in the clinics involved.

The second most important factor in obtaining good results can be summarized in the "error rate." The steps after biopsy involve fixation, FISH with a variety of potentially different protocols and probes, and cell scoring. However, the overall accuracy of these steps can be summarized in a single number, which is the error rate of a PGD laboratory. This error rate can be obtained by reanalyzing all the cells of nonreplaced embryos (abnormal embryos and arrested normal embryos) and determining if the original diagnosis was correct. Unfortunately, error rates vary widely, ranging from 2–7% [2, 15, 38] to 40–50% [22, 41] depending on the PGD laboratory. As shown in a recent review, error rates around 50% will in fact decrease implantation rates [39].

When performed using appropriate, well-validated methods, FISH can detect 90% of the chromosome abnormalities detected by CGH [16, 42], and some PGD laboratories do appear to obtain consistently good results with FISH and cleavage-stage embryo biopsy. Regardless, the field of PGD is evolving away from biopsying at this stage of embryo development and is increasingly focusing on biopsy of polar bodies from oocytes or zygotes or removal of trophectoderm cells from blastocysts. These embryonic stages may be more resilient to technical manipulation. Additionally, the limited chromosomal screening conveyed by FISH is increasingly being replaced by comprehensive methods of DNA analysis, which detect close to 100% of chromosomal abnormalities. The new wave of aneuploidy testing technologies is extremely redundant (each chromosome tested multiple times at different sites), readily automated, less subjective, and theoretically less prone to errors.

Comprehensive DNA Analysis Techniques

Here we will cover three techniques that are currently being used for PGD of chromosome abnormalities. Comparative genome hybridization (CGH) was first applied to day-3 embryo biopsies [43–47]. However, CGH is time consuming and is incompatible with day-3 biopsy and transfer by day 5, necessitating cryopreservation of embryos while testing is carried out. At the time that it was first applied, embryo freezing was a relatively inefficient technique and the low survival rate of thawed embryos likely neutralized any beneficial effects of CGH. For these reasons, CGH was temporarily abandoned and not applied again until the development of vitrification [48]. In conjunction with vitrification, CGH has been clinically applied to polar bodies [49–51] and blastocyst biopsies [5, 52]. The combination of CGH, blastocyst biopsy, and vitrification significantly improved implantation rates in a recent study, from 46.5% in controls to 72.2% in cycles with screening, with nearly 100% of blastocysts surviving biopsy [5]. However, many clinics are not yet proficient at blastocyst culture and vitrification. Furthermore, freezing adds extra cost to the cycle, and a majority of patients prefer to have a fresh cycle. Thus, for the time being, day-3 biopsy combined with comprehensive chromosome analysis remains the choice for most physicians and patients.

Two other techniques, microarray CGH (array CGH or aCGH) [53–57] and single-nucleotide polymorphism (SNP) microarrays [58–60], can be used for comprehensive chromosome analysis of single cells from day-3 biopsy and yield results in 24 h. The rapid turnaround time for these methods eliminates the need to cryopreserve embryos while testing is carried out.

Array CGH (aCGH) is already widely used for the cytogenetic analysis of prenatal and postnatal samples [61–66] since it is rapid and cost-effective and allows chromosomal regions to be screened at high resolution. Several types of aCGH platform are available for the purposes of aneuploidy screening. The variety most commonly used for the purpose of PGD utilizes bacterial artificial chromosome (BAC) probes, about 150,000 bp in length, covering all chromosome bands and giving a 4 MB or lower resolution. Even higher resolutions are achievable but not generally recommended since at that level, the difference between clinically significant duplications/deletions and normally occurring copy number variations is less clear. A microarray recently validated for PGD had 4,000 probes and thus covered ~25% of the genome sequence [58]. Microarray CGH has a similar accuracy rate to conventional CGH and should therefore be capable of producing similar results to those obtained in the promising CGH study performed by Schoolcraft et al. [5].

CGH and aCGH provide a quantitative analysis based on comparing the relative amount of DNA from two different sources, one from the clinical sample (e.g., a cell from an embryo) and another from a chromosomally normal individual. DNA samples from the two sources are differentially labeled and hybridized to either metaphase chromosomes (CGH) or probes on a microarray (aCGH). In the case of aCGH, each probe reveals the relative amounts of these two DNAs at a single chromosomal site. Since multiple copies of each probe are placed on the microarray and each chromosome is tested at many distinct loci, the diagnosis is very accurate.

Chromosome imbalances (aneuploidies, unbalanced translocations, deletions, and duplications) are easily detected using CGH and aCGH, but a limitation of these approaches is that diploidy cannot be distinguished from changes involving loss or gain of an entire set of chromosomes (e.g., haploidy, triploidy, tetraploidy, etc.). How important is this? In a recently submitted paper by Munne et al. (personal communication), about 7.7% ($n = 91,073$) of the supposedly 2PN embryos tested were polyploid or haploid but the majority of them had additional abnormalities detectable by CGH or array CGH and only 1.8% of all embryos were homogeneously polyploid or haploid. Furthermore, of those, the majority arrested by day 4, leaving only 0.2% of developing embryos uniformly polyploid or haploid. This suggests that failure to detect polyploid embryos may rarely lead to a misdiagnosis but is unlikely to have a significant impact on the clinical efficacy of the screening using aCGH or CGH.

Single nucleotide polymorphisms are areas of the genome where a single nucleotide in the DNA sequence varies within the population. Most SNPs are biallelic, existing in one of two forms, and are found scattered throughout the genome. By determining the genotype of multiple SNPs along the length of each chromosome, a haplotype (a contiguous series of polymorphisms on the same chromosome) can be assembled. This ultimately allows the inheritance of individual chromosomes or pieces of chromosomes to be tracked from parents to embryos. Current SNP microarrays simultaneously assay hundreds of thousands of SNPs, while utilizing powerful software to distinguish how many copies of each chromosome was inherited by an embryo [58, 60, 67].

All of the new generation of chromosome screening methods (CGH, aCGH, and SNP microarrays) rely on whole genome amplification (WGA) to amplify DNA from the single cell or small number of cells removed from a developing embryo

[68]. CGH can be performed in combination with a variety of WGA methods; however, SNP microarrays are more sensitive to the type of amplification technique used and are not compatible with all methods. Currently, WGA methods like multiple displacement amplification (MDA), GenomePlex, and PicoPlex are most commonly used for SNP microarrays. These amplification methods allow for better overall coverage of the genome compared with earlier WGA methods (e.g., degenerate oligonucleotide primed PCR) and are less inclined to preferentially amplify some parts of the genome while leaving others unamplified or under amplified.

Currently, a few PGD groups around the world are validating SNP microarrays and analysis software for clinical use in PGD for aneuploidy screening. It is expected that data from the clinical use of SNP microarrays will closely match the data from CGH and aCGH testing. While the technologies differ greatly, both types of arrays (CGH-based and SNP-based) are trying to answer the same question; how many copies of each chromosome is present in a sample?

The small size of the SNP array probes can lead to poor hybridization efficiencies and low signal intensities for individual probes. This factor, coupled with the failure of WGA methods to amplify the entirety of the genome, can lead to many probes yielding no result (i.e., a low "call rate"). Also, allele dropout (ADO) and/or preferential amplification (PA) of one SNP allele versus another can lead to a great deal of "noise" in the system, which requires sophisticated interpretation. Several methods for the cleaning up of data from SNP microarrays have been developed: qualitative methods, looking only at the inheritance of specific SNPs and requiring comparison with parental DNA samples; quantitative approaches, assessing only the intensity of SNP calls; and techniques combining qualitative and quantitative methods, using both SNP intensity calls and inheritance patterns.

For qualitative approaches, it is necessary to assess parental DNA prior to clinical embryo testing. The key requirement is the deduction of the four parental haplotypes for each chromosome. Embryo testing is then focused on detecting the individual parental haplotypes, revealing how many chromosomes were inherited from each parent, i.e., karyomapping [58]. This approach has the disadvantage that mitotic abnormalities, in which only two haplotypes are present in a trisomy (i.e., caused by duplication of one of the two chromosomes in the embryo after fertilization), will not be detected. This can misdiagnose a substantial amount of embryos since 30% of aneuploid embryos contain mitotic abnormalities (mosaics) [15]. A quantitative approach compares the intensity of each SNP against the other SNPs. A purely quantitative approach for aneuploidy screening may not require parental testing ahead of the cycle; however, this approach would not be compatible with combination testing of single gene defects with aneuploidy screening (discussed below). This approach is currently the least developed. A qualitative/quantitative approach has also been applied clinically, and probably can obviate the issues mentioned above for purely qualitative or quantitative approaches [60, 67]. All of the analysis approaches still share one limitation and that is the diagnosis of tetraploidies. In a tetraploid cell, only two haplotypes are present (i.e., a postmeiotic duplication of a euploid cell); therefore, all SNPs will have the same intensity.

SNP-based microarrays offer some advantages over aCGH: (a) if qualitative analysis is employed, SNP-based microarrays can also detect the parental origin of any chromosome abnormalities. This may be valuable in rare instances of young couples producing many chromosome abnormalities but of little relevance to cases of advanced maternal age where at least 90% of the aneuploidies will be maternal in origin, and those of paternal origin are most likely mitotic error where the paternal chromosome was randomly recruited as the extra chromosome. These errors offer no predictive value for other embryos in the cohort or for future cycles; (b) SNP microarrays applied to PGD for chromosome rearrangements can differentiate between normal and balanced (carrier) embryos. However, because the rate of abnormalities in translocation cases is generally very high (>80%) [69], the great majority of PGD cycles do not have a surplus of embryos with a balanced chromosome constitution. In most cases, whatever balanced embryos are available are needed for transfer; (c) SNP arrays can directly produce a fingerprint of the embryo, allowing for assessment of which of the transferred embryos led to a pregnancy. However, if a laboratory is using aCGH, a similar test can be performed by utilizing a small aliquot of the DNA produced by WGA to perform conventional DNA fingerprinting; (d) finally, qualitative SNP arrays can also detect uniparental disomy (UDP), although this is a very rare event (e.g., UDP 15 occurs in 0.001% of newborns (OMIM)).

A major disadvantage of a qualitative or combination approach to SNP array analysis is the need to assess parental DNA ahead of the PGD cycle. This complicates patient management, adds substantially to the cost of the test, and precludes ad hoc decisions on biopsy for PGD. Approximately 20% of IVF cycles with planned PGD are canceled on day 3 due to low embryo numbers. Thus, these patients would have spent money on precycle parental testing that was ultimately unnecessary.

Validation of aCGH and SNP Arrays

Due to the intrinsic and often unforeseen problems with every new technology, a novel method should always be validated against other, more established methods [70]. Assessing a new approach against itself may preclude the detection of technique-related flaws. Thus, validation by inadequate methods such as the analysis of cell lines with defined chromosome abnormalities which cannot mimic mosaicism and other peculiarities of the cell being tested; analysis of eggs or embryos by one technique with analysis of polar bodies or the remainder of the embryo by the same technique which will preclude identifying abnormalities not detectable by that technique; blindly replacing undiagnosed embryos (either by single embryo transfer or fingerprinting the embryo) and following pregnancies and clinical losses to determine the fate of each tested embryo which does not account for the status of nonimplanted embryos; or using the SNP calls in one chromosome as internal controls for other SNPs in that same chromosome [60] may lead to false assumptions. In addition, the use of analysis tools that are qualitative in nature will miss the presence of two chromosomes of the same grandparental origin, and the errors caused by mosaicism will not be taken into account in this validation mode, resulting in bogus 99.9% confidence results.

In our opinion, the optimal method for validating a new technique is to reanalyze those embryos that were not transferred to the patient, either because they underwent arrest or because they were diagnosed chromosomally abnormal. The reanalysis of these embryos should be done with another well-established technique, the "gold standard." This would discern shortcomings of the new method under evaluation and account for issues related to embryo biology, such as mosaicism. The only problem with this approach is that euploid arresting embryos may become abnormal (karyokinesis without cytokinesis) from day 3 to day 5 before reanalysis [71, 72] and there is a scarcity of nonreplaced normal embryos.

To simplify comparison between studies, an error should be classified as diagnosing an embryo as euploid when reanalysis shows that it was abnormal or vice versa. Due to the extent of mosaicism, an error rate per chromosome has questionable relevance and no clinical importance compared to an error rate per embryo.

SNP microarrays have undergone a variety of validation experiments, such as comparison of PGD results and analysis of babies born [67, 73], SNP microarray reanalysis of embryos previously analyzed by SNP arrays [59], and using data from one set of SNPs as internal controls for another set of SNPs. To date, no studies have confirmed the original diagnosis by reanalyzing the remaining embryonic cells with a different technique.

Microarray CGH for PGD has been validated by analysis of single cells from known cell lines (Dagan Wells, personal communication) and by analyzing eggs with aCGH and comparing them to the results obtained using aCGH of the corresponding PBs (Montag and Gianaroli, personal communication). In a recent study, day-3 embryos analyzed by PGD with aCGH that were not replaced because of chromosome or morphological abnormalities were reanalyzed in most of their remaining cells by FISH using 12 probes for the most common chromosome abnormalities plus probes for any chromosomes found abnormal according to aCGH. Only 1.9% of embryos were found to be incorrectly diagnosed [58]. This is even lower than the 7% error rate expected solely from mosaicism as calculated in FISH studies [15]. Most likely, analyzing all of the chromosomes leads to the ascertainment of more chaotic embryos, further lowering the overall error rate.

Clinical Results

Of the techniques discussed, CGH is the one for which the greatest quantity of clinical data is available [5, 49, 50, 52]. Sher et al. [49] detected a 74% ongoing pregnancy rate per transfer and 63% per retrieval in women with an average age of 37.5 years. For patients of a similar age, receiving blastocyst transfer, Schoolcraft et al. [5] detected a significant increase in implantation rates, from 46.5 to 72.2% ($p < 0.001$) following embryo selection using CGH. Interestingly, both studies showed high implantation rates and both avoided cleavage-stage embryo biopsy and transferred embryos that had previously been cryopreserved in a later cycle. In addition to the potential benefits of transferring euploid embryos, there may be additional advantages associated with transfer in a nonstimulated cycle [74]. Loss of blastocyst-stage embryos after devitrification in the study by Schoolcraft et al. was minimal (0.7%) [5].

Regarding day-3 biopsy followed by aCGH and day-5 replacement, our most recent data [75] showed that only 118/151 PGD cycles had normal embryos for transfer in a population 38 years of age. The pregnancy rate was 59% per transfer compared with 38% in controls with a transfer ($p < 0.001$). The ongoing pregnancy rate for the PGD group was 54% per transfer, compared with 31.1% in controls with a transfer ($p < 0.001$). These results are encouraging but not as impressive as the day-5 (blastocyst) biopsy results. It is probable that the difference between clinical results obtained using CGH and aCGH is related to the stage at which biopsy was carried out rather than to differences in the method of chromosome screening. It is very likely that aCGH will replicate the results obtained by CGH when applied in conjunction with blastocyst biopsy. In summary, although data on the clinical application of comprehensive chromosome analysis techniques is preliminary, all studies suggest a significant improvement in ART results.

Less clinical data is available from SNP-based microarrays. In presentations at ASRM, Schlenker et al. [76] reported that CGH and SNP microarrays provided the same high implantation rates after blastocyst biopsy and vitrification. Also, in an ongoing RCT using 24-chromosome analysis by qPCR, higher pregnancies rates were obtained when biopsy was performed on day 5 than in controls with no intervention [77].

Microarrays for PGD of Gene Defects

Neither CGH microarrays nor the SNP microarrays in current use can directly detect gene defect mutations. However, SNP microarrays can be used to indirectly infer the presence or absence of a chromosome segment containing a mutant gene (i.e., identification of the same SNP haplotype as the parental chromosome carrying the mutation). A diagnosis can be performed based upon this sort of information [59]; indeed, this approach has recently been applied clinically for the simultaneous detection of gene defects and chromosome abnormalities [78].

In the case of aCGH, although gene defects cannot be detected directly, enough DNA is produced during the WGA step of the procedure that an aliquot can be used for aCGH analysis of chromosome abnormalities and another taken for PCR-based analysis of gene defects.

The high levels of ADO recorded after WGA mean that direct detection of a mutation using a microarray is likely to be less reliable than existing forms of PGD. Microarray-based diagnosis will be safer using approaches such as karyomapping, where conclusions are based upon the results from multiple linked SNPs, rather than a single mutation site. While the sort of microarrays used for preconception screening are not currently suitable for PGD, it is anticipated that their use will significantly increase the identification of high-risk couples and therefore lead to an increase in the usage of genetic testing modalities such as prenatal testing and PGD.

Glossary

Allele dropout (ADO) The failure to detect an allele in a sample or the failure to amplify an allele during PCR.

Aneuploidy The condition of a cell or of an organism that has additions or deletions of a small number of whole chromosomes from the expected balanced diploid number of chromosomes.

Array comparative genomic hybridization (aCGH) A technique to detect genomic copy number variations at a high resolution level using differentially labeled DNA samples (one of unknown karyotype, one known normal karyotype) after hybridization to specific parts of the genome printed on a glass slide.

Bacterial artificial chromosome (BAC) Artificial chromosome vector derived from bacteria used for cloning relatively large DNA fragments.

Chromosome translocation A chromosomal configuration in which (usually) the ends of two nonhomologous chromosomes have become exchanged.

DNA fingerprint The derivation of unique patterns of DNA fragments obtained using a number of short repeats following polymerase chain reaction allowing discrimination between the genetic makeup of one person from another or one embryo from another.

Comparative genomic hybridization (CGH) A technique that is used to detect chromosome gain or loss by hybridizing DNA from a target cell and a normal cell that are differentially labeled with unique fluorescent dyes to a normal karyotype.

Euploidy The condition of a cell or organism that has one or more complete sets of chromosomes.

Fluorescence in situ hybridization (FISH) A cytogenetic technique that is used to detect and localize the presence or absence of specific DNA sequences on chromosomes.

Haplotype A set of closely linked genetic markers present on one chromosome that tend to be inherited together (not easily separable by recombination).

Karyotype Cytogenetic chromosome analysis with direct visualization of the chromosomes to determine chromosome number and structure/content.

Meiotic error A chromosome error arising during meiosis (reduction division) in an egg or sperm.

Microarray Sometimes called a gene chip or a DNA chip. Microarrays consist of large numbers of molecules (often, but not always, DNA) distributed in rows in a very small space. Microarrays permit scientists to study inheritance of chromosomes and gene expression by providing a snapshot of all the genes that are active in a cell at a particular time.

Mitotic error A chromosome error arising during mitosis (division) of an embryo.
Mosaicism Two or more distinct chromosomal or genetic lineages within an individual embryo.
Polyploidy A cell or an organism having three or more chromosome sets.
Preferential amplification (PA) Phenomenon that occurs during amplification from small amounts of starting DNA where one allele preferentially amplifies more than the other allele.
Preimplantation genetic diagnosis (PGD) Diagnosis of a cell from a preimplantation embryo for a specific genetic disease before embryo transfer.
Preimplantation genetic screening (PGS) Screening of a cell from a preimplantation embryo for the detection chromosomal disorders before embryo transfer.
Single nucleotide polymorphism (SNP) A variation of a single nucleotide of DNA useful in understanding and identifying a higher risk of a disease in particular people.
Whole genome amplification (WGA) The in vitro amplification of a full genome sequence, ideally with even representation of the genome in the amplified product.

References

1. Munné S, Alikani M, Tomkin G, Grifo J, Cohen J. Embryo morphology, developmental rates and maternal age are correlated with chromosome abnormalities. Fertil Steril. 1995;64: 382–91.
2. Magli MC, Gianaroli L, Ferrareti AP, Lappi M, Ruberti A, Farfalli V. Embryo morphology and development are dependent on the chromosome complement. Fertil Steril. 2007;87:534–41.
3. Bielanska M, Tan SL, Ao A. Chromosomal mosaicism throughout human preimplantation development in vitro: incidence, type, and relevance to embryo outcome. Hum Reprod. 2002; 17:413–9.
4. Munné S, Serena C, Colls P, Garrisi J, Zheng X, Cekleniak N, Lenzi M, Hughes P, Fischer J, Garrisi M, Tomkin G, Cohen J. Maternal age, morphology, development and chromosome abnormalities in over 6000 cleavage-stage embryos. Reprod Biomed Online. 2007;14: 628–34.
5. Schoolcraft WB, Fragouli E, Stevens J, Munné S, Katz-Jaffe MG, Wells D. Clinical application of comprehensive chromosomal screening at the blastocyst stage. Fertil Steril. 2010;94(5): 1700–6.
6. Hassold T, Chen N, Funkhouser J, Jooss T, Manuel B, Matsuura J, Matsuyama A, Wilson C, Yamane JA, Jacobs PA. A cytogenetic study of 1000 spontaneous abortions. Ann Hum Genet. 1980;44:151–78.
7. Daniely M, Aviram-Goldring A, Barkai G, Goldman B. Detection of chromosomal aberrations in fetuses arising from recurrent spontaneous abortions by comparative genome hybridization. Hum Reprod. 1998;13:805–9.
8. Fritz B, Hallermann C, Olert J, Fucs B, Bruns M, Aslan M, Schmidt S, Coerdt W, Muntefering H, Rehder H. Cytogenetic analyses of culture failures by comparative genome hybridization. Re-evaluation of chromosome aberration rates in early spontaneous abortions. Eur J Hum Genet. 2001;9:539–47.
9. Qumsiyeh MB, Kim KR, Ahmed MN, Bradford W. Cytogenetics and mechanisms of spontaneous abortions: increased apoptosis and decreased cell proliferation in chromosomally abnormal villi. Cytogenet Cell Genet. 2000;88:230–5.

10. Carp H, Toder V, Aviram A, Daniely M, Mashiach S, Barkai G. Karyotype of the abortus in recurrent miscarriages. Fertil Steril. 2001;75:678–82.
11. Menasha J, Levy B, Hirschhorn K, Kardon NB. Incidence and spectrum of chromosome abnormalities in spontaneous abortions: new insights from a 12-year study. Genet Med. 2005;7(4):251–63.
12. Munné S, Lee A, Rosenwaks Z, Grifo J, Cohen J. Diagnosis of major chromosome aneuploidies in human preimplantation embryos. Hum Reprod. 1993;8:2185–91.
13. Munné S, Magli C, Bahçe M, Fung J, Legator M, Morrison L, Cohen J, Gianaroli L. Preimplantation diagnosis of the aneuploidies most commonly found in spontaneous abortions and live births: XY, 13, 14, 15, 16, 18, 21, 22. Prenatal Diagn. 1998;18:1459–66.
14. Magli MC, Sandalinas M, Escudero T, Morrison L, Ferrareti AP, Gianaroli L, Munné S. Double locus analysis of chromosome 21 for preimplantation genetic diagnosis of aneuploidy. Prenat Diagn. 2001;12:1080–5.
15. Colls P, Escudero T, Zheng X, Lenzi M, Cinnioglu C, Cohen J, Munné S. Increased efficiency of preimplantation genetic diagnosis for infertility through reanalysis of dubious signals. Fertil Steril. 2007;88:53–61.
16. Colls P, Goodall N, Zheng X, Munné S. Increased efficiency of preimplantation genetic diagnosis for aneuploidy by testing 12 chromosomes. Reprod Biomed Online. 2009;19:532–8.
17. Jansen RPS, Bowman MC, De Boer KA, Leigh DA, Lieberman DB, McArthur SJ. What next for preimplantation genetic screening (PGD)? Experience with blastocyst biopsy and testing for aneuploidy. Hum Reprod. 2008;23:1476–8.
18. Verlinsky Y, Cieslak J, Frieidine M, Ivakhnenko V, Wolf G, Kovalinskaya L, White M, Lifchez A, Kaplan B, Moise J, Valle J, Ginsberg N, Strom C, Kuliev A. Pregnancies following pre-conception diagnosis of common aneuploidies by fluorescence in-situ hybridization. Hum Reprod. 1995;10:1923–7.
19. Verlinsky Y, Kuliev A. Preimplantation diagnosis of common aneuploidies in fertile couples of advanced maternal age. Hum Reprod. 1996;11:2076–7.
20. Kuliev A, Cieslak J, Ilkevitch Y, Verlinsky Y. Chromosomal abnormalities in a series of 6733 human oocytes in preimplantation diagnosis for age-related aneuploidies. Reprod Biomed Online. 2002;6:54–9.
21. Verlinsky Y, Tur-Kaspa I, Cieslak J, Bernal A, Morris R, Taranissi M, Kaplan B, Kuliev A. Preimplantation testing for chromosomal disorders improves reproductive outcome of poor prognosis patients. Reprod Biomed Online. 2005;11:219–25.
22. Coulam CB, Jeyendram RS, Fiddler M, Pergament E. Discordance among blastomeres renders preimplantation genetic diagnosis for aneuploidy ineffective. J Assist Reprod Genet. 2007;24:37–41.
23. Gianaroli L, Magli C, Ferraretti AP, Munné S. Preimplantation diagnosis for aneuploidies in patients undergoing in-vitro fertilization with a poor prognosis: identification of the categories for which it should be proposed. Fertil Steril. 1999;72:837–44.
24. Munné S, Magli C, Cohen J, Morton P, Sadowy S, Gianaroli L, Tucker M, Márquez C, Sable D, Ferraretti AP, Massey JB, Scott R. Positive outcome after preimplantation diagnosis of aneuploidy in human embryos. Hum Reprod. 1999;14:2191–9.
25. Gianaroli L, Magli MC, Ferraretti AP. The in vivo and in vitro efficiency and efficacy of PGD for aneuploidy. Mol Cell Endocrinol. 2001;183:S13–8.
26. Gianaroli L, Magli MC, Ferraretti AP, Tabanelli C, Trombetta C, Boudjema E. The role of preimplantation diagnosis for aneuploidy. Reprod Biomed Online. 2001;4:31–6.
27. Munné S, Sandalinas M, Escudero T, Velilla E, Walmsley R, Sadowy S, Cohen J, Sable D. Improved implantation after preimplantation genetic diagnosis of aneuploidy. Reprod Biomed Online. 2003;7:91–7.
28. Gianaroli L, Magli C, Ferraretti AP, Tabanelli C, Trengia V, Farfalli V, et al. The beneficial effects of PGD for aneuploidy support extensive clinical application. Reprod Biomed Online. 2004;10:633–40.

29. Munné S, Chen S, Fischer J, Colls P, Zheng X, Stevens J, et al. Preimplantation genetic diagnosis reduces pregnancy loss in women 35 and older with a history of recurrent miscarriages. Fertil Steril. 2005;84:331–5.
30. Munné S, Fischer J, Warner A, Chen S, Zouves C, Cohen J. Referring centers PGD group. Preimplantation genetic diagnosis significantly reduces pregnancy loss in infertile couples: a multi-center study. Fertil Steril. 2006;85:326–32.
31. Garrisi GJ, Colls P, Ferry KM, Zheng X, Garrisi MG, Munné S. Effect of infertility, maternal age and number of previous miscarriages on the outcome of preimplantation genetic diagnosis for idiopathic recurrent pregnancy loss. Fertil Steril. 2009;92:288–95.
32. Rubio C, Buendía P, Rodrigo L, Mercader A, Mateu E, Peinado V, Delgado A, Milán M, Mir P, Simón C, Remohí J, Pellicer A. prognostic factors for preimplantation genetic screening in repeated pregnancy loss. Reprod Biomed Online. 2009;18(5):687–93.
33. Staessen C, Platteau P, Van Assche E, Michiels A, Tournaye H, Camus M, et al. Comparison of blastocyst transfer with or without preimplantation genetic diagnosis for aneuploidy screening in couples with advanced maternal age: a prospective randomized controlled trial. Hum Reprod. 2004;19:2849–58.
34. Platteau P, Staessen C, Michiels A, Van Steirteghem A, Liebaers I, Devroey P. Preimplantation genetic diagnosis for aneuploidy screening in patients with unexplained recurrent miscarriages. Fertil Steril. 2005;83:393–7.
35. Mastenbroek S, Twisk M, Van Echten-Arends J, Sikkema-Raddatz B, Korevaar JC, Verhoeve HR, et al. Preimplantation Genetic Screening in Women of Advanced Maternal Age. New Engl J Med. 2007;357:9–17.
36. Hardarson T, Hanson C, Lundin K, Hillensjo T, Nilsson L, Stevic J, Reismer E, Borg K, Wikland M, Bergh C. Preimplantation genetic screening in women of advanced maternal age caused a decrease in clinical pregnancy rate: a randomized controlled trial. Hum Reprod. 2008;23:2806–12.
37. Munné S, Sandalinas M, Escudero T, Marquez C, Cohen J. Chromosome mosaicism in cleavage stage human embryos: evidence of a maternal age effect. Reprod Biomed Online. 2002;4:223–32.
38. Gutiérrez-Mateo C, Colls P, Sánchez-García J, Escudero T, Prates R, Ketterson K, Wells D, Munné S. Validation of microarray comparative genomic hybridization for comprehensive chromosome analysis of embryos. Fertil Steril. 2011;95(3):953–8.
39. Munné S, Wells D, Cohen J. Technology requirements for preimplantation genetic diagnosis to improve art outcome. Fertil Steril. 2010;94(2):408–30.
40. De Vos A, Staessen C, De Rycke M, Verpoest W, Haentjens P, Devroey P, Liebaers I, Van de Velde H. Impact of cleavage-stage embryo biopsy in view of PGD on human blastocyst implantation: a prospective cohort of single embryo transfers. Hum Reprod. 2009;12: 2988–96.
41. Baart E, Van Opstal D, Los FJ, Fauser BCJM, Martini E. Fluorescence in-situ hybridization analysis of two blastomeres from day-3 frozen-thawed embryos followed by analysis of the remaining embryo on day-5. Hum Reprod. 2004;19:685–93.
42. Munné S, Fragouli E, Colls P, Katz M, Schoocraft W, Wells D. An improved 12-chromosome FISH test could detect 91% of aneuploid blastocysts. Reprod Biomed Online. 2010;20:92–7.
43. Wells D, Sherlock JK, Handyside AH, Delhanty DA. Detailed chromosomal and molecular genetic analysis of single cells by whole genome amplification and comparative genome hybridization. Nucleic Acids Res. 1999;27:1214–8.
44. Voullaire L, Wilton L, Slater H, Williamson R. Detection of aneuploidy in single cells using comparative genome hybridization. Prenat Diagn. 1999;19:846–51.
45. Wells D, Delhanty JDA. Comprehensive chromosomal analysis of human preimplantation embryos using whole genome amplification and single cell comparative genomic hybridization. Mol Human Reprod. 2000;6:1055–62.
46. Wilton L, Williamson R, McBain J, Edgar D, Voullaire L. Birth of a healthy infant after preimplantation confirmation of euploidy by comparative genomic hybridization. N Engl J Med. 2001;345: 1537–41.

47. Wells D, Escudero T, Levy B, Hirschhorn K, Delhanty JDA, Munné S. First clinical application of comparative genome hybridization (CGH) and polar body testing for Preimplantation genetic diagnosis (PGD) of aneuploidy. Fertil Steril. 2002;78:543–9.
48. Kuwayama M. Highly efficient vitrification for cryopreservation of human oocytes and embryos: the Cryotop method. Theriogenology. 2007;67:73–80.
49. Sher G, Keskintepe L, Keskintepe M, Ginsburg M, Maassarani G, Yakut T, Baltaci V, Kotze D, Unsal E. Oocyte karyotyping by comparative genome hybridization provides a highly reliable method for selecting "competent" embryos, markedly improving in vitro fertilization outcome: a multiphase study. Fertil Steril. 2007;87:1033–40.
50. Fragouli E, Escalona A, Gutierrez-Mateo C, Tormasi S, Alfarawati S, Sepulveda S, Noriega L, Garcia J, Wells D, Munné S. Comparative genomic hybridization of oocytes and first polar bodies from young donors. Reprod Biomed Online. 2009;18:228–37.
51. Fragouli E, Escalona A, Gutierrez-Mateo C, Tormasi S, Alfarawati S, Sepulveda S, Noriega L, Garcia J, Wells D, Munné S. Comparative genomic hybridization of oocytes and first polar bodies from young donors. Reprod Biomed Online. 2009;18:228–37.
52. Fragouli E, Alfarawati S, Katz-Jaffe M, Stevens J, Colls P, Goodall N, Tormasi S, Gutierrez-Mateo C, Prates R, Schoolcraft WB, Munné M, Wells D. Comprehensive chromosome screening of polar bodies and blastocysts from couples experiencing repeated implantation failure. Fertil Steril. 2010;94(3):875–87.
53. Hu DG, Webb G, Hussey N. Aneuploidy detection in single cells using DNA array-based comparative genomic hybridization. Mol Hum Reprod. 2004;10:283–9.
54. Le Caignec C, Spits C, Sermon K, De Rycke M, Thienpont B, Debrock S, Staessen C, Moreau Y, Fryns JP, Van Steirteghem A, Liebaers I, Vermeesch JR. Single-cell chromosomal imbalances detection by array CGH. Nucleic Acids Res. 2006;34:e68.
55. Hellani A, Abu-Amero K, Azouri J, El-Akoum S. Successful pregnancies after application of array-comparative genomic hybridization in PGS-aneuploidy screening. Reprod Biomed Online. 2008;17:841–7.
56. Fishel S, GordonA LC, et al. Birth after polar body array CGH prediction of embryo ploidy following IVF—the future of IVF? Fertil Steril. 2009;93(3):1006–7.
57. Munné S, Gutierrez-Mateo C, Sanchez-Garcia JF, Ketterson K, Prates R, Keningsberg D (2009) Validation of microarray CGH for PGD by FISH reanalysis. Fertil Steril. 2009;92(3) Suppl S2.
58. Handyside AH, Harton GL, Mariani B, Thornhill AR, Affara NA, Shaw MA, Griffin DK. Karyomapping: a universal method for genome wide analysis of genetic disease based on mapping crossovers between parental haplotypes. J Med Genet. 2009;47(10): 651–8.
59. Treff N, Su J, Tao X, Miller KA, Levy B, Scott RT. A novel single-cell DNA fingerprinting method successfully distinguishes sibling human embryos. Fertil Steril. 2010;94(2):477–84.
60. Johnson DS, Gemelos G, Baner J, Ryan A, Cinnioglu C, Banjevic M, Ross R, Alper M, Barrett B, Frederick J, Potter D, Behr B, Rabinowitz M. Preclinical validation of a microarray method for full molecular karyotyping of blastomeres in a 24-h protocol. Hum Reprod. 2010;25(4): 1066–75.
61. Sismani C, Kitsiou-Tzeli S, Ioannides M, et al. Cryptic genomic imbalances in patients with de novo or familial apparently balanced translocations and abnormal phenotype. Mol Cytogenet. 2008;1(1):15.
62. Goobie S, Knijnenburg J, Fitzpatrick D, et al. Molecular and clinical characterization of de novo and familial cases with microduplication 3q29: guidelines for copy number variation case reporting. Cytogenet Genome Res. 2008;123(1–4):65–78.
63. Dimova I, et al. Whole genome analysis by array-based comparative genomic hybridization in patients with congenital malformations. Balkan J Med Genet. 2008;11(1):33–40.
64. Beaudet al, Belmont JW. Array-based DNA diagnostics: let the revolution begin. Annu Rev Med. 2008;59:113–29.
65. Heinrich U, et al. Array comparative genomic hybridisation in clinical diagnostics: principles and applications. J Lab Med. 2009;33(5):255–66.

66. Stejskalová E, et al. Cytogenetic and array comparative genomic hybridization analysis of a series of hepatoblastomas. Cancer Genet Cytogenet. 2009;194(2):82–7.
67. Treff NR, Su J, Kasabwala N, Tao X, Miller KA, Scott Jr RT. Robust embryo identification using first polar body single nucleotide polymorphism microarray-based DNA fingerprinting. Fertil Steril. 2009;90(Suppl):S82–3.
68. Vanneste E, Voet T, Le Caignec C, et al. Chromosome instability is common in human cleavage-stage embryos. Nat Med. 2009;15(5):577–83.
69. Munné S, Sandalinas M, Escudero T, Fung J, Gianaroli L, Cohen J. Outcome of preimplantation genetic diagnosis of translocations. Fertil Steril. 2000;73:1209–18.
70. Scott R, Treff N. Assessing the reproductive competence of individual embryos: a proposal for the validation of new "-omics" technologies. Fertil Steril. 2010;94(3):791–4.
71. Munné S, Alikani M, Grifo J, Cohen J. Monospermic polyploidy and atypical embryo morphology. Human Reprod. 1994;9:506–10.
72. Márquez C, Sandalinas M, Bahçe M, Alikani M, Munné S. Chromosome abnormalities in 1255 cleavage-stage human embryos. Reprod Biomed Online. 2000;1:17–27.
73. Scott TR (2010) Choosing the best embryo for transfer. In: 2010 Syllabus, Pacific Coast Reproductive Society, Rancho Mirage, CA, p. 51–63.
74. Shapiro BS, Daneshmand ST, Garner FC, Aguirre M, Hudson C, Thomas S. High ongoing pregnancy rates after deferred transfer through bipronuclear oocyte cryopreservation and post-thaw extended culture. Fertil Steril. 2009;92:1594–9.
75. Munné S, Surrey M, Grifo J, et al. Preimplantation Genetic Diagnosis using array CGH significantly increases ongoing pregnancy rates per transfer. Fertil Steril. 2010;94:(4)Suppl S81.
76. Schlenker T, Stevens J, Rawlins M, McCormick S, Katz-Jaffe MG, Schoolcraft WB. Clinical success with vitrification following trophectoderm biopsy for comprehensive chromosomal screening. Fertil Steril. 2009;92(Suppl):S-71.
77. Scott RT, Tao X, Taylor D, Ferry KM, Treff NR. A prospective randomized controlled trial demonstrating significantly increased clinical pregnancy rates following 24 chromosome aneuploidy screening: biopsy and analysis on day 5 with fresh transfer. Fertil Steril. 2010;94:Suppl S2(O-65).
78. Handyside A, Grifo J, Gabriel A, Thornhill A, Griffin D, Ketterson K, Prates R, Tormasi S, Fischer J, Munné S. First clinical application of karyomapping for PGD of Gaucher disease combined with 24 chromosome screening. Reprod Biomed Online. 2010;20 Suppl 1:S16.

Part V
Molecular Insights

Chapter 24
The Role of Mitochondria in the Establishment of Developmental Competence in Early Human Development

Jonathan Van Blerkom

While morphological and performance characteristics of oocytes and early human embryos during culture in vitro have long been the mainstay of clinical IVF for evaluations of developmental competence, new technologies based on genomic, proteomic, and metabolomic analysis have begun to enter assessment schemes by providing a wide array of target genes whose expression levels, measured at the mRNA and protein level with commercial and custom made microarrays, may be competence associated. The relative merits of morphology and different "omic"- related methods for competence assessment and selection remain to be determined from comparative outcome findings. Whether they can be readily incorporated into the IVF laboratory and whether quantitative measurements at the biochemical and molecular levels can provide a level of confidence that is superior to what an experienced observer would normally conclude from detailed microscopic findings. However, morphology and metabolomics are the most likely to be developmentally related and to reflect the normality of molecular and cellular functions during oogenesis and preimplantation embryogenesis.

An understanding of the biological origins of developmental competence in the oocyte and how it is maintained through the pre- and early postimplantation stages of human embryogenesis has been an ongoing theme of research in clinical IVF. More recently, the notion that mitochondria may be involved in human oocyte and preimplantation embryo competence has led to a resurgence of interest in the role of this cytoplasmic component as a central player in the regulation and normality of early human development. While the respiratory role of mitochondria as the site

J. Van Blerkom, PhD (✉)
Department of Molecular, Cellular and Developmental Biology, University of Colorado, Porter Bioscience Building, Boulder, CO 80302, USA
e-mail: Jonathan.vanblerkom@colorado.edu

of oxidative phosphorylation and ATP production is universally recognized by the common use in the literature of terms such as "the powerhouse of cells," these organelles have pleiotropic functions including β-oxidation, steroidogenesis, reactive oxygen species (ROS) generation, oxygen sensing, and participation in the regulation of calcium homeostasis, signal transduction, determination of cytoplasmic redox state, and apoptosis [1–3]. For the oocyte and embryo, specific mitochondrial parameters such as mtDNA copy number and cytoplasmic bioenergetic levels have been correlated with or related to the frequency of aneuploidy and the success of fertilization and preimplantation embryogenesis [4–12]. Given the multiple and varied roles that mitochondria have in normal cell function, it is not too surprising that they are an ideal candidate as a developmental common denominator, for competence studies in human oogenesis and embryogenesis and as such form the basis for this review.

Mitochondrial Functions and Activities in the Mammalian Oocyte and Early Embryo

Mitochondria in the mammalian oocyte and early preimplantation stage embryo, including the human, are functionally similar but structurally undeveloped when compared to forms present during the blastocyst stage or in somatic cells, such as those of the cumulus oophorus and corona radiata. Human oocyte mitochondria are usually spherical to slightly oval in shape and about 1 µm or less in diameter [13, 14]. While active in ATP synthesis, the levels of generation are assumed to be relatively low, which would be consistent with the occurrence of few short cristae located at the periphery of an electron dense matrix. Prior to cavitation, mitochondria usually become elongated and progressively develop well-formed cristae that traverse a matrix of lower electron density. By the expanding blastocyst stage, they assume forms characteristic of highly active (energetic) organelles typical of differentiated cells. An early indication that the normality of mitochondrial development may be a factor in the inability of cleavage human stage embryos to initiate cavitation comes from fine structural studies of human embryos that arrest development during cleavage, in which few, if any, stage-appropriate forms are detected [15, 16]. Although electron microscopic findings provide an intriguing correlation with developmental arrest in the human, a cause–effect relationship cannot be concluded solely on the basis of fine structure.

Developmental Significance of Mitochondrial DNA Content

More recent investigations of the involvement of mitochondria in human oocyte and embryo competence have correlated stage-appropriate development and performance in vitro with mtDNA content. In this instance, the association between mtDNA copy number and the capacity or level of ATP generation found in somatic cells is assumed to be similar. This assumption seemed to be validated in initial reports by the finding of low copy numbers in oocytes that failed to mature to metaphase II in vivo or fertilize in vitro [6, 17]. However, reported mtDNA contents range from the low ten thousands to over one million in normal appearing MII oocytes [11, 18, 19], which can be problematic in determining threshold levels that may be stage-specific or more importantly, developmentally relevant. For example, the threshold mtDNA copy number suggested to be normal for a competent MII human oocyte by Zeng et al. [12] is significantly higher than the level proposed by Santos et al. [17] for competence. Further confounding the threshold issue is that mitochondrial mass and mtDNA copy number are often used interchangeably, and if each organelle contains one or two genomes at MII [20], the expected numerical complement of mitochondria implied by these findings might be in high hundreds of thousands [19]. However, while mitochondria are the most abundant organelles in the mature oocyte, fine structural images [14] and analysis of living cells with mitochondria-specific fluorescent probes [21] suggest a normal complement in the tens of thousands. Indeed, if mtDNA copy numbers at high end of this range correlated with complement size, it would be evident at the fine structural level by virtue of a mitochondrial density that would occupy virtually the entire cytoplasm, which has not been the case in reported fine structural studies.

The simplest explanation that reconciles differences in mtDNA content and mitochondrial mass is that multiple genomes exist in each organelle, especially at MII, when most measurements have been made. This interpretation has been supported by counting individual mitochondria in each cell of fully expanded blastocyst-stage mouse and human embryos and in trophectodermal outgrowths of mouse embryos, with different mitochondria-specific fluorescent probes that target different mitochondrial sites or properties [21]. The assumption upon which these studies was based is that while mtDNA levels may fluctuate during oogenesis and preimplantation embryogenesis (see below), in aggregate, the relative number of mitochondria present in the peri-implantation-stage blastocyst should reflect the complement present in the MII oocyte because mitochondrial replication begins after implantation [22], and to date, fine structural studies of normally progressing preimplantation-stage embryos show no degenerate forms or indications of mitochondrial replication [15]. Results derived from different mitochondria-specific fluorescent probes indicate that the 100-cell human blastocyst (ICM and trophectoderm) contains approximately 18,000–25,000 mitochondria. Previous electron microscopic analyses of normal-appearing MII human oocytes suggested that a mitochondrial complement around 25K may be normal; however, mtDNA copy number derived from sibling oocytes detected genomic copy numbers between ~110,000 and ~240,000 [23].

Recent studies of mtDNA content during porcine oocyte maturation may clarify the apparent numerical discrepancy between mitochondrial complement size and mtDNA copy number. Spikings et al. [24] reported that similar to the situation in other species, a significant burst of mtDNA replication occurs during preovulatory maturation in the porcine, which results in an increase in genomic content that is several fold higher than levels measured at the germinal vesicle stage. However, such an increase is not observed in rat oocytes that matured in vitro [25], suggesting that the stage-specific upregulation of mtDNA synthesis may operate through signals transmitted to the immature oocyte at the outset of maturation through cumulus and coronal cells, which, in turn, may be responding to signal transduction cascades initiated by LH.

The above findings suggest that each mitochondrion in a normal-appearing MII-stage human oocyte likely contains multiple genomes which, if confirmed by additional studies, would go a long way in reconciling apparent differences between organelle mass and mtDNA content. The importance of reconciling mitochondrial mass and mtDNA content is not only to clarify apparent confusions in the literature but rather also to have a firmer basis for relating mitochondrial properties in the human oocyte and early embryo with competence. Low mtDNA copy numbers have been a suggested etiology of maturation and fertilization failure for human oocytes and for poor embryo performance in vitro [12, 26]. A better understanding of the extent to which fertilization or early embryo failure is related to an acute increase in mtDNA content during the terminal stages of oogenesis (i.e., preovulatory maturation), rather than to an actual organelle deficiency, could point to regulatory defects in the stage-related expansion of mtDNA. Confirmation for the human could make the signaling pathway for mtDNA expansion a focus of study for competence rather than the apparent endpoint, mtDNA content. In this regard, a potentially important finding of Spikings et al. [24] may have implications for the human: during cleavage, approximately 80% of the elevated mtDNA content measured in the mature oocyte was no longer detectable, suggesting that degradation of mitochondrial genomes (but not mitochondria) is a normal process during early development.

What could be the developmental significance of a process that rapidly increases the number of mitochondrial genomes during preovulatory maturation only to degrade them after fertilization? Given the comparatively undeveloped structure of oocyte mitochondria, a transient increase in mtDNA could alter the dynamic relationship between ATP supply and demand during certain stages of oogenesis and early embryogenesis when energy demands may be needed to support cytoplasmic remodeling, circulation, chromosomal segregation, and polar body formation [3]. In this regard, species-specific differences may exist in how differential energy demands may be supplied during the preovulatory and early embryonic stages. In the mouse, for example, spatial changes in mitochondrial density appear to be satisfied by the active translocation of mitochondria to the perinuclear region beginning around germinal vesicle breakdown [27, 28]. Van Blerkom and Runner [27] first proposed that active translocation in the mouse oocyte may be an adaptive mechanism that can elevate ambient levels of ATP in specific areas of the cytoplasm where demand is transiently higher. As discussed below, an increase in the magnitude of $\Delta\Psi_m$ or mtDNA copy number may be other strategies to achieve a similar end in species where significant cytoplasmic remodeling and redistribution of mitochondria are not apparent, such as in the human oocyte.

In certain instances, upregulation of mtDNA replication has been generally considered a compensatory mechanism to increase ATP production under conditions of reduced respiratory function resulting from the acute or chronic effects of toxic insults such as excessive superoxide production. A similar phenomenon of increased mtDNA content has also been reported for sperm and oocytes. May-Panloup et al. [10] reported that the mtDNA content of human sperm with abnormalities known to compromise fertility was significantly higher than in normospermic samples. This was confirmed by Song and Lewis [29] for asthenozoospermic individuals, who also showed that the loss of DNA integrity was higher in affected men, which most was likely due to fragmentation and guanosine oxidation (8oxyG) resulting from excessive levels of mitochondrial superoxide production. In this instance, the increase in average mtDNA content was suggested to compensate for mtDNA mutations or fragmentation that may affect the electron transport chain and therefore respiratory (ATP generation) capacity. If an increase in mtDNA copy number occurs when mature sperm are in the ejaculatory pathway, potential upregulation of ATP production would not reverse structural alterations in plasma membrane integrity and function induced by lipid peroxidation, nor would it correct nascent mutations or defects in mtDNA integrity. The notion that increased mtDNA copy number may be a natural compensatory mechanism would seem to be contradicted by the clinical finding that even if such a process occurs, the sperm are still functionally compromised with respect to motility, and the affected men are still classified as infertile or subfertile.

Wang et al. [30] reported that fully grown MII oocytes obtained from streptozotocin (STZ)-induced diabetic mice show alterations in mitochondrial fine structure such as rupture of the outer membrane, changes in internal membrane organization, and organelle swelling. These defects are consistent with reduced mitochondrial function resulting from respiratory chain defects which, depending upon extent, could activate the mitochondria-dependent apoptotic pathway. However, against a background of mitochondrial alteration and damage, the mtDNA content of diabetic oocytes measured by quantitative real-time PCR was significantly higher than levels in untreated controls [31]. Similar to what may be an adaptive survival mechanism in other cells, increased mtDNA content was postulated by these investigators to be a compensatory mechanism to maintain ATP at levels required to support oocyte maturation and early development in the presence of respiratory chain dysfunction. However, a compensatory explanation does not account for the pronounced delay in meiotic maturation to MII observed in these mouse oocytes. In this regard, reduced mitochondrial function associated with disorders in the electron transport chain, and abnormalities in stage-specific translocation and spatial remodeling of mitochondria, which have been proposed to focally balance ATP supply and demand during mouse oocyte maturation [27, 32], were suggested by Wang and Moley [31] to contribute to meiotic spindle malformations and errors in chromosomal segregation during oocyte maturation in the diabetic mouse model. The transmission of structurally or functionally compromised mitochondria would likely have toxic effects on development during the preimplantation stages that cannot be relieved by increasing mtDNA copies. Since a burst of mtDNA replication appears to be a normal feature of preovulatory maturation [24], the extent to which, if any, the mtDNA content in diabetic oocytes reflects this process, or is substantially different from levels detected in unaffected oocytes, remains to be determined. A similar issue concerns whether levels of mtDNA degradation during cleavage in STZ diabetic mice differ from controls. It seems unlikely that mitochondria in the oocytes of diabetic women are functionally compromised, as this disease is primarily associated with defects in follicular growth, ovulation, and maintenance of gestation, rather than disorders in oocyte maturation, fertilization, and early embryonic development. However, the assumption that mitochondrial function is normal in this instance remains to be investigated at the fine structural, biochemical, and mtDNA levels.

The notion that an inherent mechanism that upregulates mtDNA replication in order to compensate for bioenergetic deficiencies associated with sublethal mitochondrial dysfunction may be particularly relevant for women of advanced reproductive age. Maternal age is the foremost factor associated with the probability of natural cycle pregnancy and gestation to term birth, and it is no different with respect to outcome in assisted reproduction. A high proportion of oocytes obtained for IVF after ovarian hyperstimulation and ovulation induction in women of advanced maternal age are immature or if mature, have a high probability of being aneuploid. If fertilized, the resulting embryos often arrest or develop abnormally during the preimplantation stages and are more likely to undergo demise after implantation than is the case for younger women. The possibility that mitochondrial mutations resulting in respiratory dysfunction may contribute to an age-related reduction in fertility and fecundity first received support from the studies of mtDNA by Keefe et al. [33], who reported that the frequency of a common mitochondrial deletion, the 4,977 bp deletion (corresponding to nucleotide pairs 8,482–13,460), was increased in the oocytes of older women. This common deletion also occurs in rhesus macaque oocytes and has been suggested to contribute to impaired mitochondrial ATP production [34]. Whether the relative size of the deletion, which is larger in the rhesus (5,704 bp) than human (4,977 bp), is related to the extent of detectable respiratory dysfunction is unknown. However, Muller-Hocker et al. [16] did not detect an increased frequency of either point mutations or the 4,977 bp deletion in women of advanced maternal age (>40). These investigators did report fine structural morphometric results that indicated a significant increase in mitochondrial density occurred in older oocytes and that the diameter of mitochondria was also larger than measured in oocyte mitochondria of younger women. While the increase in mitochondria diameters may be due to slight swelling resulting from a $\Delta\Psi_m$ that is insufficient to maintain normal volume homeostasis [2, 35], their findings also showed no age-related functional defects in respiratory chain enzymes. Whether an increase in mitochondrial numbers and changes in organelle diameters indicate a compensatory mechanism to increase ATP production in the oocytes of women of advanced maternal age, as suggested by Muller-Hocker et al. [16], remains to be confirmed. However, unlike the upregulation of mtDNA content in functionally compromised sperm, a similar compensatory mechanism does not appear to occur in "older" human oocytes [36].

Correlating oocyte and embryo developmental ability with levels of mtDNA copy number, organelle complement, and bioenergetic capacity has been the basis of recent mitochondrial studies in animal models such as the bovine [37–39], pig [9], mouse [27], and human [12, 17]. For the human, a determination of threshold levels for each of these mitochondrial parameters has been suggested to represent possible analytic tools that could be used to diagnose fertilization or developmental failure. However, establishing a cause–effect relationship with regard to developmental competence may be problematic and more apparent than real. With respect to stage-specific bioenergetic thresholds, Van Blerkom et al. [4] reported that experimentally reducing net cytoplasmic ATP contents in the mouse by approximately 50% did not inhibit maturation from the germinal vesicle (GV) to MII stages, and while these treated oocytes were fertilizable in vitro, a high proportion of embryos arrested shortly after fertilization and none progressed to the blastocyst. Presumably, postfertilization developmental arrest was associated with irreversible mitochondrial damage with adverse downstream consequences. In contrast, Wai et al. [40] showed that mouse oocytes with as few as 4,000 mtDNA copies were fertilizable and capable of developing to the blastocyst stage, but died shortly after implantation. They concluded that (1) a threshold level of 40,000–50,000 mtDNA copies in the MII mouse oocyte was required to support development during the early post-implantation period and (2) high copy numbers in the mature oocyte were necessary in order to distribute mitochondria and mtDNA to the cells of the early implanting embryo prior to the initiation of mtDNA replication and organelle biogenesis. For the bovine, Chiaratti and Meirelles [39] reported no quantitative difference in mtDNA content between competent and incompetent embryos. However, in an elegant experiment, these authors removed ~64% of the mitochondria from MII oocytes after compartmentalizing these organelles to one pole of the oocyte by centrifugation. They found that oocytes, depleted of mitochondria by this extent, were fertilizable and competent to develop to the blastocyst stage. For these blastocysts, mtDNA contents were similar to nonmanipulated controls. The compensatory strategy employed by mitochondrially depleted embryos to restore normal mtDNA levels by the blastocyst stage is to upregulate the expression of TFAM and NRF1, two critical genes in mitochondrial function that control mtDNA replication and transcription, respectively. Chiaratti and Meirelles [39] reached two important conclusions for preimplantation development in the bovine: (1) an intrinsic mechanism exists in the early embryo to provide a threshold mtDNA content required for blastocyst formation, and (2) competent embryos can regulate mtDNA content regardless of copy numbers present at MII. The degradation of mtDNA detected during the cleavage stages [24] may be part of a self-regulatory mechanism to maintain a threshold mtDNA content required to support postimplantation development prior to mtDNA replication and mitochondrial biogenesis [40]. Because of the high degree of similarity between mammals with respect to the developmental biology of oocyte maturation, fertilization, and preimplantation embryogenesis, the above strategies for establishing a developmental threshold for mtDNA copy number may also apply to the human and, if confirmed, could indicate that the developmental consequences of a bioenergetic deficit may not be evident at MII or during the early stages of embryogenesis. However, testing this supposition experimentally using the same inhibitor treatments or invasive manipulations [39] to downregulate mitochondrial metabolism or reduce mitochondrial complement would require IVF and embryo culture. It is doubtful that such experiments would be considered acceptable or indeed ethical.

Although the above findings demonstrate molecular strategies used by the oocyte and early embryo to up- or downregulate mtDNA copy numbers, it is unclear how levels that may be below or in excess of a postimplantation threshold are recognized at the cellular level. As noted above, reported mtDNA contents between MII human oocytes in the same cohort can differ by over an order of magnitude, and similar differences have been reported for other species [38]. While speculative, one possibility may be related to the redox state of the cytoplasm and the influence mitochondria have on redox homeostasis, which in turn can regulate the activity of redox-dependent signaling pathways and other redox-sensitive regulatory factors (e.g., transcription factor, see below). The extent to which, if any, the redox state of the ooplasm or embryo cytoplasm can be related to mtDNA copy number and stage-specific mtDNA expansion or degradation warrants investigation.

Roles of Mitochondrial Reorganization During Early Development

Oncosis is a survival strategy that can be employed by some cells in order to adapt to transient reductions in ATP generation, such as during ischemic episodes [41]. In these instances, cytoplasmic remodeling results in mitochondrial translocation to the center of the cell, usually around the nucleus, and to balance ATP demand with reduced bioenergetic capacity, portions of the cortical cytoplasm are extruded as blebs that are largely devoid of mitochondria. The extruded cytoplasm remains connected to the underlying cell by cytoplasmic bridges. If normoxic conditions return and ATP levels rise, mitochondria disperse and the cytoplasmic extrusions are resorbed; if the restoration of normoxic conditions is within a cell type-specific tolerance, survival is indicated by the restoration of normal function. This novel mechanism of adaptation to transient anoxia or severe hypoxia has been suggested to operate in cleavage-stage human embryos that exhibit very similar cellular responses and characteristics [42]. One of the more remarkable features of human embryo performance during the early cleavage stages in vitro are instances of fragment "disappearance" during subsequent culture, resulting in embryos that appear largely morphologically normal and stage-appropriate [23, 43]. This phenomenon has been observed by time lapse, even in embryos with fragmentation levels classified as high grade, where resorption restored stage-appropriate morphology and the affected cell(s) underwent division [42].

Light microscopic [44] and fine structural analyses [42] offer a possible explanation for the restoration of apparently normal cell function—the spherical fragments occur in columns that are interconnected to one and another and to the underlying cell by cytoplasmic bridges. The fragments contain few mitochondria that are mostly high potential and derived from the subplasmalemmal cytoplasm [45]. Van Blerkom et al. [42] suggested that abnormal patterns of cytoplasmic remodeling, possibly resulting from corresponding disorders in cytoskeletal organization, could locally reduce mitochondrial density in the pericortical cytoplasm in some cleavage stage blastomeres. In contrast, remodeling does not appear to influence mitochondria in the subplasmalemmal cytoplasm, as discussed below. The compartmentalization of this cytoplasm into columns of interconnected extrusions (blebs) may be a local response to a focal ATP deficit. Restoration of a more normal distribution of mitochondria, especially in the cortical cytoplasm, was suggested to relieve the local bioenergetic deficit and return normal cell function, which is the situation when the oncosis-inducing stress is relieved. The persistence of fragments on cells that underwent a significant reduction in volume was considered to result from the failure of mitochondria to redistribute, and in these instances, high-density mitochondrial aggregates are observed in more central regions of the cytoplasm.

Whether by stage-specific up- or downregulation (degradation) of mtDNA content, active mitochondrial translocation, or perhaps an oncotic-like mechanism, adaptive strategies exist in cells to survive short-term ATP deficits and balance regional changes in the demand-supply equilibrium, and these mechanisms may also be employed by human oocytes and early embryos. The utilization of adaptive strategies is likely embryo-specific because within cohorts cultured in the same environment, not all are affected. This longstanding and consistent observation in clinical IVF demonstrates that at the blastomere level, the normality of development can differ from the embryo as a whole, which can develop progressively in the presence of cells that appear developmentally compromised owing to unique intracellular conditions, physiology, or genetics. At present, clinical and experimental findings from human IVF indicate the importance of mitochondrial function as a primary driver of normal development, although threshold levels of ATP generation and their relationship to mtDNA copy number remain unclear. This is not surprising considering that from the earliest classes one takes in biology, mitochondria are defined as the "powerhouses" of the cell, and this descriptor is still used in many scientific publications. However, what has emerged from studies of mitochondrial function in mammalian oocytes and nascent embryos is that how "power" is distributed within the cell and can be adjusted to meet local changes in demand is as important in understanding cell function during early development as is the power source [3]. Typically, studies of the bioenergetic state of the human oocyte and early human embryo have focused on ATP content at a particular stage. For example, several studies indicate that an ATP content around 1.8 pM may be a steady-state level consistent with competence for the oocyte competence and early human embryo [4, 12]. However, the values obtained represent the net cytoplasmic content at the time of measurement because rates of ATP turnover are rarely determined, and developmental competence is assumed because ATP quantitation requires cell lysis. Therefore, conclusions about developmentally significant threshold levels represent comparative values derived from oocytes that fail to mature in vivo or in vitro, or fertilize in vitro, or from embryos that arrest cell division or show apparent common performance and developmental abnormalities during cleavage, such as grossly unequal cell divisions, high-grade fragmentation, or blastomere multinucleation. If adaptive mechanisms are employed during early development to overcome bioenergetic deficits, they are apparently insufficient in a compensatory context in these instances.

Mitochondrial Inheritance After Fertilization

Although ATP measurements appear to provide a general impression of bioenergetic states that could be of clinical value if related to stage-specific threshold levels, performance defects such as those noted above cannot be assumed, a priori, to have such an etiology. For example, measurements of ATP levels in human embryos that arrest development at the pronuclear to 8-cell stage do not consistently or necessarily have ATP contents that differ significantly from their normally progressing counterparts (e.g., dispermic fertilization) or from normally fertilized siblings cryopreserved at the pronuclear stage and cultured through the cleavage stages after thawing (unpublished). In contrast, the failure to develop into a normally compacted morula that can initiate cavitation, or the inability of a cavitated embryo to progress to the expanded blastocyst stage, which is an energy-intensive process, is more likely to have an origin associated with mitochondrial structural or functional defects [15, 16]. While quantitation of the ATP content(s) of whole embryos may not be informative in a diagnostic sense, or capable of identifying a specific cause of embryo arrest or developmental abnormality, semi-quantitative assessments of mitochondrial mass in individual blastomeres may have clinical value in this regard. Van Blerkom et al. [43] showed that quantitative values for bioenergetic state and comparative mitochondrial mass could be assessed in the same blastomere(s) with highly sensitive organelle-specific fluorescent probes used for the latter. Examination of mitochondrial fluorescence alone in intact 2- and 4-cell stage embryos showed disproportionate mitochondrial segregation with subsequent performance in vitro related to stage (2–8 cell) and extent. These investigators suggested that the origin of this pattern of disproportionate mitochondrial inheritance was related to the symmetry of peripronuclear mitochondrial aggregation at the 1-cell stage. For normally developing fresh and thawed embryos between the 2- and 16-cell stages, the relative intensity of mitochondrial fluorescence and net cytoplasmic ATP content were largely similar between blastomeres. Subsequent studies have shown that blastomere-specific differences in the relative intensity of mitochondrial fluorescence are a comparatively common theme for embryos that developed no further than the 4- or 8-cell stage, with blastomere-specific differences in relative intensity up to 80% observed (unpublished). These findings suggest that a focus on noninvasive methods of assessing mitochondrial mass at the blastomere level could provide important clues related to competence for the entire embryo.

Functional Compartmentalization of Mitochondrial Activity

Several lines of investigation indicate that intracellular mechanisms that readjust ATP supply and demand within the oocyte and early blastomere may be a critical determinant of the normality of development. Local changes in ATP demand can be met by transient changes in mitochondrial distribution using active (cytoskeletal elements such as microtubules) and passive (intracellular circulation) mechanisms that affect organelle density and ambient bioenergetic state [2, 3, 46]. An increased potential across the inner mitochondrial membrane is also associated with higher levels of ATP generation, and in some cultured cell lines, changes in $\Delta\Psi_m$ have been reported to be location dependent. In certain instances, high potential mitochondria are localized to the cell margins where the plasma membrane is motile, with lower potential forms in the interior, especially around the nucleus [47]. These investigators reported that subplasmalemmal mitochondria shift from high to low potential at zones of intercellular contact, but when contact is interrupted, return to high potential where the cell margins are free. In these cells, changes in ATP demand required to support plasma membrane dynamics at the free margins of a cell appear to be met locally by increasing $\Delta\Psi_m$ rather than by mitochondrial translocation to increase organelle density. In other cells, local changes in demand are accommodated by mitochondrial aggregation, which by virtue of altering ambient cytoplasmic redox state (see below) can increase focal levels of respiration in the aggregate [46]. A similar focal change in $\Delta\Psi_m$ in subplasmalemmal mitochondria has been reported for early cleavage-stage mouse embryos [48]. At the zone of gap-junction-mediated contact between blastomeres, the corresponding mitochondria are low potential but become high potential when the cells are separated. Mitochondria at the free margins are high potential. When repositioned 180° at the 2-cell stage, such that the formerly free margins are in contact, high potential shifts to low potential, and vice versa.

Mechanisms of mitochondrial redistribution, translocation, and aggregation detected in cultured cells also occur during early development. In some species, such as the mouse [27, 28] and hamster [49], microtubule-mediated mitochondrial translocation [32] during oocyte maturation and early postfertilization development results in the formation of a relatively dense sphere of mitochondria around the developing nuclear region of the oocyte and juxtaposed pronuclei of the 1-cell embryo. Van Blerkom and Runner [27] first proposed this pattern of cytoplasmic remodeling readjusts ATP supply to accommodate higher ambient energy demands associated with the evolving nuclear region in both oocyte and nascent embryo. In the maturing mouse and human oocyte and pronuclear stage embryo, mitochondria in the subplasmalemmal cytoplasm have an apparent $\Delta\Psi_m$ that is significantly higher than exhibited by the vast majority of mitochondria within the cell [48]. It is worth mentioning that mitochondria which are actively translocated to the perinuclear region during oocyte maturation in the mouse are low potential and that the high potential forms in the subplasmalemmal region do not participate in this redistribution [48] and remain spatially stable and at a comparatively high potential from the oocyte through the cleavage stages [50].

Although the subplasmalemmal domain contains less than ~3% of the complement of mitochondria in the mature oocyte, their loss by minor fragmentation from this domain is apparently irreversible, and depending upon the degree of loss, adverse developmental effects including delayed or arrested cell division have been reported [50]. Similarly, failure to assume a high $\Delta\Psi_m$ at MII, or a domain of high potential forms that is scant and largely discontinuous, has been associated with sperm penetration failure in the human after conventional IVF [48, 51]. It has been suggested that high potential and a subplasmalemmal localization may provide higher ambient concentrations of ATP to support ATP-driven plasma membrane activities that include sperm penetration and migration of the incorporated sperm nucleus [3, 52]. Reversibly reducing $\Delta\Psi_m$ in this domain was inconsistent with penetration until high potential was restored [50].

Intracellular Free Calcium and Mitochondrial Activity

The above findings suggest that mitochondrial potential, location, and density are mechanisms by which ATP may be differentially generated, distributed, and utilized within the cytoplasm of the oocyte and early embryo, and defects in each element of this energy management system could affect competence depending on stage and extent. As noted above, the absence of high $\Delta\Psi_m$ in the subplasmalemmal domain at MII is associated with penetration failure for both fresh [48, 50] and thawed human oocytes [51]. Local changes in the concentration of intracellular free calcium is another critical element in the regulation of mitochondrial ATP production and, for the human, may be directly related to developmental abnormalities that can occur well beyond the preimplantation stages [53]. Mitochondria are excitable organelles [54] that respond to changes in ambient free calcium levels by releasing or sequestering calcium, and the level of response can be related to the magnitude of $\Delta\Psi_m$. Mitochondria respond to calcium released from intracellular stores, such as the smooth-surfaced endoplasmic reticulum (sER), through the calcium-induced calcium release pathway (CIRC) [55, 56] and from calcium released by mitochondria themselves through the mitochondrial calcium-induced calcium release (mCIRC) [57]. It has long been known that calcium is a regulator of mitochondrial ATP synthesis [58]. Dumollard et al. [59] demonstrated that by experimentally manipulating calcium release from sSER, ambient calcium levels and mitochondrial activity were tightly coupled in a regulatory manner that could up- or downregulate levels of respiration in the newly fertilized mouse oocyte. The benefit for the oocyte or early embryo of such tight coupling is that local, stage-specific ATP demands can be met without involving the entire mitochondrial complement, which has the potential of increasing levels of ROS (superoxide). In the mouse and human oocyte and early embryo, fine structural analyses show cisternae of the sER in contact with mitochondria [14], especially in the pericortical/subplasmalemmal cytoplasm where of mitochondria surround sER aggregates [23, 48]. Van Blerkom et al. [48, 60] suggested that the fertilization-induced influx of calcium may increase mitochondrial activity in the subplasmalemmal domain and

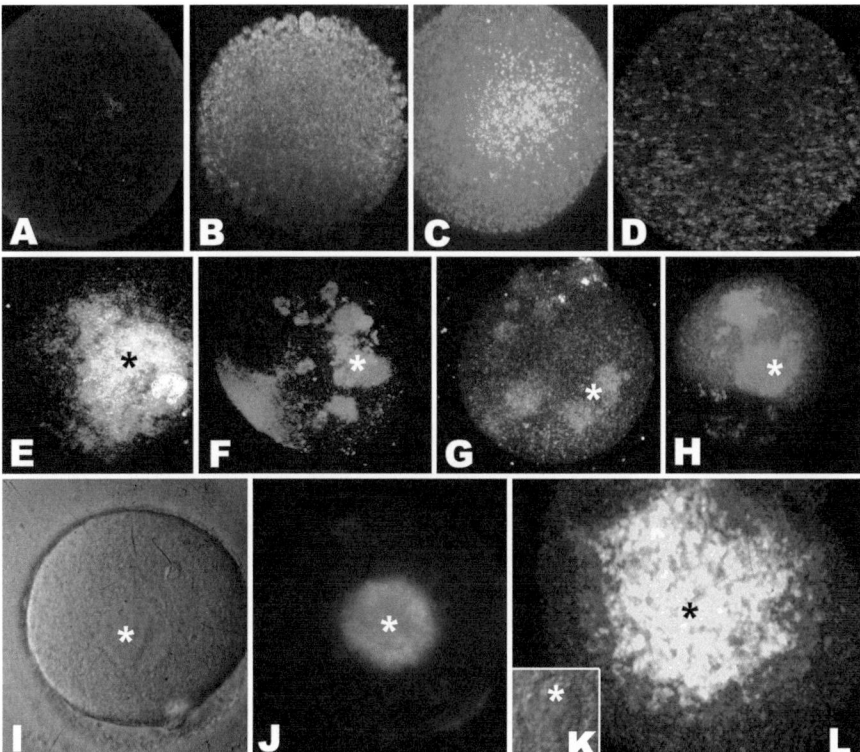

Fig. 24.1 Normal (**a–d**) and abnormal (**e–h**) patterns of increased levels of intracellular free calcium (*asterisk*) after ionophore-activation of MII human oocytes. (**j, l**) show a highly intense and prolonged flare of fluorescence, detected by a fluorescent calcium reporter, which corresponds to calcium released from a single, large aggregate of sER cisternae (*asterisk*, **i, k**). This sER aggregate defines an abnormal human oocyte phenotype, and its occurrence during IVF has been associated with unusually high levels of ATP generation and genomic imprinting disorders in newborns

possibly initiate mCIRC along the circumference of the oocyte, which could locally assist in the cortical granule exocytosis and other calcium-dependent activities associated with sperm penetration. The validity of this notion remains to be determined experimentally.

Little is known about spontaneous abnormalities in calcium release at the earliest stage of human fertilization and whether defects in calcium signaling [61] or levels could have downstream effects on mitochondrial activity or the normality of embryogenesis. Typically, studies of changes in cytoplasmic free calcium involve preloading oocytes with a fluorescent calcium reporter such as Fluo-4 AM [51, 60] followed by activation with a calcium ionophore (e.g., A23178; [3, 56]) or insemination by intracytoplasmic sperm injection (ICSI) [62, 63]. The normal pattern of free calcium fluorescence observed by scanning laser confocal microscopy after human oocyte activation is shown in Fig. 24.1a–d. Shortly after ionophore exposure, the relative intensity of fluorescence increases throughout the cytoplasm (Fig. 24.1b, c) before decaying to levels (Fig. 24.1d) that existed in reporter-labeled oocytes prior to activation (Fig. 24.1a). In contrast, within the same cohort(s) of MII oocytes activated 2–4 h after follicular aspiration and hyaluronidase-mediated corona and cumulus cell denudation, the rise in fluorescent intensity in some oocytes was regional (asterisk, Fig. 24.1e–f) rather than a uniform. In most instances, the intensity of calcium fluorescence declined to background levels at rates similar to those observed in oocytes with a uniform rise. The oocytes shown in Fig. 24.1e, h are representative examples of a pattern of cytosolic calcium fluorescence that was an exception. Fluo-4 AM fluorescence was detectable for at least 2 h after levels returned to background in similarly treated oocytes, such as those shown in Fig. 24.1d, g. The average net ATP content measured 4 h after activation in oocytes with these aberrant patterns of free calcium fluorescence was significantly higher by ~30–50% (3.3 pM, ±0.6 pM, $n = 23$) than normal for MII human oocytes [4] that exhibited a uniform calcium rise (1.8 pM, ±0.3 pM, $n = 15$). A very similar phenomenon occurs in MII human oocytes cryopreserved by programmed (slow) cooling which, after thawing, are preloaded with this calcium probe and ionophore activated. Preliminary findings indicate that while <4% of fresh oocytes display this abnormal pattern (1/27), distinct regions of intense fluorescence occurred in approximately 42% (13/31) of oocytes that were of similar (normal) appearance at cryopreservation and activated 2–4 h after thawing (similar to Fig. 24.1e–h). However, ATP levels measured at 4 h after activation were not significantly different from levels measured in similar oocytes prior to cryopreservation [51].

The above findings suggest the possibility that oocyte-specific defects in sER function may be associated with the slow cooling cryopreservation, but freezing per se does not appear to affect global cytoplasmic ATP content after thawing. In this regard, the unusual patterns of calcium rise and the corresponding increase in net cytoplasmic ATP content observed in fresh oocytes could support the notion of tight metabolic coupling between sER-derived calcium and mitochondrial ATP production discussed above. The absence of a similar increase in ATP content in thawed oocytes could indicate cryopreservation-induced damage to mitochondria that makes them less responsive to calcium at the 4-h time point or an abnormal increase in ATP demand that requires higher levels of production that is not evident when total net cytoplasm ATP content is measured. Whether oocyte cryopreservation by slow cooling irreversibly alters mitochondrial organization at the fine structural level is unclear. While some reports have described alterations that could compromise function [64], others have not [65, 66], and in our experience, mitochondria in MII human oocytes cryopreserved by slow cooling that remain intact during the first hour after thawing appear unchanged from their fresh counterparts (unpublished). This is not to say that mitochondria are not damaged during slow cooling cryopreservation, but the damage may be reversible or occur at a level that does not alter respiratory capacity reflected by net cytoplasmic ATP content. Whether calcium-dependent signaling pathways are perturbed by this method of cryopreservation is unknown, but cellular bioenergetic state seems unperturbed.

The most compelling evidence to date of an association between atypical sER calcium release and ATP production occurs in ionophore-activated MII human oocytes that contain a single, large, centrally located disk-like inclusion composed of cisternae of the sER [67] (asterisk, Fig. 24.1i, k). After preloading with the calcium reporter and exposure to A23187, activation is rapidly followed by an intense flare of fluorescence (2 min, asterisk, Fig. 24.1j) that coincides with the position of the inclusion. The intensity of fluorescence remains elevated for approximately 2–3 h (2 h, Fig. 24.1l), which is significantly longer than observed in unaffected oocytes [60]. Preliminary results indicate that net cytoplasmic ATP content measured at 1–4 h was ~2.0 to 2.5-fold higher than normal (3.3–4.6 pM) and remained elevated for at least 22 h before abruptly dropping to levels ≤50% of normal (0.6–0.8 pM).

The most remarkable characteristic of these oocytes was the behavior of the inclusion during prolonged culture as detected by time lapse. Figure 24.2 shows selected images at the indicated times after activation of an MII oocyte with a large sER inclusion. The arrows show the direction of movement of the disk, with the black arrows denoting movement detectable within the plane of focus, and the white arrows denoting the direction of movement when the disk moves out of and returns to the plane of focus. Over this 22-h period, the disk moves throughout the cytoplasm going out of and back into the plane of focus, often oscillating back and forth within a 20–35 micron region. The calculated rate of movement during this time was relatively constant at ~1.0 to 1.5 µm/min. Exposure of oocytes to inhibitors of oxidative phosphorylation [60] caused this motion to cease within minutes, but resumed when the inhibition was relieved, if the duration of inhibitor did not exceed ~30 min. A close inspection of these representative images shows that the movement of the disk (indicated by a white asterisk) is accompanied by corresponding dynamic changes in the cytoplasm immediately in front of and behind this structure (e.g., arrow, 17 min 56 s; black asterisks, 21 h 17 min 59 s to 21 h 47 min 59 s).

Time-lapse imaging has shown that after fertilization in the human, cytoplasmic motility increases in general and within the pericortical cytoplasm in particular [68]. However, a similar intensity and persistence of movement, such as displayed by these inclusions, has not been reported. It is tempting to speculate that the abnormal pattern of calcium release and the persistence of calcium-driven fluorescence affect the fluidity of the cytoplasm, perhaps by altering calcium-dependent structural elements responsible for cytoplasmic organization and circulation [2]. Together with an unusually elevated bioenergetic state, the condition of the cytoplasm may become permissive for and enhance dynamic movements of cytoplasmic components. In this regard, the behavior of the sER inclusion may be governed and directed by mechanisms similar to those that promote the movement of the sperm nucleus after penetration and pronuclear migration during the 1-cell stage [52]. In these instances, pronuclear migration is associated with normal levels of calcium release that are periodic (so-called calcium transients) and begins with an initial increase at the earliest stage of the fertilization process. Although likely, the extent to which defects in these transients (occurrence or amplitude) are associated with fertilization failures in human IVF where the sperm nucleus remains (unexpanded) in the

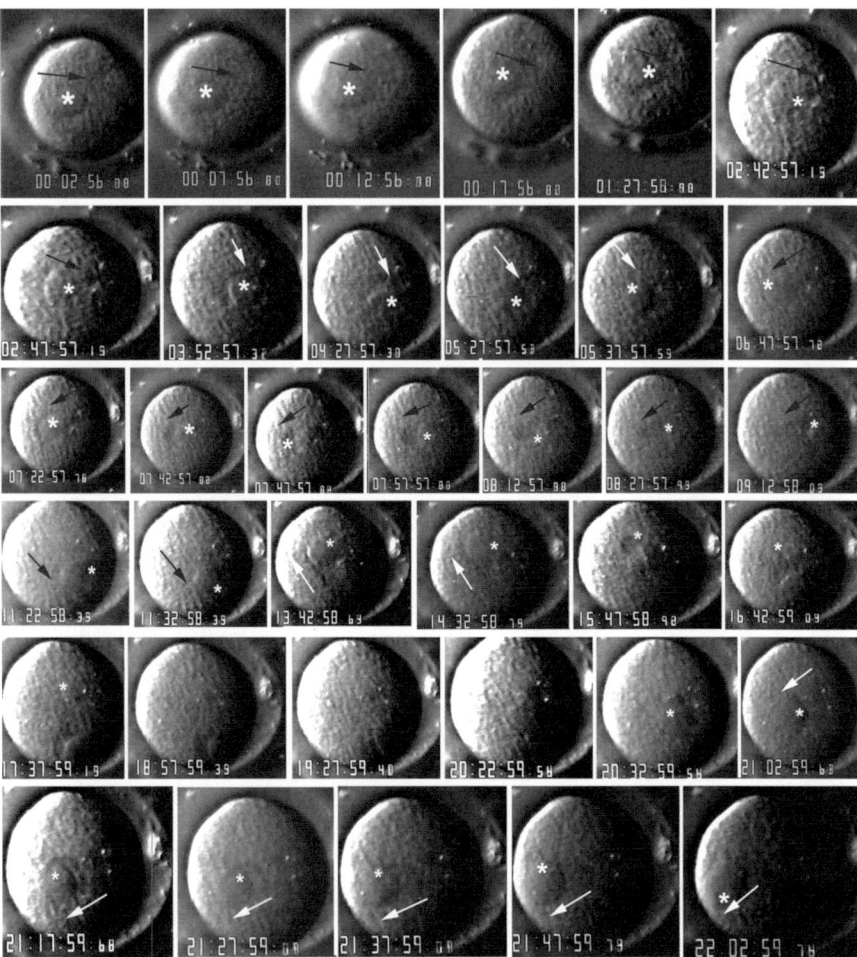

Fig. 24.2 Representative time-lapse images showing the movement of a single, larger sER inclusion (*asterisk*) in an MII human oocyte over a 22-h period. The *arrows* indicate direction at different times (indicated in *lower left*) as the inclusions move out of and into the plane of focus. This usual and persistent behavior is suggested to be supported by an enhanced cytoplasmic bioenergetic state associated with the maintenance of unusually high levels of mitochondrial ATP synthesis

pericortical cytoplasm [69], or where pronuclear migration and juxtaposition do not occur [52], remains to be determined. However, whether the abrupt cessation of the SER disk movement described above reflects reactive oxygen toxicity to mitochondria resulting from the generation of superoxide in excess of the intrinsic antioxidant capacities (e.g., mitochondrial superoxide dismutase) is one possibility under investigation.

These findings indicate that abnormalities in calcium release may have downstream developmental effects if calcium-dependent signaling pathways or processes are perturbed. Two reports, one experimental and the other clinical, strongly support this possibility. The studies of Ozil and Huneau [53] showed that the developmental consequences of increasing the level of calcium released after ionophore activation of rabbit oocytes were not evident until organogenesis, where multiple system anomalies and defects resulted in fetal demise. It is important to emphasize that preimplantation development was normal. For the human, oocytes with a large SER aggregate such as shown in Fig. 24.1i, k are fertilizable by ICSI, but few embryos develop normally during the preimplantation stages and if transferred, most cease to develop [70]. However, what is disturbing about some of the births from oocytes of this type is the occurrence of genomic imprinting disorders that have been suggested to be associated with aberrant calcium signaling at the outset of development [71]. Concerns about developmental normality and a high potential for imprinting disorders have resulted in the recent conclusion by a joint ESHRE/alpha panel of experts that human oocytes with SER inclusions, such as those described above, should never be inseminated [72].

Mitochondria and Signal Transduction Pathways

Similar to differentiated cells [73], a structural relationship between the SER and mitochondria [14, 48] in the oocyte and early likely includes regulatory functions other than calcium homeostasis and mitochondrial energetics. What is critical to understanding the extent to which abnormalities in calcium release at fertilization may affect human development is a determination of if, and how, the flow of regulatory information within the ooplasm may be perturbed and, for the early embryo, whether bidirectional information flow between the cytoplasm (e.g., transcription factors and activators) [74] and nucleus (e.g., mRNA) is altered. In this context, the identification of defects in signal transduction may provide fundamental insights into the origin of developmental competence for the oocyte and how it may be lost or compromised after fertilization. For the fresh oocyte, the occurrence of calcium release abnormalities appears to be a relatively low-frequency event, and the question remains why only some oocytes are affected. For thawed oocytes, however, the frequency is significantly higher and the extent to which this abnormality is protocol related is unclear, and the results of fine structural analyses conflict with respect to cooling and freezing protocol. While some studies report no evident alterations in sER structure or organization [65], others have described apparent swelling of the cisternae and changes in spatial organization [75] that could contribute to the atypical response to ionophore activation shown here. While it is likely that an optimized protocol of oocyte cryopreservation that minimizes damage to or alteration of sER integrity and function will be forthcoming, for some oocytes, defects in sER function may be an inherent problem associated with fertilization failure or abnormal preimplantation embryogenesis. How these defects may influence mitochondrial function, cytoplasmic bioenergetic state, and local stage-specific free energy availability are the types of developmentally significant questions that, while currently unanswered, may be fundamental to understanding the cell biology of the human oocyte and early embryo.

Mitochondria and Cytoplasmic Redox State

An important regulatory influence of mitochondria in somatic cells is their effect on the redox state of the cytoplasm. The normal state of the cytoplasm is a reducing environment, and cells employ different mechanisms to maintain redox homeostasis in the presence of mitochondria-derived oxidative stress. The pathogenesis of certain diseases is based on the inability of these mechanisms to cope with oxidative stress, such as superoxide toxicity, and at the cellular level, an inability to counter a shift toward an oxidative environment can lead to signaling disorders and bioenergetic insufficiency leading to dysfunctions in cytoplasmic bioactivities, apoptosis, or pathological cell death. Mitochondrial redistribution and localization is one means by which location-dependent ATP supply and demand requirements can be met, and potentially higher levels of superoxide production that may occur with cytoplasmic mitochondrial aggregation or remodeling are normally addressed by mitochondrial and cytoplasmic antioxidants (e.g., superoxide dismutase and glutathione).

Location-related differences in mitochondrial density that alters cytoplasmic redox potential may also regulate redox-sensitive signaling pathways and in some species, such as the sea urchin, are essential for specification of the oral-aboral axis, which involves redox-dependent signaling pathways. The establishment of this axis in the fertilized egg is regulated by an asymmetrical mitochondrial distribution in the oocyte and in the early embryo, where a redox gradient is formed by virtue of differential mitochondrial density [76, 77]. These investigators reported that the portion of the sea urchin embryo that inherits the highest density of active mitochondria is strongly biased toward oral axis specification owing to the location-specific expression of the oral axis determining transcription factor, *nodal*. According to this model, a "transcription factor" gradient is established in the blastomeres of the early embryo in which the function of different redox-sensitive transcription factors, such as *nodal*, is dependent upon a redox threshold within the redox gradient established by differential mitochondrial density. In this context, the cytoplasm of the oocyte and early blastomeres may be functionally compartmentalized as a normal consequence of relative mitochondrial density.

A similar phenomenon, albeit on a much smaller scale, has been observed in differentiated somatic cells where mitochondria aggregate in different locations in order to increase ambient ATP availability to accommodate transient changes in local energy demand [46]. Spatial remodeling of mitochondria is a dynamic process and, in active cells, may undergo continuous redistribution. Changes in mitochondrial density may also alter local cytoplasmic redox state and, as a result, locally affect bioactivities with different redox-sensitive thresholds. This form of dynamic cytoplasmic mitochondrial reorganization was suggested by Aw [46] to be a type of microzonation in which local activities could be functionally compartmentalized within the cytoplasm in response to changes in cell activity or exogenous signals such as cell contact. Changes in mitochondrial density that alter the ambient redox state may also increase respiratory activity by the aggregated mitochondria if local pH is also reduced (by ATP hydrolysis), which Aw [46] suggests, can increase the efficiency and rate of uptake of intermediately metabolites. Dynamic changes in $\Delta\Psi_m$ may be another example of mitochondrial microzonation. As described above, Diaz et al. [47] showed that the magnitude of $\Delta\Psi_m$ in mitochondria at the margins of cultured cells was cell contact dependent with a downregulation of this transmembrane potential occurring in areas of intercellular contact and communication. As previously noted, similar finding was reported for the cleavage-stage mouse embryo [48], where mitochondria in the subplasmalemmal cytoplasm corresponding to regions of intercellular contact and gap-junction-mediated intercellular communication were low potential while those beneath the free margins of the plasma membrane were high potential. In this study, experimental manipulations of early cleavage-stage embryos showed that the magnitude of $\Delta\Psi_m$ in these regions could be up- or downregulated as a function of the presence of or absence of intercellular communication and contact. It may be worthwhile to determine whether differences in redox state occur in these regions and, if confirmed, whether the absence of adequate cell contact or communication influences $\Delta\Psi_m$ and the normal functions of redox- and ROS-sensitive signaling (e.g., JAK-STAT) [78] in this region. This may be especially relevant in certain early cleavage-stage human embryos where the apparent absence of normal cell contact and communication appears to lead to aberrant development in vitro.

Findings from cultured cells and early embryos such as the sea urchin clearly demonstrate that in addition to ATP production, mitochondria have central regulatory roles in signal transduction through calcium and redox-sensitive pathways, and by creating microzones that may alter local physiology, can create cytoplasmic compartments with different functional characteristics. Evidence suggesting that similar cell biological activities occur in the mammalian oocyte and early embryo has come from the characterization of dynamic, stage-specific changes in mitochondrial distribution and from the detection of differential $\Delta\Psi_m$ that is location-based. Preovulatory cytoplasmic maturation of the oocytes of certain species, such as the mouse, involves stage-specific mitochondrial translocation to the perinuclear nuclear region [27, 28] that, in the mouse, is directed by microtubular arrays emanating from perinuclear microtubular organizing centers [32]. The formation of a relatively dense sphere of mitochondria around the developing nuclear region after germinal vesicle breakdown has been suggested to increase ambient ATP levels but may also alter the perinuclear redox state to promote formation of the first and second meiotic metaphase spindles, chromosomal segregation, and polar body abstriction [21]. Here too, the notion of thresholds may be developmentally significant as excessive or inadequate perinuclear aggregation may have coincident effects on bioenergetic and redox state that are inhibitory for maturation to MII [27, 79], or contribute to disorders in chromosomal segregation leading to aneuploidy [5, 80, 81]. In addition to the mouse [27], perinuclear aggregation has also been reported for the pronuclear and early cleavage stages in other mammals such as the pig, hamster, nonhuman primate, and the human [43, 82, 83]. Indeed, a pronounced perinuclear accumulation of mitochondria occurs in the human, and asymmetries in distribution have been related to disproportionate mitochondrial inheritance during cleavage [43]. In contrast to the mouse oocyte, mitochondrial translocation to the developing nuclear region of the maturing human oocyte is less pronounced, perhaps owing to the absence of definitive microtubular organizing centers, especially in the perinuclear region. In addition, virtually all information concerning the cytoplasmic dynamics of human oocyte maturation has come from observations made in vitro with immature oocytes, most of which had failed to reinitiate meiosis or arrested meiosis prior to MII after ovulation induction. Reliance on in vitro matured oocytes for these studies is understandable because extracting oocytes at specific stages of preovulatory maturation after ovulation induction in stimulated or natural cycles (which would be preferable) is unlikely to be the type of experiment whose inherent value can be ethically justified. However, a limited number of fine structural images of human oocytes that were at the GV stage at aspiration, or remained so during culture in vitro, often show unusually high densities of perinuclear mitochondrial aggregation [14]. Confirmation that an abnormal perinuclear redox state may be responsible for the failure of meiosis to resume or progress to MII would go a long way in providing new insights into how maturational and fertilization competence is established and, for the human, possible follicle-specific influences that promote or inhibit early development.

Mitochondrial Inner Membrane Potential and Functional Microzonation

The notions of microzonation and functional compartmentalization would be more compelling as developmentally significant aspects of oocyte maturation and early embryogenesis if they could be correlated with known abnormalities in cytoplasmic organization that have negative developmental consequences—the so-called cytoplasmic dysmorphisms described for human oocytes [67, 70]. At present, differential $\Delta\Psi_m$ appears to be one aspect of mitochondria that may support these notions [2, 21]. In the human and mouse MII oocyte, high-potential mitochondria are normally localized to the subplasmalemmal cytoplasm where they form a distinct circumferential domain detectable with $\Delta\Psi_m$-sensitive (potentiometric) fluorescent probes such as JC-1 [48, 84, 85]. In the human, the absence of high potential in this domain in fresh [48] and thawed MII stage oocytes [51] has been suggested to be a proximal cause of penetration failure in conventional IVF. A similar phenomenon has been reported for the mouse where sperm penetration is reversibly inhibited by experimentally down- and upregulating $\Delta\Psi_m$, respectively, in this domain [86].

In the mouse and human, this domain is spatially stable in the oocyte and remains so during early cleavage, and in the human, spatial stability is indicated by the absence of high-potential forms after loss by minor fragmentation [50]. While their energetic contribution to net cytoplasmic ATP levels in the MII oocyte is negligible, which would be expected considering the domain contains <3% of the total mitochondrial complement, as noted above, their loss or reduced potential in this specific region appears to have important implications for development. The possibility that this extended domain (microzone) of mitochondria may have specialized functions during early development (functional compartmentalization) is suggested by the extent of loss, either naturally occurring or experimentally induced, on the subsequent ability of the affected blastomere(s) to participate in embryogenesis. The loss of high $\Delta\Psi_m$ organelles to a few small fragments had no discernable effect on embryogenesis, whereas loss from one or more regions that significantly diminished mitochondria from this domain, or where the distribution of high-potential mitochondria was scant or discontinuous, was associated with the failure of the affected blastomere to divide. However, loss to this extent is not necessarily lethal, as the affected blastomeres typically remained undivided as the remainder of the embryo progress through the preimplantation stages. At the fully expanded blastocyst stage, the presence of a cleavage-sized cell in the perivitelline space or less commonly the blastocyst cavity may originate from an early, nonlethal, loss of high-potential mitochondria from a single blastomere.

Wilding et al. [87] reported that clusters of high-potential mitochondria occurred within the cytoplasm of arrested/degenerating human blastomeres, but not in the subplasmalemmal cytoplasm. This phenotype has been rarely observed in our experience but could be associated with a premorbid state that may lead to apoptosis, as this cell death pathway generally involves an abrupt collapse of high $\Delta\Psi_m$ leading to the release of calcium and cytochrome c. In contrast, pathological cell death usually results from a persistently low $\Delta\Psi_m$ that corresponds to a bioenergetic state that is unable to meet the minimal ATP demands required to maintain cell function. In this regard, most unfertilized human oocytes will remain intact for days in culture, and changes in mitochondrial fine structure, such as loss of cristae and changes in matrix electron density that become apparent after day 4 or 5, are consistent with a significant drop in net ATP content and scant high potential in the subplasmalemmal domain [3]. Typically, these oocytes lyse on or after day 6 or 7, indicating that cell death is likely due to an energetic deficiency associated with necrosis rather than by the induction of apoptosis [45].

While there is compelling evidence that a subplasmalemmal domain of high-potential mitochondria exists in the mature human oocyte and cleavage-stage embryo, and appears to be involved in sperm penetration, why perturbation of this microzone at the blastomere level has adverse consequences remains to be determined. One possibility suggests that higher ambient levels of ATP may be required to support dynamic membrane activities involving transporters, ion channels, and plasma membrane reorganization between the oocyte and embryonic stages. Another possibility that warrants investigation is that this domain is involved in signal transduction pathways and those that are redox- or ROS-sensitive in particular [3]. If confirmed, findings of this type may add a new dimension to our understanding of what competence entails during the earliest stages of human development. Likewise, they may provide novel diagnostic methods to assess subtle causes of fertilization failure, embryo arrest, and abnormal performance in vitro that may be related to maternal age or for some patients, to repeated negative outcomes in IVF cycles.

The role of mitochondria in the regulation of cytoplasmic redox state may be one that is unfamiliar to clinical practitioners, but is nevertheless a fundamental property that, as more information emerges, will likely become another factor to be recognized in the establishment of competence. Likewise, the relationship between mtDNA copy number at MII and whether numerical expansion occurs during the preovulatory stages may have important influences on mitochondrial activity in the oocyte and redox state and ROS/redox-sensitive signaling during fertilization and early embryogenesis. A similar activity may occur during the cleavage stages where high-potential mitochondria remain localized in the subplasmalemmal cytoplasm. It remains to be determined whether loss of these mitochondria to fragmentation, or failure to resume high potential after thawing [51], impacts the local redox state or redox-sensitive signaling at the level of the plasma membrane and subplasmalemmal cytoplasm.

A potentially important finding demonstrating that cytoplasmic redox potential can be altered by exogenous factors comes from the recent study of Dumollard et al. [88], who reported that the normality of preimplantation embryogenesis in vitro was supported by a redox potential that involved cytosolic and mitochondrial metabolism of pyruvate and lactate—the former a cytosolic oxidant and mitochondrial reductant, and the latter a strong cytosolic reductant. The potential developmental significance of these findings is that cytoplasmic redox potential can be altered by varying the concentration of intermediate metabolites normally found in embryo culture medium, such as pyruvate. In this context, seemingly minor modifications to culture medium that may change the oxidation/reduction equilibrium in a stage-dependent manner could be unrecognized factors that directly impact human embryo performance and viability during the preimplantation stages. Novel fluorescent probes that can assess intracellular redox state in living cells [89] may be sufficiently sensitive to detect local state changes that may be associated with stage-specific events such as fertilization and intercellular communication and possibly with modifications to medium composition or culture conditions. In this regard, it will be relevant to determine the extent to which, if any, metabolomic assessments of spent culture medium that have been proposed for clinical IVF [90] are detecting redox changes that could influence competence. What is particularly interesting about this possibility is that it could add redox homeostasis to the calculus of assessing outcome if differences are oocyte-/embryo-specific or cohort-wide, and perhaps suggest novel treatments that can be implemented to target functional disorders that are redox (mitochondrial)-driven.

Summary and Future Prospects

While a considerable body of evidence supports a central role of mitochondria in early human development, questions other than those discussed above are worthy of mention. What is the normal number of mitochondria in an oocyte and is there a threshold for competence? Often, mitochondrial mass and mtDNA copy number are used interchangeably, which can confound this issue as mtDNA copy numbers can vary widely, often by over an order of magnitude, between MII oocytes in the same cohort [2, 11, 18, 23]. Variations in mtDNA content between oocytes within the same and different cohorts may reflect differential levels of mtDNA expansion among mitochondria rather than numerical differences in mitochondrial complement. Resolution of this issue will require morphometric analyses, preferably with superfluous MII oocytes whose cytoplasm is characterized as normal [72]. A second question is whether mtDNA expansion occurs during preovulatory maturation, at what stage(s), and whether mtDNA degradation occurs during cleavage and how it may be regulated [24]. Whether the finding of lower mtDNA content found in rat oocytes that matured in vitro [25] pertains to the human needs to be determined if IVM is to become a standard practice in clinical IVF.

At present, while these issues are speculative, they do indicate the types of questions that may provide basic information about cell biology of the human oocyte during the terminal stages of development and at the earliest stages of embryogenesis. Against this background, the extent to which differential mitochondrial potential or activity may influence local redox state and, by extension, putative redox-sensitive or redox-dependent signaling pathways may be among the most relevant because the effects of altered signaling during embryogenesis in other developing systems, such as those described above, can be both immediate and downstream, and there is no reason to expect the human to be an exception. The basic cell biological processes and interactions discussed here for mitochondria, and emerging principals of cytoplasmic organization such as microzonation and functional compartmentalization, may be central to how developmental competence is established and maintained and, if confirmed for the human, could offer new directions for studies of the impact or regulatory influence on competence of the follicle-specific biochemical milieu. This is an exciting area of research with clear clinical implications, and it is highly likely that as investigations proceed, additional influences of mitochondrial activity and function will be recognized and incorporated into novel protocols or algorithms designed to assess developmental potential and normality.

References

1. Ramalho-Santos J, Varum S, Amaral S, Mota P, et al. Mitochondrial functionality in reproduction: from gonads and gametes to embryos and embryonic stem cells. Hum Reprod Update. 2009;15:553–72.

2. Van Blerkom J. The mitochondria in early development. Semin Cell Dev Biol. 2009;20:191–200.
3. Van Blerkom J. Mitochondrial function in the human oocyte and embryo and their role in developmental competence. Mitochondrion. 2011; 11:797–813.
4. Van Blerkom J, Davis P, Lee J. ATP content of human oocytes and developmental potential and outcome after in-vitro fertilization and embryo transfer. Hum Reprod. 1995;10:415–24.
5. Schon E, Kim S, Ferreora J, Magalhaes P, Grace M, Warburton D, et al. Chromosomal nondisjunction in human oocytes: is there a mitochondrial connection? Hum Reprod. 2000;15 Suppl 2:160–72.
6. Reynier P, May-Panloup P, Chretien M, Morgan C, et al. Mitochondrial DNA content effects the fertilizability of human oocytes. Mol Hum Reprod. 2001;7:425–9.
7. Lin WQ, Lin JJ, Ye BL, Chen YQ, Zhao JZ, Zhou Y, Chi HH. Analysis of pregnancy outcomes after in vitro fertilization-embryo transfer and intracytoplasmic sperm injection. Zhonghua Fu Chan Ke Za Zhi. 2004;39(2):108–11.
8. Brevini T, Vassena R, Francisi C, Gandolfi F. Role of adenosine triphosphate, active mitochondria, and microtubules in the acquisition of developmental competence of parthenogenetically activated pig oocytes. Biol Reprod. 2005;72:1218–23.
9. Shahinaz H, El-Shourbagy S, Spikings E, Freitas M, St John J. Mitochondria directly influence fertilisation outcome in the pig. Reproduction. 2006;131:233–45.
10. May-Panloup P, Chretien M-F, Malthiery Y, Reynier P. Mitochondrial DNA in the oocyte and the developing embryo. Curr Top Dev Biol. 2007;77:51–83.
11. Shoubridge E, Wai T. Mitochondrial DNA and the mammalian oocyte. Curr Top Dev Biol. 2007;77:87–111.
12. Zeng H, Ren Z, Yueng S, Shu Y, et al. Low mitochondrial DNA and ATP contents contribute to the absence of birefringent spindle imaged with PolScope in in vitro matured human oocytes. Hum Reprod. 2007;22:1681–6.
13. Motta P, Nottola S, Makabe S, Heyn R. Mitochondrial morphology in human fetal and adult female germ cells. Hum Reprod. 2000;15 Suppl 2:128–47.
14. Makabe S, Van Blerkom J. Human female reproductive function. Ovarian development to early embryogenesis. Boca Raton: Taylor and Francis; 2006. p. 87–177.
15. Van Blerkom J. Developmental failure in human reproduction associated with preovulatory oogenesis and preimplantation embryogenesis. In: Van Blerkom J, Motta P, editors. Ultrastructure of human gametogenesis and embryogenesis. Boston: Kluwer Academic Publishers; 1989. p. 125–80.
16. Muller-Hocker J, Shafer S, Weis S, Munscher C, Strowitzki T. Morphological, cytochemical and molecular genetic analysis of mitochondria in isolated human oocytes and reproductive age. Mol Hum Reprod. 1996;2:951–8.
17. Santos T, El-Shourbagy S, St John J. Mitochondrial content reflects oocyte variability and fertilization outcome. Fertil Steril. 2006;85:584–92.
18. Brenner C. What is the role of mitochondria in embryo competence? In: Van Blerkom J, Gregory L, editors. Essential IVF: basic research and clinical applications. Boston: Kluwer Academic Publishers; 2004. p. 273–90.
19. Steuerwald N, Barrit J, Alder R, et al. Quantification of mtDNA in single oocytes, polar bodies and subcellular components by real-time rapid fluorescence monitored PCR. Zygote. 2000;9:209–15.
20. Jansen R. Germline passage of mitochondria: quantitative considerations and possible embryological sequelae. Hum Reprod. 2000;15 Suppl 2:112–28.
21. Van Blerkom J. Mitochondria as regulatory forces in oocytes, preimplantation embryos and stem cells. Reprod Biomed Online. 2008;16:553–69.
22. Larsson N, Wang J, Wilhemsson H, Oldfors A, Rustin P, Lewandoski M, et al. Mitochondria transcription factor A is necessary for mtDNA maintenance and embryogenesis in mice. Nat Genet. 1998;18:231–6.
23. Van Blerkom J. The role of mitochondria in human oogenesis and preimplantation embryogenesis: engines of metabolism, ionic regulation and developmental competence. Reproduction. 2004;128:269–80.

24. Spikings E, Alderson J, St John J. Regulated mitochondrial DNA replication during oocyte maturation is essential for successful porcine embryonic development. Reproduction. 2007;76:327–35.
25. Zeng H, Yeung W, Cheung M, Ho P, et al. In vitro-matured rat oocytes have low mitochondrial deoxyribonucleic acid and adenosine triphosphate contents and have abnormal mitochondrial distributions. Fertil Steril. 2008;91:900–7.
26. May-Panloup P, Chretien M-F, Savagner F, Vasseur C, et al. Increased sperm mitochondrial DNA content in male infertility. Hum Reprod. 2003;18:550–6.
27. Van Blerkom J, Runner M. Mitochondrial reorganization during the resumption of arrested meiosis in the mouse oocyte. Am J Anat. 1985;171:335–55.
28. Tokura T, Noda Y, Goto Y, Mori T. Sequential observations of mitochondrial distribution in mouse oocytes and embryos. J Assist Reprod Genet. 1993;10:417–26.
29. Song GJ, Lewis V. Mitochondrial DNA integrity and copy number in sperm from infertile men. Fertil Steril. 2008;90(6):2238–44.
30. Wang Q, Ratchford A, Chi M, Schoeller E, et al. Maternal diabetes causes mitochondrial dysfunction and meiotic defects in murine oocytes. Mol Endocrinol. 2009;10:1603–12.
31. Wang Q, Moley K. Maternal diabetes and oocyte quality. Mitochondrion. 2010;10(5):403–10.
32. Van Blerkom J. Microtubule mediation of cytoplasmic and nuclear maturation during the early stages of resumed meiosis in cultured mouse oocytes. Proc Natl Acad Sci U S A. 1991;88:5031–5.
33. Keefe D, Niven-Fairchild T, Powell M, Buradagunta A. Mitochondrial deoxyribonucleic acid deletions in oocytes and reproductive aging in women. Fertil Steril. 1995;64:577–83.
34. Gibson T, Kubisch H, Brenner C. Mitochondrial DNA deletions in rhesus macaque oocytes. Mol Hum Reprod. 2005;11:785–9.
35. Van Blerkom J. The enigma of fragmentation in early human embryos: possible causes and clinical relevance. In: Van Blerkom J, Gregory L, editors. Essential IVF. Boston: Kluwer Academic Publishers; 2004. p. 377–422.
36. Barrit J, Kokot M, Cohen J, Steuerwald N, Brenner C. Quantification of human ooplasmic mitochondria. Reprod Biomed Online. 2002;4:243–7.
37. Stojkovic M, Machado S, Sktojkovick P, Zakhartchenko V, et al. Mitochondrial distribution and adenosine triphosphate content of bovine oocytes before and after in vitro maturation: correlation with morphological criteria and developmental capacity after in vitro fertilization and culture. Biol Reprod. 2001;64:904–9.
38. Tamassia M, Nuttinck F, May-Panloup P, Reynier P, et al. In vitro embryo production efficiency in cattle and its association with oocyte adenosine triphosphate content, quantity of mitochondria DNA, and mitochondrial DNA haplogroup. Biol Reprod. 2004;71:697–704.
39. Chiaratti MR, Meirelles FV. Mitochondrial DNA copy number, a marker of viability for oocytes. Biol Reprod. 2010;83(1):1–2.
40. Wai T, Ao A, Zhang X, Cry D, et al. The role of mitochondrial DNA copy number in mammalian fertility. Biol Reprod. 2010;83(1):52–62.
41. Majno G, Joris I. Apoptosis, oncosis, and necrosis: an overview of cell death. Am J Pathol. 1995;146:3–15.
42. Van Blerkom J, Davis P, Alexander S. A microscopic and biochemical study of fragmentation in stage-appropriate human embryos. Hum Reprod. 2001;16:719–29.
43. Van Blerkom J, Davis P, Alexander S. Differential mitochondrial inheritance between blastomeres in cleavage stage human embryos: determination at the pronuclear stage and relationship to micotubular organization, ATP content and developmental competence. Hum Reprod. 2000;15:2621–33.
44. Antczak M, Van Blerkom J. Temporal and spatial aspects of fragmentation in early human embryos: possible effects on developmental competence and association with the differential elimination of regulatory proteins from polarized domains. Hum Reprod. 1999;14(2):429–47.
45. Van Blerkom J, Davis P. DNA strand breaks and phosphatidylserine redistribution in newly ovulated and cultured mouse and human oocytes: occurrence and relationship to apoptosis. Hum Reprod. 1998;13:1317–24.

46. Aw T-Y. Intracellular compartmentalization of organelles and gradients of low molecular weight species. Int Rev Cytol. 2000;192:223–53.
47. Diaz G, Setzu H, Zucca A, Isola R, Diana M, et al. Subcellular heterogeneity of mitochondrial membrane potential: relationship with organelle distribution and intercellular contacts in normal, hypoxic and apoptotic cells. J Cell Sci. 1999;112:1077–84.
48. Van Blerkom J, Davis P, Mawhig V, Alexander S. Domains of high and low polarized mitochondria in mouse and human oocytes and early embryos. Hum Reprod. 2002;17:393–406.
49. Bavister B, Squirrell J. Mitochondrial distribution and function in oocytes and early embryos. Hum Reprod. 2000;15 Suppl 2:189–98.
50. Van Blerkom J, Davis P. High-polarized (DYmHIGH) mitochondria are spatially polarized in human oocytes and early embryos in stable subplasmalemmal domains: developmental significance and the concept of vanguard mitochondria. Reprod Biomed Online. 2006;13:246–54.
51. Jones A, Van Blerkom, Davis P, Toledo A. Cryopreservation of metaphase II human oocytes effects mitochondrial inner membrane potential: implications for developmental competence. Hum Reprod. 2004;19:1861–6.
52. Van Blerkom J, Davis JP, Merriam J, Sinclair J. Nuclear and cytoplasmic dynamics of sperm penetration, pronuclear formation, and microtubule organization during fertilization and early preimplantation development in the human. Hum Reprod Update. 1995;1:429–61.
53. Ozil J-P, Huneau D. Activation of rabbit oocytes: the impact of the Ca2+ signal regime on development. Development. 2001;128:917–28.
54. Ichas F, Jouaville L, Mazat J-P. Mitochondria are excitable organelles capable of generating and conveying electrical and calcium signals. Cell. 1997;89:1145–53.
55. Nassar A, Simpson W. Elevation of mitochondrial calcium by ryanodine-sensitive calcium-induced calcium release. J Biol Chem. 2000;275:23661–5.
56. Schuster S, Marhl M, Hofer T. Modeling of simple and complex calcium oscillations: from single cell to intercellular signalling. Eur J Biochem. 2002;269:1333–55.
57. Huang X, Zhai D, Huang Y. Study on the relationship between calcium-induced calcium release from mitochondria and PTP opening. Mol Cell Biochem. 2000;213:29–35.
58. Brown G. Control of respiration and ATP synthesis in mammalian mitochondria and cells. Biochem J. 1992;284:1–13.
59. Dumollard R, Hammar K, Porterfield M, et al. Mitochondrial respiration and Ca2+ waves are linked during fertilisation and meiosis completion. Development. 2003;130:683–92.
60. Van Blerkom J, Davis P, Alexander S. Inner mitochondrial membrane potential, cytoplasmic ATP content and free calcium levels in metaphase II mouse oocytes. Hum Reprod. 2003;18(2003):2429–40.
61. Cao X, Chen Y. Mitochondria and calcium signaling in embryonic development. Semin Cell Dev Biol. 2009;230:337–45.
62. Tesarik J, Sousa M, Testart J. Human oocyte activation after intracytoplasmic sperm injection. Hum Reprod. 1994;9:511–8.
63. Nakano Y, Shirakawa H, Mitsuhhashi N, Kuwabara Y, Miyazaki S. Spatiotemporal dynamics of intracellular calcium in the mouse egg injected with a spermatozoon. Mol Hum Reprod. 1997;3:1087–93.
64. Sathananthan AH. Paternal centrosomal dynamics in early human development and infertility. J Assist Reprod Genet. 1998;15(3):129–39.
65. Nottola S, Macchiarelli G, Coticchio G, Bianchi S, et al. Ultrastructure of human mature oocytes after slow cooling cryopreservation using different sucrose concentrations. Hum Reprod. 2007;22:1123–33.
66. Coticchio G, Borini A, Distratis V, Maione M, et al. Qualitative and morphometric analysis of the ultrastructure of human oocytes cryopreserved by two alterative slow cooling protocols. J Assist Reprod Genet. 2010;27:131–40.
67. Van Blerkom J, Henry G. Oocyte dysmorphism and aneuploidy in meiotically mature human oocytes after controlled ovarian stimulation. Hum Reprod. 1992;7:379–90.
68. Payne D, Flaherty SP, Barry MF, Matthews CD. Preliminary observations on polar body extrusion and pronuclear formation in human oocytes using time-lapse video cinematography. Hum Reprod. 1997;12(3):532–41.

69. Van Blerkom J, Davis P, Merriam J. A retrospective analysis of unfertilized and presumed parthenogenetically activated human oocytes demonstrated a high frequency of sperm penetration. Hum Reprod. 1994;9:2381–8.
70. Meriano J, Alexis J, Visram-Zaver J, et al. Tracking of oocyte dysmorphisms for ICSI patients may prove relevant to outcome in subsequent patient cycles. Hum Reprod. 2001;16:2118–23.
71. Otsuki J, Okada K, Morimoto Y, et al. The relationship between pregnancy outcome and smooth endoplasmic reticulum clusters in MII human oocytes. Hum Reprod. 2004;19:1591–7.
72. Balaban B, et al. Alpha scientists in reproductive medicine and ESHRE special interest group of embryology. The Istanbul consensus workshop on embryo assessment: proceedings of an expert meeting. Hum Reprod. 2011;26:1270–83.
73. Lebiedzinska M, Szabadkai G, Jones A, et al. Interactions between the endoplasmic reticulum, mitochondria, plasma membrane and other subcellular organelles. Int J Biochem Cell Biol. 2009;41:1805–16.
74. Klymkowsky M. Mitochondrial activity, embryogenesis, and the dialogue between the big and little brains of the cell. Mitochondrion. 2011;11(5):814–9.
75. Sathananthan AH, Trounson A, Freemann L, Brady T. The effects of cooling human oocytes. Hum Reprod. 1988;3(8):968–77.
76. Coffman J, McCarthy J, Dickey-Sims C, Roberston A. Oral-aboral axis specification in the sea urchin embryo II. Mitochondrial distribution and redox state contribute to establishing polarity in Stongylocentrous purpuratus. Dev Biol. 2004;273:160–71.
77. Coffman J. Mitochondria and metazoan epigenesis. Semin Cell Dev Biol. 2009;20:321–9.
78. Simon A, Rai U, Fanburg D, Cochran B. Activation of the JAK-STAT pathway by reactive oxygen species. Am J Physiol. 1998;275:C1640–52.
79. Zhang X, Wu X, Lu S, Guo Y, Ma X. Deficit of mitochondria-derived ATP during oxidative stress impairs mouse MII oocyte spindles. Cell Res. 2006;16:841–50.
80. Eichenlaub-Ritter U, Vogt E, Yin H, Gosden R. Spindles, microtubules and redox potential in ageing oocytes. Reprod Biomed Online. 2004;8(2004):45–58.
81. Eichenlaub-Ritter U, Wieczorek M, Seidel T. Age related changes in mitochondrial function and new approaches to study redox regulation in mammalian oocytes in response to age or maturation conditions. Mitochondrion. 2011;11(5):783–96.
82. Squirrell R, Schramm PD, Wokosin L, Bavister B. Imaging mitochondrial organization in living primate oocytes and embryos using multiphoton microscopy. Microsc Microanal. 2003;9:190–201.
83. Katayama M, Zhong Z, Kasi L, et al. Mitochondrial distribution and microtubular organization in fertilized and cloned porcine embryos: implications for developmental potential. Dev Biol. 2006;299:206–20.
84. Reers M, Smiley S, Mottola-Hartshorn C, et al. Mitochondrial membrane potential monitored by JC-1 dye. Methods Enzymol. 1995;260:406–17.
85. Lemasters J, Ramshesh V. Imaging of mitochondrial polarization and depolarization with cationic fluorophores. Methods Cell Biol. 2007;80:283–95.
86. Van Blerkom J, Davis P. Mitochondrial signaling and fertilization. Mol Hum Reprod. 2007;13:759–70.
87. Wilding M, Dale B, Marino M, di Matteo L. Mitochondrial segation patterns and activity in human oocytes and preimplantation embryos. Hum Reprod. 2001;16:909–17.
88. Dumollard R, Carroll K, Duchen M, Campbell K, Swann K. Mitochondrial function and redox state in mammalian embryos. Semin Cell Dev Biol. 2009;20:346–53.
89. Liu Y, Liu S, Wang Y. TEMPO-based redox sensitive fluorescent probes and their applications to evaluate intracellular redox status in living cells. Chem Lett. 2009;38:588–9.
90. Devreker F. Uptake and release of metabolites in human preimplantation embryos. In: Elder K, Cohen J, editors. Human preimplantation embryo selection. Boca Raton: Informa Healthcare; 2007. p. 179–89.

Chapter 25
Nuclear and Cytoplasmic Transfer: Human Applications and Concerns

Josef Fulka Jr. and Helena Fulka

Characteristics of Mammalian Oocytes

Mammalian oocytes are fascinating cells, and their relative big size makes them very convenient for different manipulations. In laboratory animals and also in ungulates, they can be obtained easily in sufficient number (e.g., from the slaughterhouse material). On the other hand, human oocytes are very rare. In humans, the collected oocytes are almost exclusively used for the production of test tube embryos and babies, and only minimum of IVF centers use spare oocytes for different micromanipulations, aiming to find and improve some approaches that can be used for some specific patients. Unfortunately, not all oocytes collected are morphologically and physiologically normal. When working with laboratory animals or ungulates and oocytes from a given collection are not good, we can simply discard them saying that the next collection will certainly be better. Logically, the situation in humans is completely different, and it is not so easy to discard those oocytes that are not absolutely perfect, especially in those patients where this situation is repeatedly observed. Thus, in such difficult situations the micromanipulation approaches might represent a solution. However, if we want to manipulate abnormal human oocytes we need also some normal oocytes from healthy donors. Another important aspect is that we still do not know if babies from manipulated oocytes will be absolutely normal as long-term follow-up studies are often not available. Because some very recent articles discussed the manipulations of mammalian oocytes and 1-cell stage embryos in detail in our contribution, we will outline briefly, from a general point of view, the micromanipulation possibilities that can be applied almost immediately in human-assisted reproduction [1, 2].

J. Fulka Jr., PhD (✉) • H. Fulka, PhD
Department of Biology of Reproduction, Institute of Animal Science, Prague, Czech Republic
e-mail: fulka.josef@vuzv.cz

General Morphology

The size of mammalian oocytes ranges from about 80 (mouse) to 120 μm (human, cattle, pig), so they are relatively large. But even in this case, they cannot be simply manipulated by hand. Therefore, good equipment is absolutely essential. In human-assisted reproduction, the oocytes are almost exclusively collected as mature, i.e., in metaphase II stage when they can be used directly for fertilization. However, in general, the oocytes can be collected at different stages of maturation: either as immature with intact nucleus—germinal vesicle (GV), maturing with condensed chromosomes (metaphase I)—or mature (metaphase II). The choice of maturation stage for further manipulation clearly depends on the problem that needs to be addressed.

Immature oocytes contain the GV (nucleus) that is easily visible in rodent or human oocytes. The most prominent organelle that is visible in GVs is the nucleolus. In fully maturation competent oocytes, the nucleolus is surrounded with a ring of chromatin (SN—surrounded nucleolus). On the other hand, in oocytes that are less or even not competent to mature, the chromatin is dispersed within the GV (NSN—nonsurrounded nucleolus) [3]. The oocytes are enclosed with zona pellucida and several layers of cumulus cells.

After an endogenous (exogenous) gonadotropin surge or when released from follicles and cultured under appropriate conditions, the oocytes begin to mature. Their nuclear envelope disassembles (germinal vesicle breakdown—GVBD); chromosomes condense and become gradually arranged in metaphase I. These processes are followed by a very short anaphase to telophase I transition, and the oocytes are thereafter arrested in metaphase II [4]. Two essential points must be mentioned here. First, the oocytes matured in vitro are not as good as those oocytes where this process underwent in vivo; therefore, in vitro matured oocytes usually have a lower developmental potential. Second, if we want to manipulate immature oocytes, we must remove their surrounding cumulus cells. This will even further decrease their developmental potential after fertilization [5]. However, when we need to solve, for example, the problem of absolute oocyte maturation arrest, i.e., the oocytes are unable to undergo GVBD, and we suspect that it is the cytoplasm that is responsible for this arrest, there is no other choice than to use these immature oocytes.

On the other hand, if oocytes are unable to undergo metaphase I to telophase I transition or when we suspect that their cytoplasm influences normal segregation of chromosomes (leading to aneuploidies) we can collect these oocytes from follicles at this stage (MI or shortly before). This later collection might be beneficial because the period of GVBD is essential for an establishment of oocyte developmental competence, and we may suppose that these oocytes are as good as those oocytes maturing completely in follicles. Logically, from the oocyte developmental competence point of view, best for manipulations are MII oocytes that matured completely in vivo.

Oocyte Maturation: Chromatin Modifications

As outlined above, the timing of oocyte collection might influence negatively their developmental potential. Although this might be caused by a variety of different factors and the effect of oocyte collection timing is extremely complex, it has been convincingly shown that the oocyte collection timing might influence the epigenetic status of oocytes.

The process of oocyte maturation is very dynamic from many aspects (cell cycle, distribution of organelles, etc.). This is certainly also true for different chromatin modifications. Even though the epigenetic regulation of chromatin is very complex, in this section, we will focus mainly on histone acetylation as there is growing evidence indicating that the acetylation/deacetylation processes are in a close correlation with oocyte aneuploidies. In general, when probed for acetylation at different lysine residues within histones (H3/K9, H4/K12, H4/K5, etc.), it is evident that histones are highly acetylated in GV-stage oocytes. However, as soon as GVBD occurs and chromosomes condense, the labeling signal disappears, indicating that the process of chromosome condensation is associated with histone deacetylation. During the anaphase to telophase I transition, a weak signal on chromosomes can be observed again, but at metaphase II, no labeling can be detected [6, 7]. Interestingly, if the acetylation persisted during the process of oocyte maturation, an increased number of oocytes (embryos) had chromosomal abnormalities [8]. It is also apparent that aged oocyte chromatin becomes also gradually aberrantly acetylated and in agreement with this, oocytes from older females tend to exhibit more aneuploidies than oocytes from younger females. It is commonly accepted that it is the abnormal oocyte cytoplasm that is unable to deacetylate the condensing chromatin, indicating that histone deacetylases (HDACs) are either present in insufficient quantities or are aberrantly regulated. In contrast to histone acetylation, the histone methylation pattern remains rather constant during the whole process of maturation [9]. As we mentioned above, these results were mostly obtained in the mouse, and thus, some minor differences can be expected when analyzing the oocytes from other species. To summarize, a link between the cytoplasm quality and/or oocyte collection scheme and epigenetic status of oocytes has been established; in turn, the epigenetic competence of oocytes might influence the frequency of aneuploidies. Thus, the micromanipulation techniques might solve the problem of poor oocyte cytoplasm quality; however, care should be taken when performing the oocyte collection and especially a correct timing is necessary.

Technical Aspects

Necessary Equipment

Some very recent articles describe in detail the necessary equipment, media, steps, and settings of manipulation chambers when different oocyte or embryo manipulations are performed. For this reason, we will not discuss here exhaustively everything what is necessary. Essentially, every IVF lab performing the ICSI has the very basic equipment necessary for nuclear or cytoplasmic transfer—this means the inverted microscope with manipulators and injectors and, logically, also some stereomicroscopes and incubators. To perform more sophisticated manipulations, some additional instruments are however necessary. According to our opinion, the most important is the electrofusion machine because the diameter of nuclear material (either GVs or chromosomes) is rather large and it cannot be simply injected into the host cytoplast without damage. Thus, in this case, the induced fusion between the nuclear material (karyoplast) and recipient cytoplast (cytoplast - the oocyte or zygote from which its nuclear material has been removed, enucleation) is recommended. For the visualization of chromosome groups, the PolScope optics seems to be very useful. The holding pipettes can be purchased from different companies. The injection pipettes can also be purchased, but it is our experience that it is much better if they are made directly by the person performing the manipulation. In this case, the pipette puller and microforge are necessary [1]. We strongly recommend some training with mouse or ungulate oocytes. Moreover, it is absolutely essential to study some manuals dealing with basic oocyte and embryo culture procedures and manipulations [10].

Brief Outline of Manipulation Methods

In general, and as mentioned above, the various manipulation schemes do not differ substantially from ICSI. What is however different, if we want to manipulate GVs or metaphase groups, is the composition of manipulation medium that must contain cytochalasin B (or D) to avoid the damage of biological material. However, the CB (D) is omitted from fusion media. Again, some excellent protocols describe in detail what to do and how to perform different manipulations [1, 11–13]. Logically, these protocols must be slightly modified depending on the origin of cells used and the type of manipulation. Essentially, this however only means to modify the diameter of injection pipette and possibly the fusion parameters.

Problems That Can Be Solved with Nuclear and Cytoplasmic Transfer

Possible Nuclear Transfer Combinations

In theory, the manipulation of mammalian oocytes can solve some serious problems, i.e., the inability of oocytes to begin to mature, metaphase I or metaphase II arrests, or the inability of oocytes to transform the injected sperm head into a paternal pronucleus [14]. In all those cases, we can expect that the oocyte cytoplasm is abnormal and this means to transfer the nuclear material from an abnormal cytoplasm into a normal cytoplasm from which its own nuclear material has been removed previously (cytoplast). It is also speculated that the transfer of nuclear material from the cytoplasm which is unable to induce histone deacetylation will eliminate the possible abnormal chromosome segregation, leading to prevention of aneuploidies.

It is technically relatively simple to remove the nuclear material from evidently morphologically abnormal oocytes and to transfer it into the cytoplasm that is normal. Although technically simple, this procedure might bring some serious concerns. The most often discussed method is the transfer of nuclear material from oocytes with mutated mitochondrial DNA (mtDNA) into the cytoplasts with normal mtDNA. In the next section, we will discuss the possible combinations of karyoplast-cytoplast transfer. Clearly, the choice of the combination used in the micromanipulation scheme largely depends on the problem that needs to be solved [15].

Immature Oocytes: GV Transfer

In assisted human reproduction the oocytes are mostly collected as mature—metaphase II staged—where they can be used immediately for fertilization. However, mammalian oocytes can be collected from follicles as immature (GV staged) and matured in vitro. The same is true for human oocytes. The main disadvantage is that the quality of in vitro matured oocytes is much lower when compared to oocytes matured in follicles. If we want to manipulate immature oocytes, we must free them from enclosing cumulus cells. This will further decrease their developmental potential after fertilization. It must be noted that in almost all cases mentioned below, the nuclear material is transferred into a recipient cytoplasm in the form of so-called karyoplast. This means that the isolated nucleus (chromosomes) is enclosed with a minimum volume of original cytoplasm enclosed with the plasma membrane. The oocytes without the nuclear material are called "cytoplasts."

Applications:

– Elimination of mutated mtDNA. This means that the GV is isolated from the cytoplasm containing mutated mtDNA and transferred under the zona pellucida of another oocyte that was enucleated previously and contains normal mtDNA. The introduction of GVs into cytoplasts is typically induced by electrofusion.

The reconstructed oocytes are then cultured in vitro until they reach metaphase II stage when they are fertilized. The question that remains is how to eliminate the residual karyoplast mitochondria.

- Maturation arrest. Exceptionally, the collected oocytes are immature even after hCG stimulation and they do not undergo GVBD in culture. We may suppose that their cytoplasm is defected and unable to produce some essential cell cycle regulation factor. In theory, this problem can be solved by transferring GVs from oocytes with defective cytoplasm into cytoplasm (cytoplasts) obtained by enucleation of normal oocytes. The reconstructed oocytes will be then matured in vitro. Possibly, the isolated GVs could be transferred into more maturation advanced cytoplasts, i.e., obtained by enucleation of oocytes undergoing GVBD but before the exit from MI. Under the influence of cytoplast's chromosome condensation activity (CCA), GVBD will be induced and chromosomes will condense and subsequently reach MII stage. However, it must be noted that transfer of less developmentally competent GVs with chromatin nonsurrounded nucleoli (NSN) will not increase developmental competence of reconstructed oocytes.
- Elimination of aneuploidies. The percentage of aneuploidies increases with the age of patients. Thus, it has been originally suggested that transfer of GVs from "old" oocytes into "young" oocyte cytoplasm will eliminate this problem. Experiments in the mouse however did not support this presumption.
- Repairing evidently defected oocytes. The gross morphology of some collected oocytes is sometimes evidently abnormal (e.g., their cytoplasm is not homogenous). Logically, even if these oocytes are able to mature, we cannot expect that further embryonic development will be normal. Theoretically, healthy-looking oocytes can be produced by GV transfer.

Above, we have mentioned some possible applications of GV transfer. Technically, and of course with some experience, this approach is rather simple. GVs can be located in the cytoplasm very easily without special optics (mouse, human). Moreover, GV karyoplasts can be efficiently stored in liquid nitrogen and used later on if, for example, the recipient cytoplasts are not available at the same time [16]. The main disadvantage is the fragility of immature oocytes. However, the reconstructed oocytes mature well in culture and even some offspring were obtained in the mouse. At the same time, we must bear in mind that the period of GVBD seems to be very important for very early postfertilization steps—e.g., it has been shown to be important for the demethylation of paternal DNA—and it remains to be determined how and to what extent the embryonic development and normality of offspring will be influenced if GV transfer schemes are used to produce offspring.

Maturing Oocytes

The oocytes undergoing GVBD and not yet achieving the metaphase II stage are designated as "maturing." Saying simply, these oocytes can be either at prometaphase, metaphase I, anaphase I, or telophase I. Anaphase and telophase I stages are rather short, and for this reason, their manipulations will not be discussed here. The maturing oocytes can be obtained either from stimulated follicles (i.e., in humans after approximately 20 h post-hCG) or possibly when oocytes are cultured in vitro, again after approximately 20 h postinitiation of culture. Because in this case the oocytes underwent GVBD in follicles, their quality is much higher when compared to completely in vitro matured oocytes and is essentially the same when compared to completely in vivo matured oocytes. Another important point is that the absence of cumulus cells that must be removed prior to manipulation has a minimum influence on final stages of oocyte maturation. Compared to immature oocytes, the maturing oocytes are refractory to damage. The main disadvantage is a very poor visibility of chromosome groups. This problem can be overcome, for example, when oocytes are stained with some vital DNA stains (Hoechst) and then irradiated with UV light. In human-assisted reproduction, we recommend the use of PolScope optics enabling the visualization of spindles without UV.

Applications:

- In theory, the elimination of abnormal segregation of chromosomes during the anaphase to telophase I transition due to the inability of the original oocyte cytoplasm to deacetylate histones
- To overcome the possible metaphase I arrest

It is our opinion that this approach will be used only exceptionally (i.e., to overcome metaphase I arrest). Its further use and possible justification needs additional studies not only in laboratory animals and ungulates. For example, it is critical to analyze the histone deacetylation processes in human oocytes and if the proper deacetylation can be indeed induced by transferring the chromosomes into appropriate cytoplasts.

Mature Oocytes

As mentioned above, human oocytes are mostly collected as mature, i.e., metaphase II staged. Logically, their maturation in follicles secures their best quality, although we cannot exclude that an abnormal follicular environment (hormone levels) especially in older patients is responsible for a compromised oocyte quality and the incidence of oocyte aneuploidies. As for MI, the mature oocytes (MII) are refractory to damage. Essentially, the manipulation of these oocytes is very similar to MI oocyte manipulation.

Applications:

- Elimination of mutated mtDNA by isolating metaphase II chromosome group from the cytoplasm with mutated mtDNA and its transfer into cytoplasts with normal mtDNA. This can be either done by electrofusion of karyoplasts with cytoplasts or by direct injection of a spindle with chromosomes into the cytoplast. The spindle isolation and reinjection, however, requires considerable manipulation skill as the cytoplast can be easily destroyed. On the other, the isolated spindle contains only a minimum of mitochondria (possibly with mutated DNA).
- Overcoming the metaphase II arrest. In some rare cases, the mature oocytes are not activated by fertilizing (injected) sperm for unknown reasons (not globozoospermia). If the cytoplasm is responsible for this aberrant behavior, then in theory, this problem can be solved by transferring the MII group into normal cytoplasts.
- Eventually, if ovulated oocytes are evidently morphologically abnormal, their metaphases II can be transferred into cytoplasts obtained by enucleation of high-quality mature oocytes.

The main advantage of MII oocyte manipulation is that oocytes at this stage are generally more available. The main problem is that they can be easily activated parthenogenetically, especially when they are aged. This can be eliminated by omitting calcium from the manipulation media. It must be also tested if MII karyoplasts can be stored in culture or in liquid nitrogen without considerable damage and used for transfer after thawing.

Zygotes

In fact, the transfer (exchange) of pronuclei (PNs) between mouse zygotes was the first approach demonstrating the power of micromanipulation methods [17]. From a technical point of view, it is almost similar to GV-stage oocyte manipulation. The only difference is that PNs-staged embryos are very resistant to damage and PNs karyoplasts fuse very efficiently to cytoplasts when electrofusion is used (when compared to GV karyoplasts × GV cytoplasts fusion). There is, however, one very serious ethical aspect when we consider the use of this approach in humans. For pronuclear transfer, we need the same developmental stage cytoplasts, i.e., 1-cell-stage embryos from which their own pronuclei will be removed. This actually means the destruction of the recipient embryo (possibly this might be considered by some people as to be "a new life"). This problem can be eventually overcome by transferring both pronuclei into cytoplast prepared from parthenogenetic zygotes. It is, however, our opinion that this combination will not be widely used in human ART.

Cytoplasmic Transfer

The cytoplasmic transfer in human-assisted reproduction has been pioneered by Barritt and his coworkers [18]. The primary aim was to improve developmental potential of oocytes which were evidently morphologically abnormal and to enhance their developmental potential after fertilization. Thus, a certain volume of cytoplasm from healthy oocytes has been injected into abnormal oocytes either separately or along with the fertilizing sperm. This procedure led to the production of several children, some of them with mitochondrial heteroplasmy (a situation when two or more distinct mitochondrial populations coexist within one cell). This clearly demonstrates that the injected volume of healthy cytoplasm transferred cannot secure the elimination of mutated mtDNA in the patient's oocyte. Furthermore, relatively high incidence of chromosomal abnormalities and certain birth defects led to the ban of this technique in ART.

Transfer of Organelles

Mammalian oocytes, as nearly every cell, contain many organelles, but their separate transfer or the exchange between oocytes is very difficult because they are practically invisible. The only exception is the nucleolus (nucleolus precursor body—NPB) which is well visible, for example, in human and mouse GV-staged oocytes. At this stage, typically only one nucleolus can be observed in the GV. On the other hand, pronuclei in human zygotes contain several nucleoli and this, of course, complicates their manipulation. The nucleolus becomes disassembled concomitantly with GVBD, so it cannot be detected in maturing or mature oocytes, and the nucleolar material is dispersed largely in the cytoplasm. It becomes visible again after chromosomes decondense and pronuclei are formed. In humans, it has been convincingly demonstrated that the number, distribution, and position of nucleoli can serve as an indicator of further embryonic development [19]. This brings a question whether nucleoli can be eventually transferred into zygotes with abnormal nucleolar pattern, with the aim to enhance their developmental potential [20].

The nucleolus can be relatively easily removed (enucleolation) from GVs of fully grown mouse oocytes. Similarly, mononucleolar mouse pronuclei can also be enucleolated. The oocytes or embryos without nucleoli do not develop but when the nucleolar material is reinjected into previously enucleolated oocytes (zygotes), their developmental potential is restored [21]. Interestingly, when the nucleolus is injected into an interphase cytoplasm, it is rapidly targeted into nuclei. This significantly simplifies the whole possible nucleolus transfer procedure. The nucleolus, however, is not a separated entity residing in nuclei. As we already mentioned, the close association of chromatin and nucleolus (surrounded nucleolus) is a good marker of oocyte maturation competence. This association can be also observed in zygotes. It remains to be answered if the same or equivalent association will be established after the transfer of nucleolar material and how important is this association for complete embryonic development.

Future Implications and Concerns

The aim of this chapter was not to review exhaustively the field of oocyte and embryo manipulation methods. This has been done beautifully in some recent articles and book chapters [11–13]. Thus, we rather wanted to navigate the scientists and clinicians in this field and highlight especially those articles where relevant manipulations are described in depth. Essentially, these methodological articles deal mostly with mouse oocytes and embryos but in general, the same can be performed, of course, with some minor modifications, also in human oocytes and embryos. As we mentioned above, we strongly recommend good training with laboratory animals and ungulate oocytes. From the technical point of view, the basic micromanipulation approaches are simple and they only need some skill. On the other hand, there are some important questions that need to be answered before these methods can be used in human-assisted reproduction. The key question is: how safe are these approaches? The fragmentary information we have mostly from animal experiments is clearly insufficient. However, for example, Takeuchi et al. reported a higher incidence of abnormalities in mouse offspring originating from GV transfer oocytes [22]. It is, on the other hand, well known that the mouse is very sensitive to different manipulations and culture conditions. Similarly, the increased incidence of chromosomal abnormalities and epigenetic defects has been observed in children from oocytes injected with foreign cytoplasm. Was this the effect of cytoplasmic injection, or was this the main reason that the injected oocytes were rather abnormal? Clearly, some additional experiments with the evaluation of offspring born are necessary here. In conclusion, the recent article by Tachibana et al. [23] where metaphase II chromosomes from the cytoplasm containing mutated mtDNA were transferred into cytoplasts with normal mtDNA with two healthy offspring obtained clearly demonstrate the power of micromanipulation approaches and the area of their possible clinical application in future. The first step we can find, according to our opinion, in the paper published by Craven et al. [24], is demonstrating the feasibility of pronuclear transfer in human zygotes and describing how the reconstructed zygotes further develop in culture.

Acknowledgment JFJr's lab is supported by MZE 0002701404.

References

1. Fulka H, Fulka Jr J. The use of micromanipulation methods as a tool to prevention of transmission of mutated mitochondrial DNA. Curr Top Dev Biol. 2007;77:187–211.
2. Fulka H, Langerova A, Barnetova I, et al. How to repair the oocyte and zygote? J Reprod Dev. 2009;55:583–7.
3. Tan JH, Wang HL, Sun XS, et al. Chromatin configurations in the germinal vesicle of mammalian oocytes. Mol Hum Reprod. 2009;15:1–9.
4. Trounson AO, Anderiesz C, Jones C. Maturation of human oocytes in vitro and their developmental potential. Reproduction. 2001;121:51–75.

5. Gioia L, Barboni B, Turriani M, et al. The capability of reprogramming the male chromatin after fertilization is dependent on the quality of oocyte maturation. Reproduction. 2005;130:29–39.
6. Fulka H. Changes in global histone acetylation pattern in somatic cell nuclei after their transfer into oocytes at different stages of maturation. Mol Reprod Dev. 2007;75:556–64.
7. Kim JM, Aoki F. Mechanism of gene expression reprogramming during meiotic maturation and pre-implantation development. J Mamm Ova Res. 2004;21:89–96.
8. Akiyama T, Nagata M, Aoki F. Inadequate histone deacetylation during oocyte meiosis causes aneuploidy and embryo death in mice. PNAS USA. 2006;103:7339–44.
9. Liu H, Kim JM, Aoki F. Regulation of histone H3 lysine 9 methylation in oocytes and early pre-implantation. Development. 2004;131:2269–80.
10. Hogan B, Beddington R, Constantini F, et al. Manipulating the mouse embryo: a laboratory manual. 2nd ed. New York: Cold Spring Harbor Laboratory Press; 1994. p. 497.
11. Kishigami S, Wakayama S, Thuan NV, et al. Production of cloned mice by somatic cell nuclear transfer. Nat Protoc. 2006;1: 125–38.
12. Yoshida N, Perry ACF. Piezo-actuated mouse intracytoplasmic sperm injection (ICSI). Nat Protoc. 2007;2:269–304.
13. Kawahara M, Obata Y, Sotomaru Y, et al. Protocol for the production of viable bimaternal mouse embryos. Nat Protoc. 2008;3:197–209.
14. Mrazek M, Fulka Jr J. Failure of oocyte maturation: possible mechanisms for oocyte maturation arrest. Hum Reprod. 2003;18: 2249–52.
15. Fulka Jr J, Mrazek M, Fulka H, et al. Mammalian oocyte therapies. Cloning Stem Cells. 2005;7:183–8.
16. Kren R, Fulka J, Fulka H. Cryopreservation of isolated mouse germinal vesicles. J Reprod Dev. 2005;51:289–92.
17. McGrath J, Solter D. Nuclear transplantation in the mouse by microsurgery and cell fusion. Science. 1983;220:1300–2.
18. Barritt A, Willadsen S, Brenner C, et al. Epigenetic and experimental modifications in early mammalian development: part II: cytoplasmic transfer in assisted reproduction. Hum Reprod Update. 2001;7:428–35.
19. Fulka H, Mrazek M, Fulka Jr J. Nucleolar dysfunction maybe associated with infertility in humans. Fert Steril. 2004;82:486–7.
20. Fulka H, Fulka Jr J. Nucleolar transplantation in oocytes and zygotes: challenges for further research. Mol Hum Reprod. 2010;16:63–7.
21. Ogushi S, Palmieri C, Fulka H, et al. The maternal nucleolus is essential for early embryonic development in mammals. Science. 2008;319:613–6.
22. Takeuchi T, Neri Q, Katagiri Y, et al. Effect of treating induced mitochondrial damage on embryonic development and epigenesis. Biol Reprod. 2005;72:584–92.
23. Tachibana M, Sparman M, Sritanaudomchai H, et al. Mitochondrial gene replacement in primate offspring and embryonic stem cells. Nature. 2009;461:367–72.
24. Craven L, Tuppen HA, Greggains GD, et al. Pronuclear transfer in human embryos to prevent transmission of mitochondrial DNA disease. Nature. 2010;465:82–5.

Chapter 26
Cytoskeletal Architecture of Human Oocytes with Focus on Centrosomes and Their Significant Role in Fertilization

Heide Schatten, Vanesa Y. Rawe, and Qing-Yuan Sun

In humans and most mammalian species, fertilization takes place at the MII stage (metaphase of second meiosis) in which oocytes are arrested after maturation. Oocyte quality is critically important for successful fertilization, and a variety of different criteria have been used to assess oocyte quality, although in many cases the reasons for fertilization failure remain unclear and cannot be determined based on presently available morphological and molecular/biochemical data (reviewed in ref. [1]). However, it is important to evaluate specific factors that are known to play a role in oocyte quality and affect successful fertilization. The most prominent structure of the MII oocyte is the MII spindle containing the maternal chromosomes aligned at the metaphase plate and connected to centrosomes at the opposite spindle poles by kinetochore microtubules (kMTs). Along with nucleation of kMTs from spindle pole centrosomes are pole-to-pole microtubules that are important for chromosome separation (Fig. 26.1). The integrity of the spindle fibers as well as centrosome integrity is an important criterion for oocyte quality as it reflects the general condition of the individual oocyte including oocyte aging that may occur during the process of IVF (reviewed in ref. [2]).

Spindle pole centrosomes contain numerous centrosome proteins that play a role in specific but also complex centrosome functions as will be detailed in the following sections. The sperm (Fig. 26.2), on the other hand, contains as prominent

---

H. Schatten, PhD (✉)
Department of Veterinary Pathobiology, University of Missouri-Columbia,
1600 E. Rollins Street, Columbia, MO 65211, USA
e-mail: SchattenH@missouri.edu

V.Y. Rawe, MSc, PhD
REPROTEC, Buenos Aires, Argentina

Q.-Y. Sun, PhD
State Key Laboratory of Reproductive Biology, Institute of Zoology,
Chincse Academy of Sciences, Chaoyang, Beijing, China

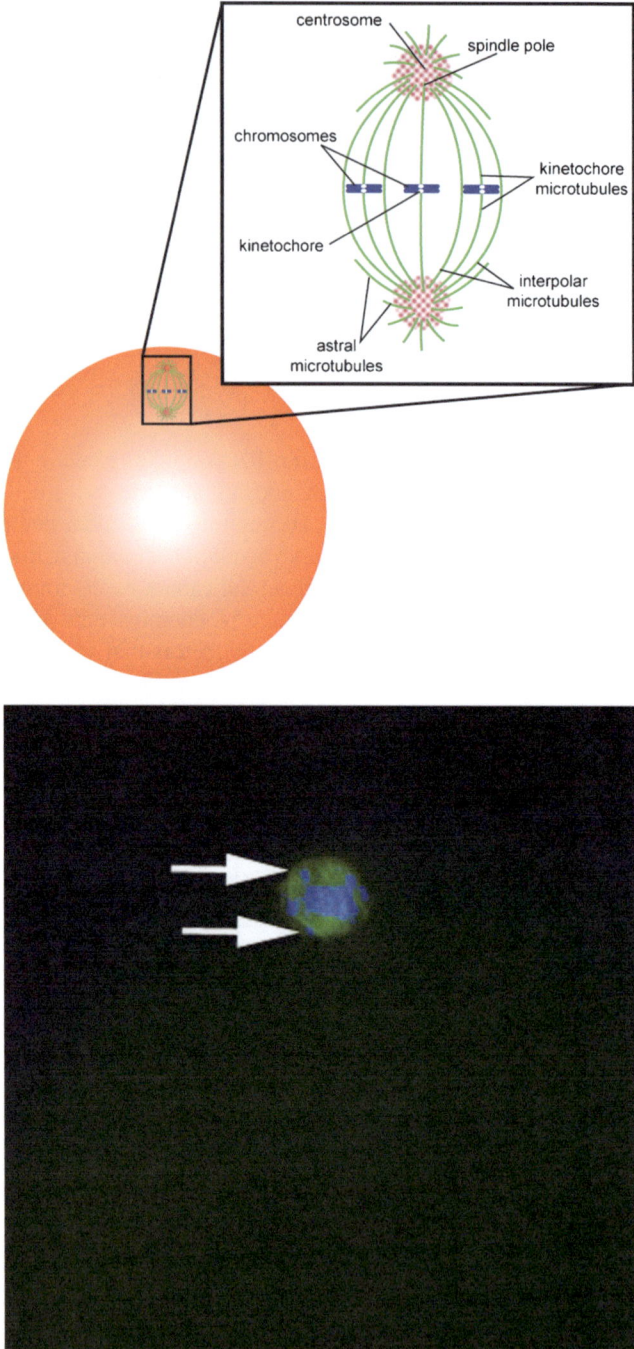

Fig. 26.1 Schematic diagram and immunocytochemistry of MII oocyte before fertilization. The MII spindle is organized from acentriolar centrosomes that nucleate kinetochore and pole-to-pole

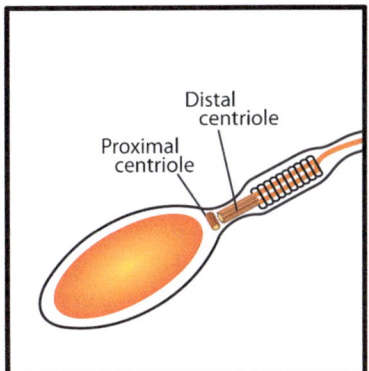 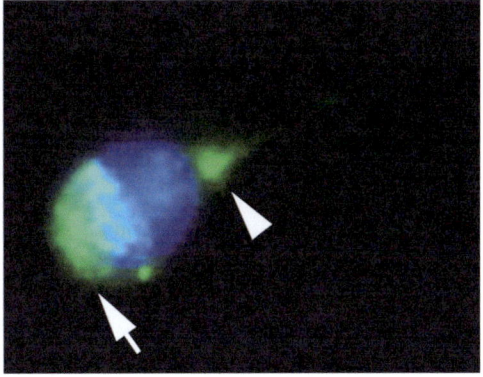

Fig. 26.2 The sperm in most mammalian species contains a proximal and a distal centriole; the proximal centriole is closely associated with the sperm nucleus and will serve as microtubule organizing center (MTOC) after fertilization while the distal centriole displays a degenerated microtubule organization and nucleates the axoneme in the sperm tail. A minimal amount of centrosomal material is associated with the sperm centrioles including gamma-tubulin and centrin. *Right panel* shows ejaculated human spermatozoa labeled with p31 antibody (against proteasome as described in text). Two populations of proteasomes can be observed on the ejaculated spermatozoa: in the acrosomal region (*arrow*) and in the sperm tail connecting piece (*arrowhead*). Release of a functional sperm centriole that acts as a zygotic microtubule-organizing center may rely on selective proteasomal proteolysis during sperm penetration, suggesting an important role of sperm proteasomes in zygotic development (from Rawe et al. [17], with permission)

microtubule cytoskeletal structure the sperm axoneme (sperm tail) and the basal body (a pair of centrioles), one of which (the proximal centriole) will be important for sperm aster formation after fertilization while the other (the distal centriole) is tightly connected to the sperm tail and serves as the nucleation material for the sperm axoneme as will be detailed below. The oocyte and sperm both contribute important cytoskeletal components that are critical for successful fertilization.

The following sections will review the centrosome and microtubule cytoskeletal organization in human oocytes and also in animal models including the pig and bovine models from post-maturation through fertilization and development to first cell division. It should be noted that while the mouse has been used for many genetic studies, it is not a useful model for cytoskeletal organization and fertilization as it differs enormously in many aspects compared to all other mammalian species and will not be included in the present chapter.

Fig. 26.1 (continued) microtubules that are regulated by a complex set of kinases to hold the MII spindle in shape and prevent deterioration. In most mammalian species, the MII spindle displays perpendicular organization to the egg cortex (parallel orientation in the mouse). Abnormal alignment of chromosomes (*blue*) can be seen with fluorescence microscopy (*arrows, bottom panel*). MII spindle microtubules can be detected using antibodies to either alpha- or beta-tubulin (*green*)

Characteristics of Centrosomes and the Microtubule Cytoskeleton in MII Oocytes, in Spermatozoa, and After Fertilization

The cytoskeleton is mainly composed of three classes of cytoskeletal fibers, i.e., microfilaments (MFs; also called actin filaments or F-actin; 5–9 nm in diameter), microtubules (MTs; 25 nm in diameter), and intermediate filaments (IFs; 10 nm in diameter) as well as numerous cytoskeleton-associated components that play a significant role in cellular functions. However, the centrosome is a critical part of the cytoskeleton and plays a major role in coordinating various cytoskeletal and cellular functions (reviewed in refs. [3–6]). This section reviews the role of centrosomes and the MT cytoskeleton in the MII oocyte and in sperm cells.

Centrosome Proteins

The structure and composition of centrosomes has been reviewed in several previous papers [3–6] and will only briefly be introduced here. The centrosome is an important microtubule organizing center (MTOC) that either directly or indirectly is responsible for multiple cellular functions. Lacking a defining membrane that is typical for other cell organelles the centrosome is a highly dynamic structure that very efficiently communicates signaling functions through its microtubule organizing capabilities. Numerous centrosome core proteins and centrosome-associated proteins play a role in centrosome functions and direct or control cell cycle-specific events.

A typical somatic cell centrosome is composed of a large number of centrosome proteins surrounding a pair of perpendicularly oriented cylindrical centrioles, therefore referred to as pericentriolar material (PCM). In reproductive cells, the oocyte's and the sperm's centrosomal material is reduced during gametogenesis (reviewed in ref. [7]), and the mature egg and sperm contain specific centrosome proteins that reconstitute a complete functional centrosome after fertilization. The oocyte does not contain centrioles, but it does contain centrosome proteins while the sperm contains the centriole surrounded by a small amount of specific centrosome proteins including γ-tubulin and centrin.

The centrosomal core material consists of a fibrous scaffolding lattice whose three-dimensional architecture is primarily maintained through specific protein–protein interactions. It is a highly dynamic structure that compacts and decompacts for cell cycle-specific requirements in which different microtubule patterns are organized depending on the centrosome shape. Highly compacted centrosomes organize focused microtubule formations while an expanded centrosome structure organizes various expanded microtubule formations. Gamma-tubulin and the γ-tubulin ring complex (γ-TuRC) are mainly responsible for the nucleation of microtubules while pericentrin plays a role in recruiting γ-tubulin to the centrosome complex. Microtubules are anchored with their minus ends to the centrosome core structure [8], and microtubule numbers and lengths are regulated and reorganized throughout the cell cycle; microtubule growth is regulated by distal plus-end addition of tubulin subunits [9]. Microtubules play a role in translocation of vesicles, enzymes, and macromolecular complexes that allow rapid modifications of centrosomal material and impact cell cycle-specific functions in which centrosomal proteins are recruited and dispersed throughout the cell cycle. Rapid microtubule growth and transport along microtubules is especially important for the rapid formation of the sperm aster after fertilization that involves microtubule motor proteins and accessory proteins to reach the female pronucleus for pronuclear movements and apposition and for the union of the pronuclei containing maternal and paternal genomes.

MII Oocytes

The MII oocyte is the end result of a complex process of oocyte maturation that is critical for MII-stage oocyte quality (reviewed in refs. [7, 10–12]). During oogenesis, centrioles that are present in oogonia become lost, and the mature oocyte is devoid of centrioles in most species. However, centrosomal components are present in the MII spindle and in reduced amounts in the cytoplasm (reviewed in Manandhar et al. [7]) that can be visualized in parthenogenetically activated oocytes [4, 5, 13].

As the oocyte has lost centrioles during gametogenesis, the MII spindle is organized by acentriolar centrosomes consisting of numerous centrosome proteins including the well-known centrosome proteins γ-tubulin, centrin, and the nuclear mitotic apparatus (NuMA) protein. In most species (not in the mouse), the MII spindle is localized perpendicular to the cell surface, and it is a barrel shape to pointed spindle structure (parallel to the egg surface in the mouse which along with many other features reemphasizes the differences in mouse oocytes compared to most other mammalian species; reviewed in Schatten and Sun [4, 5]).

Although it appears static in immunofluorescence and transmission electron microscopy (TEM) images, the MII spindle is a highly dynamic structure that maintains its shape by a complex set of regulatory kinases and other regulatory proteins (reviewed in Miao et al. [2]). The main functions of the MII spindle is to precisely separate chromosomes and extrude one set of chromosomes into the polar body so that a diploid chromosome set is restored after fertilization during which the sperm contributes the paternal set of chromosomes. Any failure in MII spindle functions can result in cell and developmental abnormalities resulting in abortion, disease, or developmental defects (reviewed in Miao et al. [2]). The MII spindle is therefore an important key structure that requires precise regulation, receiving signals from the surrounding cells, the ooplasm, and the sperm during fertilization. An intact MII spindle as shown in Fig. 26.1 (top panel) is an important criterion to assess oocyte quality. Misaligned chromosomes (arrow in bottom panel of Fig. 26.1) can be visualized as result of dysfunctional microtubules and molecular motor proteins associated with spindle abnormalities.

Spermatozoa

The components involved in sperm centrosomal functions have previously been reviewed in detail [4–7, 14–16]. Briefly, when spermatids transform into mature sperm, a partial reduction of the sperm centrosome occurs in that the proximal centriole (PC) is retained completely in the sperm localized proximal to the nucleus, while the distal centriole (DC) becomes partially reduced, and it becomes associated with the sperm axoneme in the midpiece and tail (Fig. 26.2). This distal centriole becomes restructured in that it loses the triplet MT organization while a central pair of MT doublets becomes apparent, as is characteristic for the axoneme (reviewed in Schatten and Sun [4–6]). Sperm aster organization during human fertilization requires a sperm-derived centriole that must first disengage from the sperm tail connecting piece. Release of the proximal centriole is carried out by sperm (and oocyte) proteasomes during fertilization (right panel Fig. 26.2; Rawe et al. [17]).

The Importance of Centrosomes for Fertilization and Implications for ICSI

As stated above, the precise formation of the sperm aster is critically important for pronuclear movements and for the union of male and female pronuclei as diagrammed in Fig. 26.3. The sperm centriole and surrounding centrosome material is particularly important as it provides the dominant structure onto which oocyte centrosome proteins accumulate to form a functional zygotic centrosome for the formation of the zygote aster. After release of the proximal centriole by proteasomes [17], precise nucleation of microtubules includes precise amounts of γ-TuRCs composed of γ-tubulin and accessory proteins that are associated with the centrosome core structure and nucleate precise amounts of microtubules in the rapidly changing sperm aster. γ-Tubulin needs to be recruited from the oocyte to increase sperm aster size and length in a cell cycle-specific manner that results in the functional zygote aster important for pronuclear apposition. Overrecruitment of γ-tubulin will result in nucleation of too many microtubules while underrecruitment of γ-tubulin will result in reduced aster formation that both may result in aster formation abnormalities and decreased developmental potential. Studies in the bovine system have revealed that sperm aster formation and size correlated to in vitro embryonic development to the blastocyst stage in which the degree of sperm-derived centrosome and aster organization affected male fertility and early development in a bull-dependent variation [18]. We do not yet know the full range of requirements for optimal sperm and zygote aster formation, but we do know that various factors require precise orchestration that involves phosphoproteins [19] and a variety of other

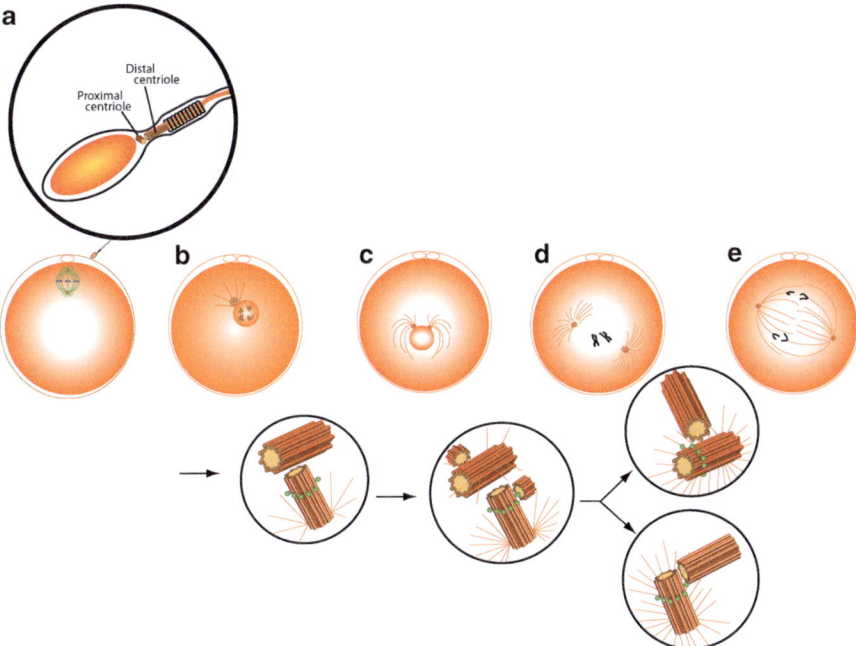

Fig. 26.3 Schematic diagram of the centriole–centrosome complex from fertilization to first cell division. (**a**) Sperm before fertilization contains a proximal and distal centriole. The meiotic spindle in the MII stage oocyte contains acentriolar centrosomes; (**b**) sperm aster formation from the sperm's proximal centriole–centrosome complex; (**c**) after pronuclear apposition, replication of the centriole at pronuclear stage; (**d**) after syngamy, the duplicated centriole–centrosome complex migrates around the zygote nucleus and relocates to opposite poles to form the centers of the mitotic spindle poles; (**e**) mitosis of the first cell cycle. Enlarged centriole complex: prior to fertilization, spermatozoa display two distinct centriolar structures with the proximal centriole located within the connecting piece next to the basal plate of the sperm head. This centriole displays a pinwheel structure of nine triplet microtubules surrounded by pericentriolar components. The degenerated distal centriole is organized perpendicular to the proximal centriole and aligned with the axoneme or sperm tail. (**b**) Shortly after sperm incorporation into the oocyte, a sperm aster is formed from the proximal centriole that allows pronuclear apposition. (**c**) After pronuclear apposition, the sperm centrioles duplicate during the pronuclear stage (in subsequent cell cycles during the G1/S phases); mother and daughter centrioles form procentrioles, fibrous material that is associated with the proximal region and grows into daughter centrioles (in subsequent cell cycles during the S and G2 phases), resulting in two pairs of centrioles that indicate duplication of centrosomal material. This pattern of centriole duplication is termed semiconservative duplication, as each daughter cell retains one of the mother's centrioles while a new daughter centriole is formed. Centriole and centrosome cycles are tightly coupled and centrosome duplication occurs at the time centrioles duplicate. (**d**) The duplicated centrioles separate and migrate around the zygote nucleus to form the opposite poles of the first mitotic spindle (modified from Schatten and Sun [6], with permission)

centrosome-associated components that have been studied to a better degree in somatic cells (reviewed in Schatten and colleagues [3–6]). In somatic cells, perhaps more than 100 different proteins play a role in centrosome and centrosome-directed cell cycle regulations including numerous regulatory components (kinases, phosphatases, and others) that associate with centrosomes during various cell cycle stages. The studies in somatic cells may indicate that over 100 different types of centrosome proteins may be involved in the dynamically changing centrosome composition during aster formation in the fertilized egg. Further studies are needed on basic and molecular levels to determine the full range of requirements for sperm and zygote aster formation to potentially improve in vitro fertilization.

Specific centrosome proteins that we know to play a critical role in centrosome and sperm functions during fertilization include pericentrin and centrin. In somatic cells, pericentrin along with several other proteins plays a role in centrosome and spindle organization [20–22]. Pericentrin forms a complex with γ-tubulin and depends on dynein for assembly onto centrosomes [22]; pericentrin gene mutation results in recruitment loss of several other centrosomal proteins. Centrins are members of a highly conserved subgroup of the EF-hand superfamily of Ca^{2+}-binding proteins. They are important for centriole functions and play an essential role in centrosome duplication ([23–25]; reviewed in Manandhar et al. [7]; Salisbury et al. [26]). Progress is being made to characterize other centrosome proteins that play a role in centrosome functions during fertilization, but our knowledge on this aspect of fertilization is still very limited.

One other protein that has proven critical for reproduction is the nuclear mitotic apparatus (NuMA) protein that is localized to the MII spindle in the mature oocyte. As NuMA is a nuclear matrix protein during interphase, it is detected in the decondensing sperm nucleus after fertilization (Rawe et al., unpublished results). Dispersion of NuMA into the cytoplasm occurs after nuclear envelope breakdown (NEBD), followed by NuMA association with mitotic centrosomes (reviewed in Sun and Schatten [30]). NuMA is never associated with the interphase centrosome; NuMA localization in the decondensing sperm nucleus after fertilization has clearly been shown for human oocytes (Rawe et al., in preparation) and for pig oocytes [27]. Studies in cloned pig and mouse embryos revealed that NuMA contributed by the donor nucleus plays a role in the formation of the mitotic apparatus during first cell division ([27–29]; reviewed in Sun and Schatten [30]). In aging or deteriorating oocytes, NuMA becomes dislocated from the MII spindle. NuMA abnormalities have previously been reported for cloning failures in rhesus monkeys [31].

Intracytoplasmic Sperm Injection and Assays for Centrosome Functions in ART

Intracytoplasmic sperm injection (ICSI; first reported by Palermo et al. [32]) has allowed a novel treatment overcoming male factor infertility primarily related to sperm motility or other unknown factors. The benefits and possible complexities associated with ICSI are important to know (reviewed by Hewitson [33]), as 50% of IVF cycles are now employing ICSI in many IVF clinics. Some of the benefits using ICSI include the possibility to coinject factors that may be causes of male factor infertility problems which has already been attempted in exploratory studies using the cat as model by coinjecting centrosomal material to restore complete centrosome function (detailed below). Future studies are needed to determine specific factors that are required to restore specific sperm functions after ICSI. Clearly, assessment of centrosomal material in sperm is important.

As the important role of centrosomes in ICSI has been recognized, possible therapies have been proposed to restore defective centrosome functions. One of the most frequently used assays to determine sperm centrosomal integrity and functioning comes from indirect studies using heterologous fertilization models in which human sperm and bovine oocytes are used to assess sperm aster formation indicative of centrosome functions [18, 34]. Several heterologous ICSI systems have been employed by various investigators (reviewed in Hayasaka et al. [35]; Terada [36]) in which human sperm were microinjected into either rabbit [37, 38] or bovine [39–43] oocytes. These assays established a relationship between infertility and sperm centrosomal dysfunction [38]. Such assays have especially been useful to asses centrosome functions in globozoospermia (characterized by sperm with round heads and lack of an acrosome and acrosomal enzymes and a disorganized midpiece [44]) in which low rates of sperm aster formation was seen when heterologous ICSI with bovine oocytes was used (15.8%). Understanding the cellular events during mammalian fertilization is a major challenge that is important to pursue for improving future infertility treatments in humans [42, 45]. Figure 26.4 shows several examples of fertilization failures in human zygotes assessed by immunocytochemistry (ICC) and confocal microscopy. Studies in the domestic cat [46] revealed short or absent sperm asters after ICSI with testicular spermatozoa compared to ejaculated spermatozoa that produced large sperm asters after ICSI. The diminished pattern of aster formation from the testicular sperm centrosome was associated with delays in first cleavage and reduced development to morulae and blastocyst stages, indicating that the size of the sperm aster may predict developmental competence. Replacement of testicular sperm centrosome by a centrosome from an ejaculated spermatozoon resulted in higher rates of embryo development comparable to data from ejaculated spermatozoa which indicates that it may be possible to restore centrosome functions with donor centrosomes although ethical questions need to be addressed before proposing such therapies for couples in which infertility is a result of centrosome-related sperm dysfunctions. These studies also point to the possibility that sperm-related centrosome dysfunctions may be associated with incomplete centrosome maturation that is important for centrosome functions and sperm aster formation. Immature sperm centrosomes may play a role in the failure of injection of round spermatids into oocytes (ROSI) that has been unsuccessful when used in IVF procedures [47]. Taken together, these studies reveal a significant role for centrosomes in fertilization indicating developmental potential.

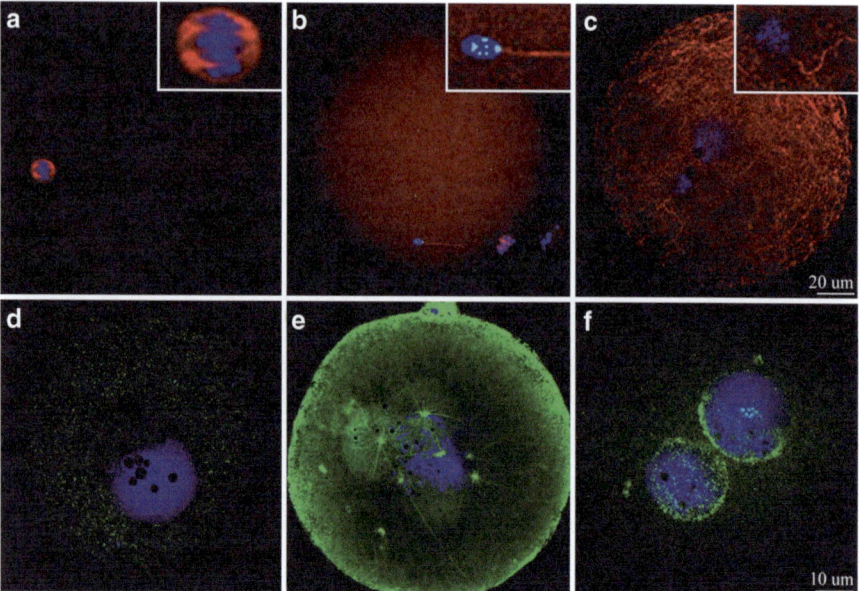

Fig. 26.4 Cytoskeletal organization and DNA configuration after failure and abnormal fertilization during IVF and ICSI. (**a**) Oocyte meiotic spindle (*red*: microtubules) with chromosomes (*blue*: DNA) at the metaphase plate. Inset in the *upper right corner* displays higher magnification detail. No sperm penetration is visualized. (**b**) The sperm head failed to form the male pronucleus, and the female chromosomes are still condensed at the meiotic spindle (lack of oocyte activation). Interestingly, fragmented sperm head is visualized after processing sample using TUNEL staining (see detail in the upper right corner, *green*). (**c**) Example of failure or incomplete male pronuclear formation at 18 h of ICSI. Microtubules (*red*) are extended through the entire oocyte cytoplasm as a result of oocyte activation. Male DNA was not completely decondensed (detail at the *upper right corner*), while female pronucleus underwent decondensation (asynchronous pronuclear development). (**d**) Formation of one pronucleus following ICSI (*blue*: DNA), presumably due to the lack of extrusion of the second polar body. (**e**) Development of three pronuclei after IVF due to polyspermy. Multiple MTOCs are shown in *green* as detected with antitubulin immunofluorescence staining for microtubules. (**f**) Arrested formation of two pronuclei. Male and female pronuclei are in close apposition at the center of the oocyte's cytoplasm. Nuclear envelopes are seen in *green*

Technical Aspects and Practical Considerations

The best characterized centrosomal core protein is γ-tubulin. In *oocytes*, its accurate distribution indicates spindle integrity, as it becomes displaced from the poles when spindles become deteriorated as is the case in aging oocytes (reviewed in Miao et al. [2]). While no definitely reliable noninvasive methods are available to assess spindle integrity, PolScope imaging has been applied to evaluate human oocyte MII spindle quality [48, 49]. In other test model species including the pig and bovine, immunofluorescence microscopy is typically used to evaluate spindle integrity using antitubulin antibodies for microtubules and antibodies to the MII centrosomal

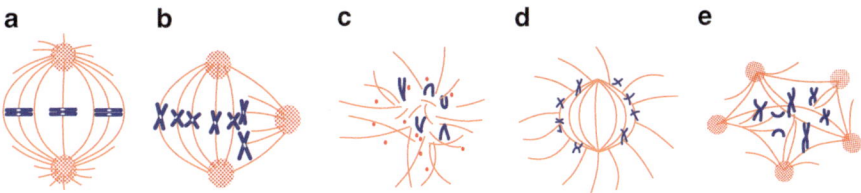

Fig. 26.5 Differences in MII spindle shapes between fresh and aged oocytes. Aged oocytes can display close to normal spindles (**a**) or highly abnormal spindles (**b–e**). (**b**) Tripolar spindle. (**c**) Highly disorganized spindle with scattered centrosomes and chromosomes. (**d**) Large irregular spindle in transverse view exhibiting dense staining for tubulin with chromatin attached to the outer edges of the spindle in a rosette formation. (**e**) Multipolar spindle. *Red* centrosomes; *green* microtubules; *blue* chromosomes (modified from Miao et al. [2], with permission)

proteins γ-tubulin, centrin, and NuMA. Images of an abnormal and normal human oocyte MII spindle is shown in Fig. 26.1 bottom panel and Fig. 26.4a, respectively. It is also important to observe that oocyte aging does not occur during the process of in vitro fertilization. In the pig model, several patterns of oocyte aging have been observed which are shown in Fig. 26.5. In humans, such patterns have been observed in deteriorated oocytes, and it has been shown that γ-tubulin and NuMA both dissociate from the spindle poles causing spindle abnormalities (Rawe et al., in preparation). Except for MII spindle evaluation using PolScope optics, future studies may consider live cell imaging with fluorescent centrosome labels such as GFP-centrin which has already been shown effective in pig studies [29].

One other aspect to assess oocyte quality for live cell noninvasive nonharmful imaging is imaging of mitochondrial distribution using multiphoton microscopy that has been employed in hamster oocytes and resulted in successful production of offspring [50]. Such approaches have not yet been used for human oocytes because of ethical considerations but may be possible.

Assessment of sperm is easier compared to oocytes, as abundant material is available that does not fall under ethical constraints. In sperm, γ-tubulin and centrin are both localized to the basal body and can be analyzed by immunofluorescence or immunoblotting in test sperm samples. Conventional EM can easily be applied to assess sperm morphology [14, 16] and immunoEM can be applied to determine the accurate localization of γ-tubulin and centrin on ultrastructural levels.

To evaluate sperm aster functions after fertilization, still the best indirect assays for centrosome functions available so far are studies of heterologous fertilization in which human sperm is tested for its fertilizing capabilities using bovine eggs as test material. Fertilization can be assessed reliably well in bovine oocytes in which the sperm forms an aster that is indicative of successful fertilization. As mentioned above, the different sizes of sperm asters indicate the sperm's fertilization capabilities and developmental potential. This assay also provides an indirect test for the sperm's centrosomal contributions; its functions can be assessed independent of the human oocyte's centrosomal components that may be a contributing factor for infertility, as the oocyte provides γ-tubulin and other regulatory factors that are essential for accurate sperm and zygote aster formation. The heterologous sperm aster tests will allow predictions on sperm or oocyte centrosomal defects. It indicates the sperm's potential to contribute to the fertilization success. If subsequent sperm aster formation is unsuccessful in human oocytes, defects in the oocyte's centrosomal components may need to be considered among other oocyte components that contribute to centrosome and sperm aster regulation. Theoretically, various regulatory factors can be coinjected along with ICSI, although we currently only know little about factors that play a role in sperm and zygote aster regulation in human oocytes. Experimental manipulation is possible in the heterologous human-sperm-bovine oocyte system such as activation by changing pH and calcium factors. While the bovine system has been used for heterologous studies, the pig is increasingly being used as it displays many similarities with human fertilization (reviewed in Schatten and Sun [4–6]).

As mentioned above, cellular organization of mitochondria has been used by Squirrell et al. [50] to select oocytes for analysis with multiphoton microscopy, a safe method to evaluate live oocytes, and follow development. The observed fertilized oocytes were implanted into a hamster and resulted in subsequent live birth of healthy offspring. Live cell imaging of mitochondria in human oocytes might be worth consideration, as accurate distribution patterns have been associated with positive developmental potential (reviewed by Schatten et al. [51]).

The methods for immunofluorescence microscopy to analyze the microtubule cytoskeleton in human sperm and oocytes have been described in extensive detail by Rawe and Chemes [52]; the following sections in the present chapter are focused on centrosome detection and builds on the previous descriptions for microtubules in which media/chemicals, antibodies and staining, consumables and disposables, equipment, and tools have been described in detail. For the centrosome studies of human nonfertilized oocytes and zygotes by electron microscopy (EM), ICC, and fluorescence microscopy in sperm and during ICSI, oocytes and zygotes of cells from couples undergoing ICSI provided the test material for our studies after written consent (described in Rawe and Chemes [52]). Briefly, for the study of human nonfertilized oocytes and zygotes by ICC and fluorescence microscopy during ICSI, cumulus cells are removed, followed by removal of the zona pellucida, formaldehyde fixation, permeabilization, antibody labeling, and mounting and visualization of formaldehyde-fixed samples [52]. Examples of applying these methods are shown in Fig. 26.4.

Analysis of Sperm by Electron Microscopy and Immunofluorescence

Sperm pathologies comprise a variety of structural and functional abnormalities that are among the many criteria underlying male factor infertility. Abnormally shaped flagella are among the clearly visible pathologies in severely asthenozoospermic men as reviewed by Rawe and Chemes [52] in which dysplasia of the fibrous sheath is most common. Sperm abnormalities can easily be determined with TEM of a sperm sample to determine the degree of abnormalities. Centrosomal components can be determined by immunofluorescence microscopy to centrosomal proteins present in sperm before fertilization. Comparison with control sperm samples is recommended. Currently known sperm centrosomal markers are γ-tubulin, MPM2 (phosphoprotein marker), and centrin. Reduced amounts of centrin have been reported in male factor-related fertilization failures.

To analyze sperm, a fresh sample of ejaculated sperm is centrifuged and washed in PBS for 5 min. After removing supernatant, the pellet is resuspended in PBS. For EM, these samples can now be processed using routine TEM methods as available in electron microscopy facilities.

The *procedures for TEM* include dilution of sperm in PBS (0.1 M, pH 7.4) (1:4 = sperm/PBS) at room temperature followed by thorough mixing. Next, sperm solution is transferred to a conical tip centrifuge tube and centrifuged at 1,500–2,000 rpm for 10 min. For fixation, 3% glutaraldehyde in PBS is added at 4°C for a fixation time of 3–5 h, followed by two rinses in PBS for 30 min each. For second fixation, 1.3% osmium tetroxide is added at 4°C for a 2-h incubation time and two subsequent rinses for 30 min each in PBS. Dehydration follows in an ascending series of ethanol at room temperature (50, 70, 90, 95%, 4 × 100%) for 20 min each followed by three rinses in propylene oxide (20 min each) as transition fluid. Embedding is performed in Epon-Araldite with steps including a mix of 1:1 propylene oxide/Epon-Araldite (2 h), fresh Epon-Araldite changes followed by curing for 24–48 h in EM molds. The materials are available from EM companies and include detailed instructions. Thin sectioning with an ultramicrotome and analysis in a TEM instrument is typically performed in electron microscopy facilities.

Routine TEM methods can be followed by *ultrastructural ICC* to determine the presence of cytoskeletal and centrosome components related to ultrastructure. For the ultrastructural ICC procedure, sperm pellets are fixed for 1 h at 4°C in 5% formaldehyde in PBS (0.1 M, pH 7.4), rinsed in buffer, and dehydrated in an increasing series of ethanol as described for conventional TEM. Infiltration and embedding is performed using LR-White Resin, medium grade for polymerization at 60°C for 24 h. Sections are mounted on 300-mesh nickel grids and dried at room temperature. Blocking buffer consists of TBS and 10% normal goat serum. Incubation in first antibody is performed by floating grids on a drop of antibody solution and left overnight at 4°C making sure the samples are not dried out by keeping them in a humidified chamber. Three washes in TBS for 1 h at 4°C is followed by incubation for 1 h at 4°C with blocking buffer containing 15 nm colloidal gold-labeled secondary antibody. Sections on grids are then counterstained with 1% osmium tetroxide followed by 1:1 aqueous uranyl acetate/acetone. For negative controls, primary antibodies are either omitted or replaced with primary antibody preadsorbed with excess antigen.

For *immunofluorescence microscopy*, 100 µL of sperm suspension is placed on a poly-L-lysine-coated cover slip on a slide warmer at 37°C. After 15 min, sperm are settled and attached to the cover slip which allows easy transfer into fixative (either 2% paraformaldehyde [PFA] in PBS at room temperature pH 7.2–7.3 or 100% methanol chilled to −20°C) for 40 min. Next, cover slips containing sperm are carefully placed into 6-well dishes (face up) containing 2% PFA in PBS and 1% Triton X-100 to permeabilize sperm cells. Next, for antibody staining, several technical approaches are possible, and one easy approach is to remove the cover slips containing sperm from the six-well plates and place each one on the center cross of a four-well Petri dish. A blocking solution is applied for 40-min incubation to bind residual-free aldehyde groups. After carefully removing the blotting solution, primary and secondary antibodies are applied as described for oocytes and zygotes. Antibodies for centrosomal proteins include γ-tubulin and centrin.

Conclusions and Future Perspectives

Centrosomes are critically important for sperm and oocyte functions and for successful fertilization after insemination in physiological, IVF, and various ART procedures such as ICSI. Numerous fertilization failures are associated with centrosome dysfunctions and can either relate to sperm centrosomal defects, oocyte centrosome defects, or to regulatory failures after fertilization. Heterologous fertilization models with human sperm and bovine or porcine oocytes will be most useful to more fully analyze sperm and egg centrosomal functions resulting in successful sperm aster and zygote aster formation. Assessing the dysfunctional factors will be important for therapeutic advances. Exploratory studies performed in the cat already revealed that it is possible to restore functional centrosomes in centrosome-related fertilization failures, although detailed basic research as well as functional studies is still needed to provide promising new therapies to possibly increase IVF and ICSI procedures related to centrosome dysfunctions.

Acknowledgment The authors gratefully acknowledge Donald Connor's professional help with the illustrations.

References

1. Swain JE, Pool TB. ART failure: oocyte contributions to unsuccessful fertilization. Hum Reprod Update. 2008;14(5):431–46.
2. Miao Y-L, Sun Q-Y, Zhang X, Zhao J-G, Zhao M-T, Spate L, Prather RS, Schatten H. Centrosome abnormalities during porcine oocyte aging. Environ Mol Mutagen. 2009;50(8):666–71.
3. Schatten H. The mammalian centrosome and its functional significance. Histochem Cell Biol. 2008;129:667–86.
4. Schatten H, Sun Q-Y. The role of centrosomes in mammalian fertilization and its significance for ICSI. Mol Hum Reprod. 2009;15(9):531–8.
5. Schatten H, Sun Q-Y. The functional significance of centrosomes in mammalian meiosis, fertilization, development, nuclear transfer, and stem cell differentiation. Environ Mol Mutagen. 2009;50(8):620–36.

6. Schatten H, Sun Q-Y. The role of centrosomes in fertilization, cell division and establishment of asymmetry during embryo development. Semin Cell Dev Biol. 2010;21:174–84.
7. Manandhar G, Schatten H, Sutovsky P. Centrosome reduction during gametogenesis and its significance. Biol Reprod. 2005;72:2–13.
8. Bornens M. Centrosome composition and microtubule anchoring mechanisms. Curr Opin Cell Biol. 2002;14:25–34.
9. McIntosh JR, Euteneuer U. Tubulin hooks as probes for microtubule polarity: an analysis of the method and an evaluation of data on microtubule polarity in the mitotic spindle. J Cell Biol. 1984;98:525–33.
10. Sun Q-Y, Schatten H. Regulation of dynamic events by microfilaments during oocyte maturation and fertilization. Reproduction. 2006;131:193–205.
11. Tosti E. Calcium ion currents mediating oocyte maturation events. Reprod Biol Endocrinol. 2006;4:74.
12. Grøndahl C. Oocyte maturation. Dan Med Bull. 2008;55:1–16.
13. Schatten H, Walter M, Biessmann H, Schatten G. Activation of maternal centrosomes in unfertilized sea urchin eggs. Cell Motil Cytoskeleton. 1992;23:61–70.
14. Chemes HE. Phenotypes of sperm pathology: genetic and acquired forms in infertile men. J Androl. 2000;21(6):799–808.
15. Sathananthan AH, Ratnasooriya WD, de Silva PK, Menezes J. Characterization of human gamete centrosomes for assisted reproduction. Ital J Anat Embryol. 2001;106(2 Suppl 2):61–73.
16. Chemes HE, Rawe VY. Sperm pathology: a step beyond descriptive morphology. Origin, characterization and fertility potential of abnormal sperm phenotypes in infertile men. Hum Reprod. 2003;9(5):405–28.
17. Rawe VY, Sutovsky P, Díaz S, Abdelmassih R, Wójcik C, Morales P, Chemes HE. The role of sperm proteasomes during early zygote development: implications for fertilization failure in humans. Hum Reprod. 2008;23:573–80.
18. Navara CS, First NL, Schatten G. Phenotypic variations among paternal centrosomes expressed within the zygote as disparate microtubule lengths and sperm aster organization: correlations between centrosome activity and developmental success. Proc Natl Acad Sci U S A. 1996;93:5384–8.
19. Palermo GD, Colombero LT, Rosenwaks Z. The human sperm centrosome is responsible for normal syngamy and early embryonic development. Rev Reprod. 1997;2:19–27.
20. Doxsey SJ, Stein P, Evans L, Calarco P, Kirschner M. Pericentrin, a highly conserved protein of centrosomes involved in microtubule organization. Cell. 1994;76:639–50.
21. Dictenberg J, Zimmerman W, Sparks C, Young A, Vidair C, Zheng Y, Carrington W, Fay F, Doxsey SJ. Pericentrin and gamma tubulin form a protein complex and are organized into a novel lattice at the centrosome. J Cell Biol. 1998;141:163–74.
22. Young A, Dictenberg JB, Purohit A, Tuft R, Doxsey SJ. Cytoplasmic dynein-mediated assembly of pericentrin and γ tubulin onto centrosomes. Mol Biol Cell. 2000;11:2047–56.
23. Levy YY, Lai EY, Remillard SP, Heintzelman MB, Fulton C. Centrin is a conserved protein that forms diverse associations with centrioles and MTOCs in *Naegleria* and other organisms. Cell Motil Cytoskeleton. 1996;33:298–323.
24. Salisbury JL. Centrin, centrosomes, and mitotic spindle poles. Curr Opin Cell Biol. 1995;7:39–45.
25. Lutz W, Lingle WL, McCormick D, Greenwood TM, Salisbury JL. Phosphorylation of centrin during the cell cycle and its role in centriole separation preceding centrosome duplication. J Biol Chem. 2001;276:20774–80.
26. Salisbury JL, Suino KM, Busby R, Springett M. Centrin-2 is required for centriole duplication in mammalian cells. Curr Biol. 2002;12:1287–92.
27. Liu ZH, Schatten H, Hao YH, Lai L, Wax D, Samuel M, Zhong Z-S, Sun Q-Y, Prather RS. The nuclear mitotic apparatus (NuMA) protein is contributed by the donor cell nucleus in cloned porcine embryos. Front Biosci. 2006;11:1945–57.
28. Zhong Z-S, Zhang G, Meng X-Q, Zhang Y-L, Chen D-Y, Schatten H, Sun Q-Y. Function of donor cell centrosome in intraspecies and interspecies nuclear transfer embryos. Exp Cell Res. 2005;306:35–46.

29. Zhong Z, Spate L, Hao Y, Li R, Lai L, Katayama M, Sun QY, Prather RS, Schatten H. Remodeling of centrosomes in intraspecies and interspecies nuclear transfer porcine embryos. Cell Cycle. 2007;6(12):1510–21.
30. Sun Q-Y, Schatten H. Multiple roles of NuMA in vertebrate cells: review of an intriguing multi-functional protein. Front Biosci. 2006;11:1137–46.
31. Simerly C, Dominko T, Navara C, Payne C, Capuano S, Gosman G, Chong KY, Takahashi D, Chace C, Compton D, Hewitson L, Schatten G. Molecular correlates of primate nuclear transfer failures. Science. 2003;300:297.
32. Palermo G, Joris H, Devroey P, Van Steirteghem A. Pregnancies after intracytoplasmic sperm injection of single spermatozoon into an oocyte. Lancet. 1992;340:17–8.
33. Hewitson L. Primate models for assisted reproductive technologies. Reproduction. 2004;128:293–9.
34. Tachibana M, Terada Y, Ogonuki N, Ugajin T, Ogura A, Murakami T, Yaegashi N, Okamura K. Functional assessment of centrosomes of spermatozoa and spermatids microinjected into rabbit oocytes. Mol Reprod Dev. 2009;76(3):270–7.
35. Hayasaka S, Terada Y, Morita J, Tachibana M, Shima-Morito Y, Kakoi-Yoshimoto T, Nakamura S, Murakami T, Yaegashi N, Okamura K. Post-ICSI cytoskeletal dynamics during fertilization. J Mamm Ova Res. 2006;23:21–6.
36. Terada Y. Functional analyses of the sperm centrosome in human reproduction: implications for assisted reproductive technique. Soc Reprod Fertil Suppl. 2007;63:507–13.
37. Terada Y, Simerly CR, Hewitson L, Schatten G. Sperm aster formation and pronuclear decondensation during rabbit fertilization and development of a functional assay for human sperm. Biol Reprod. 2000;62:557–63.
38. Terada Y, Nakamura S, Hewitson L, Simerly CR, Horiuchi T, Murakami T, Okamura K, Schatten G. Human sperm aster formation after intracytoplasmic sperm injection with rabbit and bovine eggs. Fertil Steril. 2002;77:1283–4.
39. Nakamura S, Terada Y, Horiuchi T, Emuta C, Murakami T, Yaegashi N, Okamura K. Human sperm aster formation and pronuclear decondensation in bovine eggs following intracytoplasmic sperm injection using a Piezo-driven pipette. Biol Reprod. 2001;65:1359–63.
40. Nakamura S, Terada Y, Horiuchi T, Emuta C, Murakami T, Yaegashi N, Okamura K. Analysis of the human sperm centrosomal function and the oocyte activation ability in a case of globozoospermia, by ICSI into bovine oocytes. Hum Reprod. 2002;17:2930–4.
41. Nakamura S, Terada Y, Rawe VY, Uehara S, Morito Y, Yoshimoto T, Tachibana M, Murakami T, Yaegashi N, Okamura K. A trial to restore defective human sperm centrosomal function. Hum Reprod. 2005;20(7):1933–7.
42. Rawe VY, Terada Y, Nakamura S, Chillik CF, Brugo Olmedo S, Chemes HE. A pathology of the sperm centriole responsible for defective sperm aster formation, sygamy and cleavage. Hum Reprod. 2002;17:2344–9.
43. Yoshimoto-Kakoi T, Terada Y, Tachibana M, Murakami T, Yaegashi N, Okamura K. Assessing centrosomal function of infertile males using heterologous ICSI. Syst Biol Reprod Med. 2008;54(3):135–42.
44. Dam AHDM, Feenstra I, Westphal JR, Ramos L, van Golde RJT, Kremer JAM. Globozoospermia revisited. Hum Reprod Update. 2007;13(1):63–75.
45. Rawe VY, Brugo Olmedo S, Nodar F, Doncel G, Vitullo A, Acosta A. Cytoskeletal organization defects and abortive activation in human oocytes after IVF and ICSI failure. Mol Hum Reprod. 2000;6:510–6.
46. Comizzoli P, Wildt DE, Pukazhenthi BS. Poor centrosomal function of cat testicular spermatozoa impairs embryo development in vitro after intracytoplasmic sperm injection. Biol Reprod. 2006;75(2):252–60.
47. Yanagimachi R. Intracytoplasmic injection of spermatozoa and spermatogenic cells: its biology and applications in humans and animals. Reprod Biomed Online. 2005;10:247–88.

48. Moon J-H, Hyun C-S, Lee S-W, Son W-Y, Yoon S-H, Lim J-H. Visualization of the metaphase II meiotic spindle in living human oocytes using the Polscope enables the prediction of embryonic developmental competence after ICSI. Hum Reprod. 2003;18(4):817–20.
49. Wang WH, Meng L, Hackett RJ, Oldenbourg R, Keefe DL. The spindle observation and its relationship with fertilization after intracytoplasmic sperm injection in living human oocytes. Fertil Steril. 2001;75:348–53.
50. Squirrell JM, Wokosin DL, Bavister BD, White JG. Long-term multiphoton fluorescence imaging of mammalian embryos does not compromise viability. Nat Biotechnol. 1999;17:763–7.
51. Schatten H, Prather RS, Sun QY. The significance of mitochondria for embryo development in cloned farm animals. Mitochondrion. 2005;5(5):303–21.
52. Rawe VY, Chemes H. Exploring the cytoskeleton during intracytoplasmic sperm injection in humans. In: Carroll DJ, editor. Microinjection: methods and applications, vol. 518. New York: Humana Press; 2009.

Chapter 27
Molecular Mining of Follicular Fluid for Reliable Biomarkers of Human Oocyte and Embryo Developmental Competence

Jonathan Van Blerkom

Current advances in the development and application in clinical IVF of microanalytical imaging, genetic, and biochemical technologies lead to the interesting possibility that in the near future, competence assessments of human oocytes and embryos will be algorithm-based rather than operator-based. In such a future, selection for insemination and single embryo transfer would rely on a combination of findings assessed at selected phases of oocyte and early embryonic developmental. For the embryo, quantifiable biometric characteristics of developmental performance in vitro obtained by time-lapse imaging would include pronuclear morphology and nucleolar organization, the timing and uniformity of cleavage divisions, the presence of micro- and multinucleation in blastomeres, and an accurate value for the degree of cytoplasm lost to fragmentation, if any [1]. Biochemical criteria for competence selection could come from a variety of current methods such as microanalysis of spent culture medium to detect molecular signatures [2–4], levels of gene expression by cumulus cell [5, 6], and genetic status determined by high-resolution genomic analyses from blastomere and trophectoderm biopsies [7]. In this future, the human factor is necessarily relegated to ovum pickup, perhaps fertilization, and most likely, embryo transfer.

Whether this scenario is a realistic one remains to be seen, as earlier and sanguine predictions of biochemical or physiological biomarkers of oocyte competence have yet to be fulfilled [8, 9]. However, the need for competence assessment, whether driven by instrumentation or observer, arises from an undeniable biological fact; namely, that with respect to outcome, each human oocyte and each human embryo has a unique developmental potential, and that often, competence is already

J. Van Blerkom, PhD (✉)
Department of Molecular, Cellular and Developmental Biology,
University of Colorado, Boulder, CO, USA
e-mail: Jonathan.vanblerkom@colorado.edu

compromised in the mature and fertilizable oocyte [10]. This notion has been repeatedly validated by millions of IVF cycles performed over the past 3 decades. Although not unexpected, the results of the chromosomal assessments of meiotically mature (metaphase II, MII) human oocytes and early cleavage-stage embryos with different high-resolution methods have consistently demonstrated high frequencies of aneuploidy, often with multiple chromosomal anomalies (trisomies and monosomies) affecting the same oocyte [11], and for the early embryo, aneuploidy and other developmentally lethal chromosomal segregation disorders (e.g., mosaicism [12, 13]). The occurrence of these defects still comes as a surprise to even the most experienced observer when morphologically normal and stage-appropriate oocytes and preimplantation-stage embryos are found to be chromosomally abnormal.

If computerized biometric analyses of oocytes were to become standard methods to select oocytes for insemination and embryos for transfer, the underlying causes of differential competence, such as aneuploidy, would need to be detectable in observer-free systems. It is doubtful that morphological characteristics that may be associated with competence (e.g., polar body volume, zona birefringence, cellular debris in perivitelline space [1]) can identify aneuploidies and other chromosomal defects either in the oocyte or in the early embryo. Likewise, there is no compelling clinical or experimental evidence to date which suggests that early embryos carrying specific chromosomal or single gene defects produce unique molecular signatures detectable in spent culture medium or, for that matter, can be identified by the over- or underexpression of specific mRNAs or proteins in a biopsied blastomere. This may change as human embryos with known chromosomal and genetic defects are subjected to highly sensitive analytical methods that can characterize biochemistry in microliter volumes or the molecular biology of a single cell (see below).

Follicular Fluid Biomarkers of Oocyte Developmental Competence

The efficacy and sensitivity for competence selection at the human oocyte and early embryo stages that may be afforded by molecular and metabolomic analyses remain to be demonstrated. In this regard, their use for purposes of selection may be problematic as both activities represent dynamic processes that can be subject to the conditions of culture. As discussed in detail by Menezo and Guerin [14], levels of gene expression, metabolism, and other bioactivities are not only oocyte and embryo specific but can also be significantly influenced by culture medium composition (e.g., amino acids) and the conditions of culture (e.g., oxygen tension). It can be concluded from this report that because of the dynamic nature of the interaction between the environment and the cellular processes that produce potential competence biomarkers, each needs to be evaluated critically in general and for embryos in particular, as early development from fertilization through the preimplantation stages is entirely in vitro. In addition, cost vs. benefit calculations need to be taken into account based on unambiguous demonstrations of improved outcome, as well as the ease with which genetic microarray, metabolomic, proteomic, and time-lapse imaging methodologies can be incorporated into the routine clinical IVF laboratory.

It has long been thought that competence biomarkers should exist in the follicular fluid given the differences in maturational state, fertilizability, and development competence observed in oocytes aspirated from follicles that show equivalent patterns of growth and development under exogenous gonadotropin stimulation (controlled ovarian hyperstimulation, COHS). The underlying issue in the search for competence markers in follicular fluid is related to the relative contribution of external influences that can be demonstrated to be developmental regulators or drivers for the oocyte vs. intrinsic differences that occur in oocytes themselves (i.e., at the molecular, cellular, and chromosomal levels). In this case, adverse downstream developmental consequences that may occur after fertilization would be expected to be independent of the biochemical environment within the follicle.

The search for external influences on competence has logically focused on the intrafollicular environment to which the oocyte is exposed. However, the fluid obtained for analysis may not represent conditions that could influence competence during the relatively prolonged FSH-dominated phase of follicular growth and development, but rather what occurs some 36 h after ovulation induction, typically with HCG rather than LH. Further complicating this type of analysis is that the vast majority of IVF cycles are hyperstimulated and comparisons to natural (spontaneous) are virtually nonexistent and COHS treatment could distort relative concentrations of regulatory factors, especially when fluids are pooled rather than analyzed individually for each follicle.

With these caveats in mind, what has made the follicular fluid so appealing for investigations of regulatory influences on human oocyte developmental potential is that the biochemistry is both dynamic and extraordinarily complex, a mixture of steroid hormones, growth factors, gonadotropins, cytokines, ions, amino acids, lipids, reactive oxygen species, enzymes, and other bioactive molecules that are produced in situ from the mural and cumulus granulosa or which pass through the blood follicle barrier as transudates from the perifollicular capillary bed [15–33]. It is clear even from this relatively short list of reports that qualitative and quantitative analyses of human follicular fluid demonstrate no shortage of molecules that could be biomarkers of competence, including those with regulatory and signaling functions. One of the foremost challenges in undertaking this type of investigation is the necessity to distinguish between potential targets for investigation that (a) actually influence or regulate oocyte processes and lead to competence, (b) those whose bioactivity is specific to the somatic cells of the follicle, or (c) are secretory products of the cumulus and mural granulosa destined to enter systemic circulation and whose activity is extrafollicular. However, since the beginning of clinical IVF in 1978, and despite a relatively enormous literature on this subject, few have been shown to have meaningful predictive value for selection, and at present, follicular fluid is not used for analytical purposes and is discarded by most programs. Another basic question that is rarely addressed in reports of the utility of follicular fluid for competence assessment is whether a potential biomarker can be shown to function through a signaling cascade that operates in the oocyte. In this regard, the presence of a particular growth or regulatory factor cannot be assumed, a priori, to be targeted to the oocyte, however appealing such a notion may be to those involved in competence studies. Perhaps, this is why so many reports of suggested biomarkers have been contradictory with respect to competence and outcome.

Further complicating the identification and characterization of bioactive molecules and regulatory factors that may be clinically useful as competence biomarkers in clinical IVF is whether they directly influence the developmental biology of the human oocyte or the cumulus and coronal cells. The presence of an intervening acellular zona pellucida is both a physical barrier between the oocyte and the follicular milieu and a biological filter that limits the diffusion of molecules to those up to ~60,000–70,000 Daltons. Here, the relevant issue is the particular manner by which they enter the perivitelline space (the immediate environment of the oocyte) or pass into the cytoplasm directly from the corona radiata and proximal cumulus oophorus (the somatic cell compartment) by means of gap junctions between the oolemma and the transzonal processes (TZPs, see below).

The likely pathway for the transmission of potential regulatory molecules is by means of TZPs, which arise early in oogenesis (coincident with zona pellucida formation) and occur as dense circumferential network of slender extensions of the corona radiata, the cells that reside on the zona pellucida and, to a lesser extent, from cells of the cumulus oophorus in proximity to the corona radiata [34]. These processes permit bidirectional communication between the developing and fully grown oocyte and its somatic cell component by means of gap junctions formed by connexin 37 hexamers. Transmission electron microscopic images of the TZPs show longitudinal arrays of microfilaments that extend from the cell body to the site of contact with the oolemma, and it has been suggested that they provide an internal architecture to facilitate directional transport [35]. More recently, the presence of mitochondria in TZPs has been demonstrated in living cumulus-oocyte complexes stained with mitochondria-specific fluorescent probes [36] with elongated, high-potential organelles detected along the entire length of the TZPs. Mitochondria located in proximity to the TZP terminus on the oolemma could supply ATP directly to the oocyte through gap junctions and supplement the endogenous bioenergetic capacity of the GV-stage ooplasm in the subplasmalemmal and pericortical cytoplasm, where the demand for ATP may be higher than in more interior regions [36].

While intercellular communication by the TZP pathway persists up to the luteinizing hormone (LH)-induced resumption of arrested meiosis, gap junctions are primarily involved in metabolic and electrical coupling between cells and function in this regard by regulating the flow of small molecules that act as secondary messengers. These junctions generally restrict passage of molecules to those approximate 1,000 Daltons, such as cyclic AMP, ATP, ions (e.g., calcium), and small polypeptides, but not proteins the size of most growth factors, including gonadotropins. Therefore, the potential developmental influences of regulatory proteins and other factors suggested to affect oocyte competence that exceed the molecular weight limitation of gap junctions are unlikely to do so by this direct pathway of intercellular communication. So what does the oocyte actually "see" at its surface, and how do extrinsic regulatory signals or developmental cues arrive in the perivitelline space, given the notion of the zona pellucida as a selective molecular filter, if not a barrier to certain macromolecules? For proteins excluded by gap junctions to affect the oocyte, receptor-mediated signal transduction at the level of the oolemma and uptake by endocytosis are the obvious means.

The central issue here that is worth repeating is that investigations of follicular fluid designed to identify molecules that may be involved in the acquisition of developmental competence need to consider the mechanism by which they can directly or indirectly affect the biology of the oocyte. For example, despite the withdrawal of TZPs from the oolemma at the outset of resumed meiotic maturation, the processes and the cells from which they originate remain intact and functional, as indicated for the latter by the presence of mitochondria that retain high potential [36]. Scanning electron microscopy of the underside of the zona pellucida in maturing and mature human oocytes shows a dense circumferential network of residual processes in the perivitelline space that in the native state, remain in close proximity to the oolemma [34]. Therefore, synthetic and secretory activity by the corona radiata and proximal cumulus granulosa likely continues during preovulatory maturation and putative influences from the follicular fluid on cumulus and coronal cells that could influence the oocyte likely persist. However, it remains to be determined whether biosynthetic activities that could affect the human oocyte change qualitatively or quantitatively in vivo under the influence of LH during the ~36-h-long preovulatory period. If such changes are confirmed, the long held notion that termination of TZP-mediated communication at the GV-stage signals a fundamental shift from maternal to oocyte regulation of development may need to be reconsidered.

The persistence of information flow between residual somatic cells and the oocyte during preovulatory maturation may be a currently unrecognized aspect of how competence is established, especially if the molecular nature of this information flow changes as maturation progresses to ovulation. At present, there is no evidence to suggest that as long as granulosa cells continue to secrete proteins into the perivitelline space during the preovulatory period, uptake by the oocyte (receptor mediated or endocytotic) is not functional during its maturation [37].

The intent of the preceding discussion was to emphasize that the presence alone of well-characterized growth factors and other regulatory molecules in human follicular fluid is insufficient to assume that the oocyte is the target or that they influence developmental competence. It may be for these reasons that despite the complex array of potential regulatory factors in follicular fluid noted above, to date, unambiguous evidence for developmentally significant effects on oocyte competence has remained elusive. It may well be that the principal target for growth factors in follicular fluid is the granulosa compartment, first by upregulating cell proliferation and steroidogenesis by mural granulosa and subsequently, to prepare both mural and residual cumulus granulosa for the transition to a vascular corpus luteum [38]. This is likely the function of angiogenic factors such as VEGF [39] and leptin [16], which occur at relatively high concentrations in preovulatory human follicular fluid.

While the follicular fluid can be a "gold mine" of potential regulatory factors, the fluid is discarded by virtually all IVF programs. Further complicating any scheme of molecular analysis is the unavoidable fact that follicular aspiration is not a "clean" process, and for analytical purposes, each follicle must be aspirated individually and with rinses of the aspiration needle between punctures to prevent cross-contamination with residual fluid and blood. The collection of neat aspirates can be time-consuming and can significantly extend the length of the ovum pickup procedure, especially when numerous follicles require puncture. The collection of individual aspirates also entails the tracking of the corresponding oocyte from fertilization through transfer, which, while feasible, adds considerable time and effort to the laboratory routine. Therefore, the selection of potential biomarkers of competence requires some degree of confidence that based on the known bioactivities of a candidate molecules, there is a high probability that its function, either through the cumulus and coronal cells or on the oocyte directly, will be developmentally significant.

With the possible exception of Mullerian inhibiting hormone (see below), no single component of the follicular fluid has met these criteria to date, and reports that some might, such as VEGF and leptin, have not been proven or are controversial [40–43]. Likewise, it remains to be determined whether mRNA profiles of cumulus cells, collected either free floating in aspirated follicular fluid or mechanically detached from the oocyte in vitro, are sufficiently predictive of outcome as to warrant the additional infrastructure required for microarray analysis and, more importantly, meaningful interpretation. Comparisons of mRNA expression profiles that can show differences between individual oocyte-cumulus complexes from the same or different ovaries offer a promising approach to competence selection, but whether it is clinically applicable will only become apparent when a core set of genes with known functions is identified and, on the basis of outcome, demonstrated to consistently distinguish between mature oocytes.

Recent studies of Mullerian inhibiting hormone (AMH) concentrations in follicular fluid and outcome results after IVF suggest that this molecule may indeed be a competence biomarker. AMH is a dimeric glycoprotein member of the transforming growth factor (TGF)-β superfamily whose expression by granulosa cells in large preantral and small antral follicles is upregulated at the transcriptional and posttranscriptional levels. Serum levels of AMH have received considerable attention as an indicator of ovarian reserve and for predicting the unique response of women to controlled ovarian stimulation, as well as biomarker of oocyte developmental competence [44, 45]. There is accumulating evidence that follicle-specific levels measured in aspirates at ovum retrieval may indeed be related to outcome after transfer (reviewed by Van Blerkom and Trout [9]). Based on IVF outcomes, Eldar-Geva et al. [46] proposed that of all the factors indentified in follicular fluid up to that date, only AMH appeared to be a reliable biomarker of developmental competence for the oocyte and resulting embryo.

While the collection and preparation of follicular aspirates imposes special requirements to assure the validity of AMH quantitation, the availability of commercial ELISA-based assays permits rapid results than can be used as an independent variable in oocyte and embryo selection schemes that include such traditional parameters as stage-appropriate development, performance, and morphology during in vitro culture. However, despite the growing evidence of the value of follicular AMH determinations, confirmation of optimistic reports that this protein hormone can be a highly meaningful predictor of outcome will become evident only after more IVF programs combine follicle-specific AMH concentration with outcome results from the corresponding oocyte. It may take some time to confirm or reject AMH in this regard, as most IVF centers adopt a new protocol only after sufficient confirmation is forthcoming, which is typically not from their own independent studies but from the often laborious efforts of a very few investigators.

AMH is an attractive candidate as a biomarker of competence because it is likely that levels within a specific range reflect the normality of granulosa cell development and function, which, in turn, would be expected to influence the normality of the oocyte as the follicle develops and enters the preovulatory pathway. As a member of a signaling cascade (TGF-β superfamily) that has been extensively investigated in multiple species, AMH represents an ideal candidate for detailed gene expression and function studies designed to characterize precisely how it may regulate or influence the acquisition of human oocyte competence.

A **Holistic** *Approach to Follicular Fluid in Competence Selection*

Analytical methods that offer a detailed molecular profile of neat follicular fluid have the real potential to provide a detailed biochemical "picture" of the intrafollicular milieu that may ultimately be of greater clinical utility as a biomarker of competence than are levels of individual molecules, including AMH. Methodologies such as mass spectroscopy, nuclear magnetic resonance (NMR), and Raman spectroscopy (near infra red spectroscopy, NIR) can display molecular profiles or signatures of a wide array of molecules (e.g., amino acids, metabolites small bioactive peptides, and proteins) whose levels can be correlated with embryo performance in vitro and outcome after transfer [47–50]. Similar to the rationale upon which metabolomic analysis of spent culture medium has been proposed for purposes of preimplantation-stage human embryo selection [2, 4], this "holistic" approach to follicular fluid analysis looks at both the end products of cellular activities and the presence of molecules that enter the follicle during its growth. Because instrumentation to perform NMR and NIR analysis can be adapted for use in the clinical IVF laboratory, it is likely that yet another algorithm will ultimately replace the observer for both oocyte and embryo selection, assuming that predictability levels are ultimately found to be robust. This should not be considered a negative in clinical IVF because current empirical assessments of competence based on cumulus characteristics (size, degree of expansion, the presence of foci of red blood cells, cytoplasmic density) are all that can be effectively noted, but their relevance with respect to outcome is unclear, controversial, and in some instances, more apparent than real

[1]. While the human element becomes the means by which an analytical end is achieved, the potential for establishing standard, objective criteria for selection based on molecular profiles derived from the high-resolution methods noted above should be welcomed in clinical IVF laboratory. However, only the continued accumulation of outcome-based findings will demonstrate whether the current optimism that they can indeed be robust and reliable predictors of competence is justified.

Perifollicular Blood Flow as a Noninvasive Predictor of Oocyte Competence

Interest in Doppler ultrasonographic analysis of perifollicular blood flow rates to assess the normality of follicular growth and oocyte competence has been episodic since it first introduced in clinical IVF in the late 1980s and early 1990s (see reviews by Gregory [51]; Van Blerkom and Trout [9]; Van Blerkom [52]). While most of the early reports were generally positive with respect to oocyte and embryo selection, few clinical IVF programs incorporated Doppler analysis in their follicular monitoring schemes, even when the capacity to obtain spectral imaging and quantitative values of follicle-specific blood flow was available in their instrumentation. Renewed interest in this noninvasive method of follicular analysis may be attributed in part to two factors: (a) the need for oocyte selection criteria that are independent of cumulus morphology at aspiration, especially where the number of oocytes that can be inseminated (or embryos transferred) is mandated by law and (b) the introduction of new generations of ultrasound equipment that produce high-resolution, 3D digital images that can be manipulated in real time. The ability to digitally isolate individual follicles and view blood flow patterns along the entire circumference of the follicle wall may be an important diagnostic tool and is in contrast to older 2D imaging modes, in which blood flow images and quantitative parameters (e.g., resistivity index) were obtained from selected cross-sections.

The physiological basis for assuming that perifollicular blood flow measurements offer some insight into the normality of follicular development and the competence of the corresponding oocyte is that expansion of the existing perifollicular vascular bed is normal aspect of folliculogenesis in follicles in the ovulatory pathway. Expansion of the microvasculature network appears to involve specific angiogenic growth factors such as VEGF and leptin (see above) produced by cumulus granulosa cells under the influence of FSH and LH [53]. VEGF also increases the permeability of capillaries (it was originally termed vascular endothelium and permeability factor) that might enhance the transduction of blood-borne regulatory factors into the follicle. Higher rates of blood flow would also increase rates of oxygen diffusion into the follicle, as well as the rate at which follicular components (steroids, growth factors, etc.) enter systemic circulation. Increased follicular oxygenation may be an important regulatory influence for the steroidogenic activity of the mural granulosa cells that line the follicular wall and are in close proximity to the perifollicular microvasculature. Despite numerous studies of follicular vascularity and steroidogenesis, it remains to be determined whether the level of estradiol measured in serum during follicular growth, or of progesterone after ovulation induction, can be related to follicular blood flow characteristics in general or whether high-flow follicles contribute disproportionately to levels measured in serum.

Differences in blood flow rates detected by Doppler imaging have been positively correlated with corresponding differences in the dissolved oxygen content of follicular fluid measured in neat aspirates obtained after ovulation induction in COHS cycles for IVF [54]. Although the reported differences are relatively small (i.e., between ~1 and ~4%), they may be physiologically significant insofar as reducing the extent of hypoxia that normally exists within the follicle [53] which, in turn, could influence the bioactivity of both mural and cumulus granulosa cells [54]. Molecular studies indicate that follicle-specific levels of VEGF in follicular fluid appeared to be related to corresponding expression levels of elements of the hypoxia-inducible transcription factor-signaling pathway (HIF) [9, 53], which regulates levels of VEGF expression [55]. It has been suggested that the activation of HIF may be associated with FSH stimulation of granulosa cell expansion and that the level of dissolved oxygen within the early antral follicle could be rate limiting for both granulosa cell proliferation and steroidogenic function [53]. Although speculative, one indirect action of FSH on granulosa cells could be at level of the mitochondria, which, as the oxygen sensors of a cell, could respond by increasing superoxide production to levels that are regulatory with respect to the activation of the HIF pathway [56]. Collectively, progressive increases in dissolved oxygen content during the early follicular phase may regulate granulosa cell proliferation, levels of steroid production by the mural granulosa, and protein growth factor synthesis and secretion by the cumulus granulosa. This notion is supported by the findings of Shrestha et al. [57], who distinguished between "good" and "poor" beginners on the basis of perifollicular blood flow rates measured during the early stages of follicular growth in cycles of controlled ovarian stimulation for IVF. Based on outcomes after embryo transfer, they concluded that flow rate, implantation potential, and developmental competence were related to such an extent that a poor beginning could justify cycle treatment cancelation during the early stages of stimulation.

It is worth noting that while increased intrafollicular oxygen tension levels seems relatively small (<1% to approximately 4%) [54], they may be of a magnitude sufficient to influence the function and activity (e.g., gene expression levels) of the mural and cumulus granulosa cells during follicular growth. For the cumulus granulosa in particular, levels of biosynthetic activity during the follicular phase could indirectly influence the normality cytoplasmic, nuclear, and oolemmal maturation during preovulatory period. In this regard, significantly lower frequencies of aneuploidy at MII have been reported when the dissolved oxygen content measured at aspiration was approximately 4%, as compared to similar sized follicles with poor flow characteristics and an oxygen contents $\leq\sim1\%$ [54].

One of the more unexpected findings to come from the early studies of perifollicular blood flow was the extent to which follicles of equivalent size at the time of aspiration, including those adjacent follicles, exhibited completely different quantitative flow values and in some reports, high-flow follicles occurred in one ovary, in a single follicle on one ovary, or in multiple follicles on one or both ovaries. Thus, blood flow rate could not be predicted on the basis of follicle size or location without Doppler analysis [54]. In order to quantify perifollicular blood flow rates, relatively simple grading systems were proposed using a score (A, B, C; 1–4) or grade (high or low grade) that was based on degree to which flow could be measured, either in a midline section or at multiple points, along the circumference of the follicle [51]. Correlations between blood flow characteristics, fertilization, embryo performance in vitro, and outcome indicated that oocytes from high (type A; class 3 or 4) grade follicles were more likely to result in pregnancy than those from low-flow (grade) follicles (see reviews by Gregory [51]; Van Blerkom and Trout [9]). However, while usually positive correlations between outcome and perifollicular blood flow rates appeared in the literature (see above), indicating that this metric could be used as an independent factor for oocyte and embryo selection [58], Doppler ultrasonographic analysis of perifollicular blood flow characteristics has not been widely incorporated in infertility assessment and treatment. In the past, the apparent lack of interest in this methodology may be due to the requirements for instrumentation that could perform Doppler studies, the added time, and expertise needed to obtain accurate values with conventional 2D imaging, or that the association with outcome was not sufficiently high as to warrant a significant change in protocol.

Renewed interest in blood flow measurements largely parallels the introduction of digital 3D ultrasonographic imaging in which Doppler software is often included with the instrument. Many, but not all studies, have confirmed an association with outcome and for some significant reductions in spontaneous miscarriages, supporting earlier findings that aneuploidy may be less likely in oocytes that mature in high-grade follicles (reviewed by Van Blerkom and Trout [9]; Van Blerkom [52]). While not all reports have been sanguine with respect to the utility of Doppler imaging in IVF treatments, reports of improved outcomes, including higher ongoing pregnancy rates and reduced frequencies of miscarriage, do suggest that its inclusion in ovarian monitoring and oocyte and embryo selection schemes is beneficial and can provide a quantitative measure of follicular development that is independent of growth rate. What 3D imaging has shown however is that in comparison to single cross-sectional 2D views, perifollicular blood flow in high-grade follicles cannot be assumed to involve the entire circumference of the follicle [9]. In these instances, high flow can be focal and discontinuous with relatively large regions of the follicular wall showing little, if any, significant velocity. While these follicles would likely be classified as high grade by 2D Doppler ultrasonography, they are more likely moderate to low grade; whether the corresponding oocytes have a lower competence with respect to implantation and outcome than their counterparts from follicles where blood flow is largely continuous and circumferential remains to be determined. Therefore, the simple follicular classification schemes noted above might need to be revised and standardized in order to account for subtle differences in perifollicular blood flow in apparently high-grade follicles that may be significant with respect to competence selection.

Perhaps, the most convincing evidence for the use of Doppler analysis of follicles will come from the type of NMR and NIR profiles of follicular fluid noted above, assuming that such studies will be able to show molecular signatures and levels that can produce algorithms that clearly correlate with outcome. In the meantime, where this technology exists, its use for follicular assessment should be considered as the first step in sequential assessments of competence that after fertilization, include the usual morphological characteristics of pronuclear through blastocyst stage embryos [1].

The notion that subjective observations of early human development commonly used to assess embryo viability will be succeeded by objective criteria that can be expressed in a numerical form that is predictive of outcome, such as proposed for NIR values obtained from spent embryo culture medium, is an appealing one because it would be derived from quantitative measurements of follicular characteristics (e.g., blood flow rate and pattern assessed by 3D Doppler imaging) and biochemical profiles of neat follicular fluid [59]. A change of this type in how the clinical IVF laboratory is engaged in competence assessments should be viewed positively and in terms of the potential to improve outcome and, more importantly, equalize outcomes among programs.

Summary and Perspectives

The search for biomarkers of oocyte and embryo developmental competence has been ongoing since IVF was combined with COHS to become a practical and widespread treatment for human infertility. The early optimism that measures of follicle-specific steroid hormone, protein growth factor, cytokine, and other bioactive molecules detected in the complex biochemical mix that is the follicular fluid could be biomarkers of gamete and embryo competence has not been supported by a large body of research. Thus, the biochemical and physiological environment to which the cumulus-oocyte complex is exposed to prior to ovulation is represented by the fluid discarded by most clinical IVF laboratories. Whether the current enthusiasm for some factors, such as AMH, may prove to be the exception remains to be determined. In the same respect, whether molecular surveys of gene expression in cumulus cells, either at the mRNA or at the protein levels, have sufficient predictive power to warrant adoption as a routine protocol for assessment remains to be seen. While there is no shortage of potential targets for analysis, and studies to screen targets and identify a core set of proteins or genes that may be related to competence are ongoing in this field, it is unclear at present whether they will have sufficient predictive power for oocyte and embryo selection to justify the considerable increase in expense (e.g., custom microarrays, equipment, and technical expertise) and effort (e.g., biopsy and preparation of cumulus cells) that may be required.

The "holistic" or spectrophotometric approach to competence assessment with NMR, NIR, or similar analytical methodologies is intended to obtain a comprehensive molecular snapshot of the intrafollicular milieu at the time the oocyte is retrieved. In this instance, it is the "big picture" that is relevant rather than whether the function of a putative biomarker is on the somatic cells or female gamete or both. The appeal of this line of investigation is twofold: first, the results can be both qualitative and quantitative, and second, the molecular profile displayed should be consistent with the intrafollicular biochemistry in which the oocyte matured to MII and achieved fertilization competence. In this respect, its utility lies in the fact that the analysis is done at a critical developmental endpoint for the oocyte, the transition from intrafollicular life, where the components in the follicular fluid are those derived from serum or produced in situ, to a different biochemical milieu within the Fallopian tube, where fertilization will occur.

The importance of obtaining quantitative values is that if specific components are shown to be competence associated, it may well be that it is their concentration rather than simply their presence that is associated with the acquisition of developmental viability. What will determine the success of this approach is whether comparative analysis of individual follicles reveals a relatively small number of biomarkers that can reliably distinguish oocytes that develop into embryos that progress from gestation to birth from those that do not.

In an ideal world, follicular biochemistry and the competence of the corresponding oocyte would be equivalent, which is more likely the situation in litter-bearing mammals such as rodents and rabbits, where the number of newborns is usually equivalent to the number follicles that develop in natural cycles. However, this is clearly not the situation in the human, and it has been long known that developmental competence is embryo specific, and more recent evidence demonstrates that this specificity arises in the preovulatory oocyte. This gives reason for optimism that investigations capable of displaying a comprehensive picture of the biochemistry of each follicle's fluid will be informative and clinically beneficial in infertility treatment. This might also suggest new avenues of study related to the site(s) and function of potential competence determining biomarkers that would increase significantly our understanding of the developmental biology of the human oocyte and the dynamic changes at the nuclear, cytoplasmic, and plasma membrane levels that lead to viability.

Protocols and procedures evolve in science and medicine and clinical IVF will not be exempted from the inevitable forces of change that can be envisaged for this field in the near term. If outcomes are universally improved, then basing the most fundamental of all decisions in clinical IVF, namely, which oocyte to inseminate and which embryo to transfer, on algorithms rather than empirical criteria should be welcomed, even if the longstanding and central role of the human observer is diminished or eliminated.

References

1. Balaban B, et al. Alpha scientists in reproductive medicine and ESHRE special interest group of embryology. The Istanbul consensus workshop on embryo assessment: proceedings of an expert meeting. Hum Reprod. 2011;26:1270–83.
2. Botros L, Sakkas D, Seli E. Metabolomics and its application for non-invasive embryo assessment in IVF. Mol Hum Reprod. 2008;14:679–90.

3. Scott R, Seli E, Miller L, et al. Noninvasive metabolomic profiling of human embryo culture medium using Raman spectroscopy predicts embryonic reproductive potential: a prospective blinded pilot study. Fertil Steril. 2008;90:77–83.
4. Seli E, Botros L, Sakkas D, Burns D. Noninvasive profiling of embryo culture media using proton nuclear magnetic resonance correlates with reproductive potential of embryos in women undergoing in vitro fertilization. Fertil Steril. 2008;90:2183–9.
5. McKenzie LJ, Pangas SA, Carson SA, et al. Human cumulus granulosa cell gene expression: a predictor of fertilization and embryo selection in women undergoing IVF. Hum Reprod. 2004;19: 2869–74.
6. Cillo F, Tiziana A, Brevini L, et al. Association between human oocyte developmental competence and expression levels of some cumulus genes. Reproduction. 2007;134:645–50.
7. Jones G, Cram D, Song B, et al. Novel strategy with potential to identify developmentally competent IVF blastocysts. Hum Reprod. 2008;23:1748–59.
8. Michael A. Do biochemical predictors of outcome exist? In: Van Blerkom J, Gregory L, editors. Essential IVF: basic research and clinical applications. Boston: Kluwer Academic; 2004. p. 81–110.
9. Van Blerkom J, Trout S. Oocyte selection in contemporary clinical IVF: do follicular markers of oocyte competence exit? In: Elder K, Cohen J, editors. Human preimplantation embryo selection. London: Informa Press; 2007. p. 301–24.
10. Edwards R. Causes of early embryonic loss in human pregnancy. Hum Reprod. 1986;1: 85–98.
11. Kuliev A, Cieslak J, Llkevitch Y, Verlinsky Y. Chromosomal abnormalities in a series of 6,733 human oocytes in preimplantation diagnosis for age-related aneuploidies. Reprod Biomed Online. 2003;6:54–9.
12. Kalousek D. Pathogenesis of chromosomal mosaicism and its effect on early human development. Am J Med Genet. 2000;91: 39–45.
13. Ambartsumyan G, Clark A. Aneuploidy and early human embryo development. Hum Mol Genet. 2008;17(R1):R10–5.
14. Menezo Y, Guerin P. Preimplantation embryo metabolism and embryo interaction with the in vitro environment. In: Elder K, Cohen J, editors. Human preimplantation embryo selection. London: Informa Press; 2007. p. 191–200.
15. Tam P, Ng T, Mao K. Beta-endorphin levels in preovulatory follicles and the outcome of in vitro fertilization. J In Vitro Fertil Embryo Transf. 1988;5:91–5.
16. Cioffi JV, Blerkom JA, et al. The expression of leptin and its receptors in preovulatory human follicles. Mol Hum Reprod. 1997;3: 467–72.
17. Oosterhuis G, Vermes I, Lambalk C, et al. Insulin-like growth factor (IGF)-1 and IGF binding protein-3 concentration in follicular fluid from human stimulated follicles. Fertil Steril. 1998;90:60–4.
18. Mendoza C, Cremades N, Ruiz-Requena E, et al. Relationship between fertilization results after intracytoplasmic sperm injection, and intrafollicular steroid, pituitary hormone and cytokine concentrations. Hum Reprod. 1999;13:863–8.
19. Mendoza C, Ruiz-Requena E, Ortega E, et al. Follicular fluid markers of oocyte developmental potential. Hum Reprod. 2002;17: 1017–22.
20. Michael A, Collins T, Norgate D, Gregory L, et al. Relationship between ovarian cortisol:cortisone ratios and the clinical outcome of in vitro fertilization and embryo transfer (IVF-ET). Clin Endocrinol. 1999;51:535–40.
21. Sabatini L, Wilson C, Lower A, Al-Shawaf T, Grudzinskas J. Superoxide dismutase activity in human follicular fluid after controlled ovarian hyperstimulation in women undergoing in vitro fertilization. Fertil Steril. 1999;72:1027–34.
22. Lee K, Joo B, Na Y, et al. Relationships between concentrations of tumor necrosis factor-alpha and nitric oxide in follicular fluid and oocyte quality. Fertil Steril. 2000;17:222–8.
23. Oyawoye O, Abdel Gadir A, Garner A, et al. Antioxidants and reactive oxygen species in follicular fluid of women undergoing IVF: relationship to outcome. Hum Reprod. 2003; 18:2270–4.

24. Antczak M. The synthetic and secretory behaviors (nonsteroidal) of ovarian follicular granulosa cells: parallels to cells of the endothelial lineage. In: Van Blerkom J, Gregory L, editors. Essential IVF: basic research and clinical applications. Boston: Kluwer Academic; 2004. p. 1–42.
25. Ocal P, Aydin S, Cepni I, et al. Follicular fluid concentration of vascular endothelial growth factor, inhibin A and inhibin B in IVF cycles: are they markers for ovarian response and pregnancy outcome? Eur J Obstet Gynecol Reprod Biol. 2004;115:194–9.
26. Pasqualotto E, Agarwal A, Sharma R, et al. Effect of oxidative stress in follicular fluid on the outcome of assisted reproduction procedures. Fertil Steril. 2004;81:973–6.
27. Wunder D, Mueller M, Birkhauser M, Bersinger N. Steroids and protein markers in the follicular fluid as indicators of oocyte quality in patients with and without endometriosis. J Assist Reprod Genet. 2005;22:257–64.
28. Wu Y, Chang C, Cai J, et al. High bone morphogenetic protein-15 level in follicular fluid is associated with high quality oocyte and subsequent embryonic development. Hum Reprod. 2007;22: 1526–31.
29. Ledee N, Lombroso R, Lombardeli L, Selva J, et al. Cytokines and chemokines in follicular fluids and potential of the corresponding embryo: the role of granulocyte colony-stimulating factor. Hum Reprod. 2008;23:2001–9.
30. Sinclair K, Lunn L, Kwong Y, et al. Amino acid and fatty acid composition of follicular fluid as predictors of in-vitro embryo development. Reprod Biomed Online. 2008;16:859–68.
31. Godard NM, Pukazhenthi BS, Wildt DE, Comizzoli P. Paracrine factors from cumulus-enclosed oocytes ensure the successful maturation and fertilization in vitro of denuded oocytes in the cat model. Fertil Steril. 2009;91(5 Suppl):2051–60.
32. Revelli A, Delle Piane L, Casano S, et al. Follicular fluid content and oocyte quality: from single biochemical markers to metabolomics. Reprod Biol Endocrinol. 2009;7:40–53.
33. Rodgers R, Irving-Rodgers H. Formation of the ovarian follicular antrum and follicular fluid. Biol Reprod. 2010;82:1021–9.
34. Makabe S, Van Blerkom J. Human female reproduction: ovarian development to early embryogenesis. New York: Taylor and Francis; 2006.
35. Van Blerkom J, Motta P. The cellular basis of mammalian reproduction. Baltimore: Urban and Schwartenberg; 1979.
36. Van Blerkom J. Mitochondrial function in the human oocyte and embryo and their role in developmental competence. Mitochondrion. 2011;11:797–813.
37. Antczak M, Van Blerkom J. Oocyte influences on early development: the regulatory proteins leptin and STAT3 are polarized in mouse and human oocytes and differentially distributed within the cells of the preimplantation stage embryo. Mol Hum Reprod. 1997;3:1067–86.
38. Antczak M, Van Blerkom J, Clark A. A novel mechanism of vascular endothelial growth factor, leptin and transforming growth factor beta2 sequestration in a subpopulation of human ovarian follicle cells. Hum Reprod. 1997;12:2226–34.
39. Monteleone P, Giovanni A, Simi G, et al. Follicular fluid VEGF levels directly correlate with perifollicular blood flow in normoresponder patients undergoing IVF. J Assist Reprod Genet. 2008;25:183–6.
40. Barroso G, Barrioneuvo M, Rao O, Graham L, et al. Vascular endothelial growth factor, nitric oxide, and leptin follicular fluid levels correlate negatively with embryo quality in IVF patients. Fertil Steril. 1999;72:1024–6.
41. Mantzoros C, Cramer D, Liberman R, Barbieri R. Predictive value of serum and follicular fluid leptin concentrations during assisted reproductive cycles in normal women and in women with polycystic ovarian syndrome. Hum Reprod. 2000;15:539–44.
42. Tsai E, Yang C, Chen S, et al. Leptin affects pregnancy outcome of in vitro fertilization and steroidogenesis of human granulosa cells. J Assist Reprod Genet. 2002;19:169–76.
43. DePlacido G, Alviggi C, Clariza R, et al. Intra-follicular leptin concentration as a predictive factor for in vitro oocyte fertilization in assisted reproductive techniques. J Endocrinol Invest. 2006;29:719–26.

44. Hazout A, Bouchard P, Seifer D, et al. Serum anti-mullerian hormone/mullerian-inhibiting substance appears to be a more discriminatory marker of assisted reproductive technology outcome than follicle-stimulating hormone, inhibin B, or estradiol. Fertil Steril. 2004;82: 1323–9.
45. Silberstein T, MacLaughlin D, Shari I, et al. Mullerian inhibiting substance levels at the time of HCG administration in IVF cycles predicts both ovarian reserve and embryo morphology. Hum Reprod. 2006;21:159–63.
46. Eldar-Geva T, Ben-Chetrit A, Spitz I, et al. Dynamic assays of inhibin B, anti-mullerian hormone and estradiol following FSH stimulation and ovarian ultrasonography as predictors of IVF outcome. Hum Reprod. 2005;20:3178–83.
47. Bayer S, Armant D, Dlugi A, Seibel M. Spectrophotometric absorbance of follicular fluid: a predictor of oocyte fertilizing capability. Fertil Steril. 1988;49:442–6.
48. Aharoni A, Ric de Vos C, Verhoeven H, et al. Nontargeted metabolome analysis by use of Fourier transform ion cyclotron mass spectrometry. OMICS. 2002;6:217–34.
49. Singh R, Sinclair K. Metabolomics: approaches to assessing oocyte and embryo quality. Theriogenology. 2007;68 Suppl 1:S56–62.
50. Piñero-Sagredo E, Nunes S, de Los Santos MJ. NMR metabolic profile of human follicular fluid. NMR Biomed. 2010;23(5):485–95.
51. Gregory L. Peri-follicular vascularity: a marker of follicular heterogeneity and oocyte competence and a predictor of implantation in assisted conception cycles. In: Van Blerkom J, Gregory L, editors. Essential IVF: basic research and clinical applications. Boston: Kluwer Academic; 2004. p. 59–80.
52. Van Blerkom J. An overview of determinants of oocyte and embryo developmental competence: specificity, accuracy and applicability in clinical IVF. In: Gerris J, Racowsky C, et al., editors. Single embryo transfer. New York: Cambridge University Press; 2009. p. 17–52.
53. Van Blerkom J. Follicular influences on oocyte and embryo competence. In: De Jonge C, Barratt C, editors. Assisted reproductive technology. Cambridge: Cambridge University Press; 2002. p. 81–105.
54. Van Blerkom J, Antczak M, Schrader R. The developmental potential of the human oocyte is related to the dissolved oxygen content of follicular fluid: association with vascular endothelial growth factor levels and perifollicular blood flow characteristics. Hum Reprod. 1997;12(5):1047–55.
55. Semenza G. Regulation of mammalian O_2 homeostasis by hypoxia-inducible factor 1. Annu Rev Cell Dev Biol. 1999;15:551–78.
56. Bruick R. Oxygen sensing in the hypoxic response pathway: regulation of hypoxia-inducible transcription factor. Genes Dev. 2003;17:2614–23.
57. Shrestha S, Costello M, Sjoblom P, et al. Power Doppler ultrasound assessment of follicular vascularity in the early follicular phase and its relationship with outcome in in vitro fertilization. J Assist Reprod Genet. 2006;23:1610169.
58. Robson S, Barry M, Norman R. Power Doppler assessment of follicular vascularity at the time of oocyte retrieval in in vitro fertilization cycles. Fertil Steril. 2008;90:2179–82.
59. Malamitsi-Puchner A, Sarandakou A, Baka S, et al. Concentrations of angiogenic factors in follicular fluid and oocyte-cumulus complex culture medium from women undergoing in vitro fertilization: association with oocyte maturity and fertilization. Fertil Steril. 2001;76:98–101.

Index

A
aCGH. *See* Array comparative genomic hybridization (aCGH)
AH. *See* Assisted hatching (AH)
AMH. *See* Mullerian inhibiting hormone (AMH)
Aneuploidy screening
 CGH, 298–299
 FISH, 297–298
 IVF programs, 291–292
 risks, 289, 291
Array comparative genomic hybridization (aCGH)
 BAC, 306
 clinical data, 309, 310
 cytogenetic analysis, 305–306
 limitation, 306
 validation, 308–309
ART. *See* Assisted reproduction technology (ART)
Assisted hatching (AH)
 benefits, 255
 complications, 254
 definition, 246
 embryo hatching, 246
 embryo stages
  blastocyst stage, 253
  early, 251–252
  fragment removal, 252
  frozen-thawed embryos, 253
  necrotic material removal, 253–254
 indications, 246–247
 micromanipulation techniques, 246
 monozygotic twinning, 254
 partial zona drilling, 247

procedure
 chemical zona drilling, 249
 enzymatic zona digestion, 250
 laser technologies, 250–251
 mechanical partial zona dissection, 248–249
 RI micromanipulation systems, 174
 ZP (*see* Zona pellucida (ZP))
Assisted reproduction technology (ART)
 centrosomes and ICSI, 366–367
Aster formation, centrosomes, 364, 366, 370
Asthenozoospermia, 183
ATP generation and mtDNA, 320, 327
Automated intracytoplasmic sperm injection
 hamster testing model, 206, 207
 immobilization, 205–206
 maximum intensity region algorithm, 205
 microrobots, 200
 mouse embryo tests, 206
 oocyte/sperm manipulation devices
  motorized rotational stage, 204–205
  motorized syringe, 204
  precision vacuum pump, 203–204
  vacuum-based cell holding device, 203, 204
 operation sequence, 201–203
 robotic microinjection, 199–200
 sperm cell tail tracking, 205–206
 success rate, 206, 207
 survival rate, 206
 system architecture, 201, 202
 vision-based contact detection, 205
Azoospermia
 Eppendorf micromanipulator, 181

B

Biomarkers
  molecular mining, 387–388
  sperm testing, 93–94
Birefringence, ICSI
  definition, 146
  enhanced magnification, 151, 152
  postacrosomal region, localization of, 149, 150
  sperm head, 146–147
  sperm sample parameters *vs.* spermatozoa, 147, 148
  TEM analysis, 149–147
Blastomere removal
  aspiration, 275–276
  extrusion method, 276
  fluid displacement, 276

C

Centrin, 366
Centrosomes
  characteristics of, 362
  ICSI, 364–367 (*see also* Intracytoplasmic sperm injection (ICSI) centrosomes)
  microtubule formations, 362
  MII oocytes, 362–363
  proteins, 362–363
  spermatozoa, 364
  technical aspects and practical considerations, 368–370
    heterologous sperm aster tests, in bovine oocytes, 370
    MII spindle shapes, fresh and aged oocytes, 369
    mitochondria, 370
CGH. *See* Comparative genomic hybridization (CGH)
Chromatin modifications, oocyte maturation, 349
Cleavage-stage embryo biopsy
  advantages, 269, 270
  blastomere removal
    aspiration, 275–276
    extrusion method, 276
    fluid displacement, 276
  cell removal, 277–278
  cell selection, 279–280
  definition, 269
  disadvantages, 269, 270
  embryo cryopreservation, 282
  mosaicism, 280, 281, 283
  non-contact laser, 273–274

prior preparation, 276–277
reliability, 278
safety, 280–282
success rates, 278–279
timing of, 277
whole genome amplification, 282
zona pellucida penetration
  chemical, 272
  mechanical, 270, 272
COC. *See* Cumulus–oocyte complex (COC)
Comparative genomic hybridization (CGH)
  embryo biopsy, PGD, 298–299
  PGD, chromosome abnormalities, 305–306
Computer-assisted sperm analysis.
  See Sperm assessment
Corona radiata, 210
Cryopreservation
  mammalian oocytes
    (*see* Mammalian oocytes)
  oocyte morphological abnormalities, 19–20
  spindle imaging, in oocytes, 32
Cryptozoospermia, 183
Cumulus cell gene expression
  cell biology, 39–40
  gene expression studies, 40–42
Cumulus–oocyte complex (COC)
  cell biology, 39–40
  gene expression studies, 40–42
  processing, ICSI, 210
Cytoplasmic redox state, mitochondrial role, 340
  dynamic process, 336
  location-related differences, in density, 336
  nodal, 336
  perinuclear aggregation, 337–338
Cytoplasmic transfer, 355
Cytoskeletal architecture, human oocytes
  centrosomes
    characteristics of, 362
    ICSI, 364–367
    infertility, 366, 367, 369
    integrity, 359, 367
    microtubule formations, 362
    MII oocytes, 362–363
    proteins, 362–363
    spermatozoa, 364
    technical aspects and practical considerations, 368–370
  immunocytochemistry, of MII oocyte before fertilization, 359–361
  oocyte quality, 359

sperm
    electron microscopy and immunofluorescence, 370–372
    proximal and distal centriole in, 359, 361

D

Defective sperm–zona pellucida binding (DSZPB), 68–69
DFI. *See* DNA fragmentation index (DFI)
Disordered zona pellucida-induced acrosome reaction (DZPIAR), 69
Distal centriole, 359, 361
DNA fragmentation index (DFI), 65
Doppler ultrasonographic analysis, perifollicular blood flow, 384–387
DSZPB. *See* Defective sperm–zona pellucida binding (DSZPB)
DZPIAR. *See* Disordered zona pellucida-induced acrosome reaction (DZPIAR)

E

Electronic micromanipulators. *See* Eppendorf micromanipulator
Electron microscopy (EM), sperm analysis, 370–372
Electrophoretic sperm separation
    clinical applications, 127–128
    development of, 122–123
    equipment setup and separation parameters
        cleaning, 126
        current and voltage setting, 125
        electrophoresis buffers and temperature settings, 125
        separation cartridges and sample handling, 123–125
    principles of, 121
    spermatozoa, electrophoretic properties, 122
    validation method
        sample recovery and purity, 126
        sperm vitality and motility, 126–127
Embryo(s)
    aneuploidy screening
        CGH, 298–299
        FISH, 297–298
        IVF programs, 291–295
        risks, 289, 291
    development, 287–289
        and implantation, 5–6
        and pregnancy outcome, zona, 34–35

Enzymatic zona digestion, AH, 250
Eppendorf micromanipulator
    advantages, 181
    description
        components, 180, 181
        control board, 180–182
        motor module unit, 180, 182
    ICSI procedure
        preparation, 181–183
        technique description, 184
    sperm swim-up technique, 183
Extracytoplasmic abnormalities, 13–14

F

Failed fertilization. *See* Human oocyte activation mechanism
FISH. *See* Fluorescent in situ hybridization (FISH)
Fluo-4 AM, intracellular free calcium, 331, 332
Fluorescent in situ hybridization (FISH)
    embryo biopsy, PGD, 297–298
    polar body biopsy, 266
Follicular fluid. *See* Molecular mining, follicular fluid

G

Gene expression, 40–42
Genetic constitution, 20–22
Germinal vesicle (GV) transfer, immature oocytes
    aneuploidies elimination, 352
    evidently defected oocytes, repairing, 352
    maturation arrest, 352
    mutated mtDNA, elimination of, 351–352
Giant oocytes evaluation, 17–18
Globozoospermia
    Eppendorf micromanipulator, 183
    human oocyte activation, 231

H

HA binding. *See* Hyaluronic acid (HA) binding
Hamster oocyte penetration test, 66
Holistic approach, to follicular fluid, 383–384
HOST. *See* Hyposmotic swelling test (HOST)
Human oocyte activation mechanism
    activation stimulus, 229–230
    artificial activation
        factors, 228–229

Human oocyte activation mechanism (cont.)
	failure mechanisms, 227–228
	indications, 229
	sperm-activating ability test, 228
	Ca^{2+} factor, 228–229
	GSH, 226
	human chorionic gonadotropin administration, 230
	initial sperm nucleus swelling, 226
	PLC zeta, 227
	PVP effect, 226
	specific protocols, 230–232
	sperm plasma membrane damage, 225–226
	thiol-reducing agents, 226
	touching tail, 225, 226
Human sperm–oocyte interaction, 66–68
Human sperm–oolemma binding, 69
Hyaluronic acid (HA) binding. *See also* Sperm testing
	aneuploidy frequency, 106
	DNA integrity, 105–106
	FISH analysis, 106–108
	ICSI sperm selection, 106–108
	IVF-ICSI data, 110–111
	vs. sperm binding, 102
	sperm development, 99–102
	using PICSI dishes, 109–110
Hydraulic manipulators, ICSI
	control unit, 159–160
	drive unit, 161–162
	joysticks, 161
	maintenance, 165
	microtool alignment, 162–166
	role, 157
	universal joint design, 161, 162, 164, 165
Hyposmotic swelling test (HOST), 64

I

ICSI centrosomes. *See* Intracytoplasmic sperm injection (ICSI) centrosomes
Immunocytochemistry, of MII oocyte before fertilization, 359–361
Immunofluorescence microscopy, sperm analysis, 371
IMSI. *See* Intracytoplasmic morphologically selected sperm injection (IMSI)
IntegraTi™
	air assisted microinjectors, 172
	heated stages, 173
	installation, 168–169
	mechanical stages, 173–174
	micromanipulators, 169

	micropipettes, 169–172
	PL30 tool holders, 169–171
	SAS microinjectors, 172–173
Intracellular free calcium, mitochondrial role, 330–335
Intracytoplasmic morphologically selected sperm injection (IMSI). *See also* Leica (AM 6000) workstation
	blastocyst absence, 79
	ICSI candidates, 79–80
	implantation failure/DNA fragmentation, 78–79
	limiting factors, 80
	unexplained infertility, 79
Intracytoplasmic sperm injection (ICSI) centrosomes
	abnormal spermatozoa injection effect, 77–78
	application, 238
	centrosomes
		in ART, 366–367
		aster formation, 364, 366
		centriole–centrosome complex, 365
		cytoskeletal organization and DNA configuration, 368–369
		fertilization and implications for, 364–366
		nuclear mitotic apparatus (NuMA) protein, 366
		pericentrin and centrin, 366
	COC processing, 210
	corona radiata, 210
	DNA damage effect, 83
	failure, 217–218
	fertilization mechanism, 227
	human oocyte activation mechanism
		artificial activation, 227–230
		initial sperm nucleus swelling, 226
		PVP effect, 226
		specific protocols, 230–232
		sperm-associated oocyte-activating-factor release, 227
		sperm plasma membrane damage, 225–226
	hyaluronic acid, 214
	hyaluronidase, 210–211
	hydraulic manipulators
		control unit, 159–160
		drive unit, 161–162
		joysticks, 161
		maintenance, 165
		microtool alignment, 162–166

Index	397

universal joint design, 161, 162, 164, 165
immotile sperm, 215–216
IMSI indications
   blastocyst absence, 79
   ICSI candidates, 79–80
   implantation failure/DNA
      fragmentation, 78–79
   limiting factors, 80
   unexplained infertility, 79
laser-assisted approach, 218
Leica (AM 6000) workstation, 194–196
long-term safety, 87–88
modified technique, 218–219
MSOME
   with ICSI, 74
   normalcy, 74–75
   nuclear morphology, sperms, 74
   routine laboratory semen analysis,
      81–82
   sperm classification, 76–77
oocyte denudation, 210–211
polyvinylpyrrolidone, 211
procedure, Eppendorf micromanipulator,
    181–185
RI micromanipulation systems, 175
selection (*see also* Sperm testing)
   benefits of, 113–114
   sperm charge properties, 112
spermatozoa
   catching, 211–213
   immobilization, 213–214
   selection, 214–215
spermatozoa selection
   IMSI, 75–76
sperm selection without vacuoles, 82
standardized procedure, 216
suboptimal pronuclear formation, 217
technical aspect, 88–89
temperature and time schedule, 209
vacuoles
   blastocyst formation, 85
   DNA damage-repairing factors, 86–87
   effect, 83
   endogenous and exogenous ROS, 86
   location, 86
   types of, 85–86

L
Laser-assisted ICSI, 218
Laser-assisted polar body biopsy, 263–265
Leica (AM 6000) workstation
   description, 188–189

preparation of
   components, switching on, 188, 189
   dish preparation, 190–191
   ICSI, 194–196
   motile sperm selection, 192–194
   pipette installation, 188, 189
   preliminary settings, 191
switch off, 196
vacuoles, 192–195
Livestock production via micromanipulation
   to engineer livestock genomes, 240–241
   ICSI, large animal xenografting, 241–242
   intracytoplasmic sperm injection
      application, 238
   overcoming technical difficulties,
      238–240

M
MACS. *See* Magnetic-activated cell sorting
    (MACS)
Magnetic-activated cell sorting (MACS)
   apoptosis and ROS, 132–133
   in clinical application, 138–139
   cryobiology of, 138
   density gradient centrifugation, 134
   efficiency of, 137
   embryo cleavage rate, 139
   nanoparticles, cell separation
      biocompatible, 131
      in research and clinical protocols, 132
   principles of, 135–136
   in sperm selection, 140
   swim-up, 135
Male fertility. *See* Sperm assessment
Male infertility, 183
Mammalian cryobiology.
    See Mammalian oocytes
Mammalian embryology.
    See Mammalian oocytes
Mammalian ICSI, 241–242
Mammalian oocytes, 347
   and early embryo, mitochondrial functions
      and activities, 320
Mechanical partial zona dissection, AH,
    248–249
Mechanical zona pellucida penetration,
    270, 272
Metaphase II (MII) oocytes, 8
Metaphase of second meiosis (MII oocytes),
    359, 362–363, 368–369
Microinjection. *See* Intracytoplasmic sperm
    injection (ICSI) centrosomes

Micromanipulation. *See also* Livestock
        production via micromanipulation
    livestock genomes, 240–241
    system, ICSI
        antivibration systems, 158
        description, 158
        electrical coarse control manipulator,
            159, 160
        hydraulic micromanipulators
            (*see* Hydraulic manipulators, ICSI)
        maintenance, 165
        on microscopes, 158
        microtool alignment, 162–166
        universal joint design, 161, 162,
            164, 165
Microzonation and mitochondrial inner
        membrane potential, 338–340
Mitochondrial role, in human developmental
        competence
    cell biology of, 341
    cytoplasmic redox state, 340
        dynamic process, 336
        location-related differences,
            in density, 336
        nodal, 336
        perinuclear aggregation, 337–338
    DNA content
        mitochondrial mass, 321
        mtDNA copy number and ATP
            generation, 320–321
        oocyte and embryo developmental
            ability, 324–325
        porcine oocyte maturation, numerical
            discrepancy, 321
        preimplantation development, in
            bovine, 325
        preovulatory maturation, 322
        replication, 321–323
        STZ-induced diabetic mice, alteration
            and damage, 323
    functional compartmentalization, 329–330
    functions of, 320
    genomic, 319
    inheritance, after fertilization, 328
    inner membrane potential and functional
        microzonation, 338–340
    intracellular free calcium
        ATP content measurement, 332, 333
        Fluo-4 AM, oocytes, 331, 332
        ionophore-activated MII human
            oocytes, 333
        signaling pathways or processes, 335
        slow cooling cryopreservation, 332
        smooth-surfaced endoplasmic
            reticulum (sER), 330
        time-lapse images, sER inclusion,
            333, 334
    in mammalian oocyte and early
        embryo, 320
    morphology and metabolomics, 319
    proteomic, 319
    reorganization, during early
        development, 326–328
    signal transduction pathways, 335–336
    threshold for, 341
Molecular mining, follicular fluid
    competence selection
        embryo, 377
        holistic approach, 383–384
        oocyte, 377, 378
    follicular biochemistry, 388
    genetic and biochemical technologies
        in, 377
    microanalytical imaging, 377
    oocyte developmental competence
        challenges, 379–380
        follicular aspiration, 382
        gap junctions, 380–381
        growth factors, 381
        Mullerian inhibiting hormone (AMH),
            382, 383
        transzonal processes (TZPs), 380
        zona pellucida, 380, 381
    perifollicular blood flow, oocyte
        competence
        Doppler ultrasonographic analysis,
            384–387
        grading systems, 386
        HIF, 385
        physiological basis, 384–385
        qualitative and quantitative, 388
        search for biomarkers, 387
Motile-sperm organelle morphology
        examination (MSOME), 187.
        See also Intracytoplasmic sperm
        injection (ICSI) centrosomes
    with ICSI, 74
    normalcy, 74–75
    nuclear morphology, sperms, 74
    routine laboratory semen analysis, 81–82
    sperm classification, 76–77
MSOME. *See* Motile-sperm organelle
        morphology examination
        (MSOME)
mtDNA. *See* Mutated mitochondrial DNA
        (mtDNA)
Mullerian inhibiting hormone (AMH),
        382, 383
Mutated mitochondrial DNA (mtDNA),
        351–352, 354–356

Index

N
Nonviable testicular sperm, 232
Normozoospermic patient, 230, 231
Nuclear and cytoplasmic transfer
  combinations, 351
  human applications, 356
  immature oocytes, GV transfer, 351–352
  of mammalian oocytes, characteristics, 347
  mature oocytes, 353–354
  maturing oocytes, 353
  morphology, 348
  oocyte maturation, chromatin modifications, 349
  organelles transfer, 355
  technical aspects
    equipment, 350
    manipulation methods, 350
  zygotes, 354
Nuclear mitotic apparatus (NuMA) protein, 366
NuMA protein. See Nuclear mitotic apparatus (NuMA) protein

O
Oocyte(s)
  developmental competence, follicular fluid biomarkers, 378–383
  immature, germinal vesicle (GV) transfer, 351–352
  in mammals, characteristics, 347
  maturation, chromatin modifications, 349
  mature, 353–354
  maturing, 353
Oocyte–cumulus–corona complex, 6–8
Oocyte denudation
  ICSI, 210
Oocyte quality assessment
  cumulus cell gene expression
    cell biology, 39–40
    gene expression studies, 40–42
  cytoplasmic abnormalities, 8–9
  cytoplasmic granularity and viscosity, 9–10
  embryo development and implantation, 5–6
  extracytoplasmic abnormalities, 13–14
  first polar body morphology evaluation, 14–15
  genetic constitution, 20–22
  giant oocytes evaluation, 17–18
  metaphase II (MII) oocytes, 8
  morphological abnormalities
    developmental competence, 18–19
    oocyte–cumulus–corona complex morphology, 6–8
  oocyte morphological abnormalities, cryopreservation, 19–20
  perivitelline space abnormalities, 17
  quality and morphological appearance, 4–5
  shape abnormalities, 15
  smooth endoplasmic reticulum clusters appearance, 11–13
  vacuolization, 10–11
  zona pellucida abnormalities, 15–17
Oocyte/sperm manipulation devices
  motorized rotational stage, 204–205
  motorized syringe, 204
  precision vacuum pump, 203–204
  vacuum-based cell holding device, 203, 204

P
Partial zona dissection (PZD), 174
Partial zona drilling, AH, 247
PCR technique
  polar body biopsy, 266–267
Pericentrin, 366
Perifollicular blood flow, oocyte competence, 384–387
Perivitelline space abnormalities, 17
PGD. See Preimplantation genetic diagnosis (PGD)
Polar body biopsy
  chemical ZP opening, 262
  FISH analysis, 266
  laser-assisted ZP opening, 263
  mechanical ZP opening, 262–263
  PCR, 266–267
  pitfalls, 265–266
  polar body
    description, 261
    isolation of, 266
  polarization microscopy, 263–265
  procedure, 263–265
  timing, 262
Polarization microscopy
  in assisted reproduction, 29–30
  spindle imaging
    cryopreserved oocytes, 32
    in vitro matured oocytes, 32
    and laboratory parameters, 32–33
    meiotic cell cycle, 31
    presence and location, 31
  zona imaging
    embryo development and pregnancy outcome, 34–35
    as prognostic factor, 33
    zona birefringence and architecture, 33

Polscope-based sperm selection, ICSI
 aneuploidy, 146, 151–152
 azoospermia, 146
 birefringence
  definition, 146
  enhanced magnification, 151, 152
  postacrosomal region, localization of, 149, 150
  sperm head, 146–147
  sperm sample parameters *vs.* spermatozoa, 147, 148
  TEM analysis, 146–147
 clinical validity, 147–151
 DNA integrity, 151–152
 embryo viability, 145
 oligoasthenoteratospermia (OAT), 145–146
 use of, 149, 151
Polyvinylpyrrolidone (PVP), 211
Preimplantation genetic diagnosis (PGD)
 chromosome abnormalities
  aCGH, 307–309
  CGH, 305–306
  SNP microarrays, 305–307, 309, 310
 cleavage-stage embryo biopsy (*see* Cleavage-stage embryo biopsy)
 definition, 303
 DNA analysis techniques, 305–308
 embryo biopsy
  aneuploidy, 289, 291–292, 296–297, 299
  chromosomal translocation testing, 293–295
  development, 287–289
  FISH analysis, 303–304
  gene defects, microarrays, 310–311
Protein tyrosine phosphorylation, 70
Proximal centriole, 361
PVP. *See* Polyvinylpyrrolidone (PVP)
PZD. *See* Partial zona dissection (PZD)

R
Research instruments (RI) micromanipulation systems
 assisted hatching, 174
 biopsy micropipettes, 176
 blastocyst/oocyte/embryo biopsy, 175–176
 foundation and development, 167
 instrumentation principles, 167–168
 integraTi™
  air assisted microinjectors, 172
  heated stages, 173
  installation, 168, 170

 mechanical stages, 173–174
 micromanipulators, 169
 micropipettes, 169–172
 PL30 tool holders, 169–171
 SAS microinjectors, 172–173
 intracytoplasmic sperm injection, 175
 PZD, 175
 SUZI, 175
 troubleshooting, 176–177
 zona drilling, 174
 zona pellucida (ZP), 168, 174, 176
RI micromanipulation systems. *See* Research instruments (RI) micromanipulation systems
Robotic intracytoplasmic sperm injection. *See* Automated intracytoplasmic sperm injection
Round-headed spermatozoa, 230

S
SAS microinjectors. *See* Screw-actuated syringes (SAS) microinjectors
Screw-actuated syringes (SAS) microinjectors, 172–173
sER. *See* Smooth-surfaced endoplasmic reticulum (sER)
Short culture. *See* Embryo(s)
Signal transduction pathways and mitochondria, 335–336
 threshold for, 341
Single nucleotide polymorphisms (SNP) microarray
 advantages, 308
 clinical data, 309, 310
 disadvantage, 307, 308
 qualitative methods, 307
 size, 307
 validation, 308–309
Smooth-surfaced endoplasmic reticulum (sER), 330–335
SNP microarray. *See* Single nucleotide polymorphisms (SNP) microarray
SOD. *See* Superoxide dismutases (SOD)
Sperm assessment
 automated sperm morphology, 65–66
 biochemical evaluation, 58–59
 chromatin normality, 64–65
 concentration, 56
 DFI, 65
 DNA normality, 64–65
 electron microscopy and immunofluorescence, 370–372
 hypoosmotic swelling test, 64

IVF/ART, application to, 59
liquefaction and appearance, 52–54
logistic regression analysis, 64
macroscopic evaluation, 52
microscopic evaluation, 55
morphology, 56–57
motility, 55–56
motility measurements, 65
non-sperm cellular elements, 58
pH, 55
proximal and distal centriole in, 359, 361
sample collection, 51–52
sperm function tests
  DSZPB, 68–69
  DZPIAR, 69
  hamster oocyte penetration test, 66
  human sperm–oocyte interaction, 66–68
  human sperm–oolemma binding, 69
  hyperactivation, 70
  protein tyrosine phosphorylation, 70
  sperm–zona pellucida binding, 70
  sperm–zona pellucida-induced acrosome reaction, 70
sperm vitality, 57–58
standard semen analysis, 50–51
total sperm count, 63
viscosity, 54
volume, 54–55
Spermatozoa, cytoskeletal architecture, 364
Sperm biomarkers, 93–94
Sperm cell tail tracking algorithm, 205–206
Sperm testing
biomarkers, 93–94
development of, 99–102
excessive semen ROS production, 103–104
genetic integrity, 98–99
HA binding
  aneuploidy frequency, 106
  DNA integrity, 105–106
  FISH analysis, 106–108
  ICSI sperm selection, 106–108
  IVF-ICSI data, 110–111
  using PICSI dishes, 109–110
  vs. hyaluronic acid binding, 102
ICSI selection
  benefits of, 113–114
  sperm charge properties, 112
male fertility and semen parameters, 94–95
semen chamber device, 102–103
sperm chromatin maturation, 104–105
spermiogenetic events and sperm fertilizing function, 95–96

structure and function, 97–98
Sperm–zona pellucida binding, 70
Sperm–zona pellucida-induced acrosome reaction, 70
Spindle
cryopreserved oocytes, 32
in vitro matured oocytes, 32
and laboratory parameters, 32–33
meiotic cell cycle, 31
presence and location, 31
Sub-zonal insemination (SUZI), 175
Superoxide dismutases (SOD), 40
SUZI. *See* Sub-zonal insemination (SUZI)

T
TEM. *See* Transmission electron microscopy (TEM)
Teratozoospermia
Eppendorf micromanipulator, 183
human oocyte activation, 231
Tertiary care ART center. *See* Assisted reproduction technology (ART)
Transcriptome, 41
translocation testing
balanced, 293, 294
monogenic diseases, 295
reciprocal, 293, 294
Robertsonian, 293, 294
STR-based molecular strategies, 295–296
Transmission electron microscopy (TEM)
sperm analysis, 370–372
Transzonal processes (TZPs), oocyte developmental competence, 380
γ-Tubulin, 362–364, 366, 368–369

U
Ultrastructural immunocytochemistry, sperm analysis, 371

V
Vacuoles
blastocyst formation, 85
DNA damage-repairing factors, 86–87
effect, 83
endogenous and exogenous ROS, 86
location, 86
types of, 85–86
Vacuolization, 10–11
Vision-based contact detection, automated ICSI, 205

X
Xenograft-ICSI technique, 241–242

Z
Zona
  birefringence and architecture, 33
  drilling
    AH, chemical, 249
    RI micromanipulation systems, 174
  polarization microscopy
    birefringence and architecture, 33
    embryo development and pregnancy outcome, 34–35
    as prognostic factor, 33
Zona pellucida (ZP)
  abnormalities, 15–17
  artificial manipulation, 254
  chemical penetration
    cleavage-stage embryo biopsy, 272
  description, 245
  embryo hatching, 246
  freezing-thawing process, 253
  function of, 245
  laser photoablation, 250–251
  removal, 248
  RI micromanipulation systems, 168, 174, 176
  thinning, 247–248
ZP. *See* Zona pellucida (ZP)
Zygote(s)
  nuclear and cytoplasmic transfer, 354

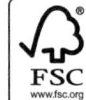

MIX
Papier aus verantwortungsvollen Quellen
Paper from responsible sources
FSC® C105338

If you have any concerns about our products,
you can contact us on
ProductSafety@springernature.com

In case Publisher is established outside the EU,
the EU authorized representative is:
**Springer Nature Customer Service Center GmbH
Europaplatz 3, 69115 Heidelberg, Germany**

Printed by Libri Plureos GmbH
in Hamburg, Germany